W9-AYQ-965

Computers in Health Care

Kathryn J. Hannah   Marion J. Ball
Series Editors

Marion J. Ball   Kathryn J. Hannah
Ulla Gerdin Jelger   Hans Peterson
Editors

Nursing Informatics
Where Caring and Technology Meet

With 18 Illustrations

Springer-Verlag
New York Berlin Heidelberg
London Paris Tokyo

Marion J. Ball
Associate Vice Chancellor
University of Maryland
Baltimore, MD 21201
USA

Kathryn J. Hannah
Professor, Faculty of Nursing
University of Calgary
Calgary, Alberta T2N 1N4
Canada

Ulla Gerdin Jelger
Health Care Information Systems
Stockholm County Council
Stockholm S-10272
Sweden

Hans Peterson
Director, Health Care Information Systems
Stockholm County Council
Stockholm S-10272
Sweden

Library of Congress Cataloging-in-Publication Data
Nursing informatics.
  (Computers in health care)
  Includes bibliographies and index.
  1. Nursing—Data processing. 2. Information
storage and retrieval systems—Nursing. I. Ball,
Marion J. II. Series: Computers in health care
(New York, N.Y.) [DNLM: 1. Computers. 2. Information
Systems. 3. Nursing. WY 26.5 N974]
RT50.5.N87 1988   610.73'028'5   87-32200

© 1988 by Springer-Verlag New York Inc.
All rights reserved. This work may not be translated or copied in whole or in part without the
written permission of the publisher (Springer-Verlag, 175 Fifth Avenue, New York, NY 10010,
USA), except for brief excerpts in connection with reviews or scholarly analysis. Use in connection with any form of information storage and retrieval, electronic adaptation, computer software, or by similar or dissimilar methodology now known or hereafter developed is forbidden.
The use of general descriptive names, trade names, trademarks, etc. in this publication, even if the
former are not especially identified, is not to be taken as a sign that such names, as understood by
the Trade Marks and Merchandise Marks Act, may accordingly be used freely by anyone.
While the advice and information in this book are believed to be true and accurate at the date of
going to press, neither the authors nor the editors nor the publisher can accept any legal
responsibility for any errors or omissions that may be made. The publisher makes no warranty,
express or implied, with respect to the material contained herein.

Copyright is not claimed for works by U.S. Government Employees: Section 2, Unit 4,
Chapter 5.

Typeset by Asco Trade Typesetting Ltd., Hong Kong.
Printed and bound by R.R. Donnelley & Sons, Harrisonburg, VA.
Printed in the United States of America.

9 8 7 6 5 4 3 2 1

ISBN 0-387-96639-0 Springer-Verlag New York Berlin Heidelberg
ISBN 3-540-96639-0 Springer-Verlag Berlin Heidelberg New York

To the profession of nursing

Foreword

Nursing, like other health-related professions, is information-intensive. The quality of care a patient receives is based on the soundness of judgment exercised by the health care team. Underlying sound judgment is up-to-date information. Unless nurses have access to accurate and pertinent information, the care being rendered will not be of the highest standard.

What is required is not necessarily more rapid and efficient information services. Modern technology can process immense amounts of data in the blink of an eye. What we in the health professions need are information systems that are more *intelligent*, systems that can integrate information from many sources, systems that analyze and synthesize information and display it so that it may be applied directly in patient care—in other words, information that answers a question or even gives practical advice.

In order to accomplish such objectives, work is needed to establish the scientific and theoretical basis for the use of computing and information systems by health professionals. This is the research component. In addition, there is the need for continued development and evaluation of practical information systems.

Implicit in this volume are the questions: Which of the present systems will help most in nursing? Which areas in nursing could most benefit from future informatics developments? Computer-based aids to learning and to continuing education have always been important areas of emphasis for information system developments, likewise systems that enhance access to the scientific literature. Yet in nursing, especially, one may safely place the highest value on papers and systems that improve patient care. The nurse has always taken the role of advocate for the patient; in the information age this may well be even more critical.

There is no question in my mind that future progress in health care will depend as much on how *well* we communicate what we know as on how *much* we know. This volume presents a comprehensive overview of the fast growing field of nursing contributions to automated information systems.

Donald A. B. Lindberg, M. D.
Director
National Library of Medicine
Bethesda, Maryland

Series Preface

This series is intended for the rapidly increasing number of health care professionals who have rudimentary knowledge and experience in health care computing and are seeking opportunities to expand their horizons. It does not attempt to compete with the primers already on the market. Eminent international experts will edit, author, or contribute to each volume in order to privide comprehensive and current accounts of innovations and future trends in this quickly evolving field. Each book will be practical, easy to use, and well referenced.

Our aim is for the series to encompass all of the health professions by focusing on specific professions, such as nursing, in individual volumes. However, integrated computing systems are only one tool for improving communication among members of the health care team. Therefore, it is our hope that the series will stimulate professionals to explore additional means of fostering interdisciplinary exchange.

This series springs from a professional collaboration that has grown over the years into a highly valued personal friendship. Our joint values put people first. If the Computers in Health Care series lets us share those values by helping health care professionals to communicate their ideas for the benefit of patients, then our efforts will have succeeded.

Kathryn J. Hannah
Marion J. Ball

Preface

This book represents for us the potential of the new information technologies in health care and especially in nursing. In describing the evolution now occurring in the field, the book presents its material in two major divisions—Nursing Informatics and Where Caring and Technology Meet.

The content and format of the book are represented by the illustration on its cover. The wheel is made up of two concentric circles, joined together by four spokes. The inner circle stands for the patient, always the hub for nursing. The linking spokes are the four functional aspects of nursing—Clinical, Administration, Research, and Education—whose first letters form the acronym CARE. The outer ring portrays nursing informatics, the subject of this book and the field which integrates caring and technology.

Information technology brings with it new capabilities and new opportunities for the professions. Nursing and computing professionals have begun to form a variety of alliances and to assume a variety of new roles. In their 1984 book, *Using Computers in Nursing*, Ball and Hannah included selected network contacts at the conclusion of each chapter, illustrating the principle they stated in their Preface:

> One important aim of the book is to encourage networking among all nurses who are charting new ground in their individual efforts to apply the computer to the field of nursing. Each chapter . . . is dedicated to an acknowledged expert who has indicated a willingness to share his or her special expertise.
>
> The authors urge the reader to join the network and "come on line" with the leaders in health care computing! (p. xii)

Readers of the 1984 book took the invitation to heart and many new bonds, both technical and personal, were formed. Such networking is illustrated by the relationship of the four author/editors of this book with each other and with their more than thirty contributors. In this volume, Ball and Hannah join with their European colleagues, Gerdin

Jelger and Peterson, to serve at the center of a much wider network. These four are joined by fellow professionals from nursing, business, medicine, computer science, and health information—literally a host of professional fields and disciplines all concerned with the delivery of the highest quality health care. Networked together, they can provide more extensive and more current content, as they strive to integrate information technology and nursing CARE.

This book itself was assembled through technical networking. The four author/editors corresponded by international electronic mail, exchanging text and discussing key decisions regarding the book with what were often same-day responses. Manuscripts submitted by authors around the world were either transmitted electronically or translated by optical scanner into electronic form by the editors who then loaded them into a standard file for formatting and editing.

The nursing informatics scene is moving rapidly, and many exciting applications have developed since the publication of *Using Computers in Nursing*. Technology links the microcomputer to the mainframe, the operating room with the admissions office. It links the nurse in Australia with the National Library of Medicine's Medline in the United States and provides a means for a nurse to communicate electronically with colleagues around the world. It links the clinician with research data, the practitioner with expert systems. The capabilities are enormous and, even more exciting, they are being realized in actual working conditions!

Reflecting the new world that these linkages create, the book intertwines the language of computing with the language of health care. The connectivity of computer hardware and software is linkened to the human nervous system. Making this connectivity an integral component of applied information technology brings the power of computing to the nursing profession. Health care computing capabilities and applications not only integrate and extend nursing functions, but also raise technical, legal, and ethical issues.

This new power and its implications are the concern of nursing informatics, a field which will play a critical role in realizing the full potential of nursing to contribute to patient care. For nurses to realize this potential, nursing informatics must be integrated into educational curricula for nurses at the entry-to-practice level and the continuing-education level. This book is designed to be used as a tool for that integration. Prepared with the assistance of the innovators in nursing and information technology, it exemplifies the exponential growth of information in all aspects of nursing.

No one, two, three, or four individuals can cover the excitement of integrating computers into health care. Only a large network of experts can provide a snapshot of nursing informatics as it is at the time of publication. The picture will continue to change as the field evolves and grows and even further integration and connectivity bind the computer into nursing CARE. We again invite readers to join the Nursing Informatics Network.

Marion J. Ball
Kathryn J. Hannah
Ulla Gerdin Jelger
Hans Peterson

Acknowledgments

The purpose of this undertaking is to further the nursing profession's need to understand the relationship of nursing and computers, or nursing informatics. We emphasize that the field of nursing informatics embodies the use of computers in nursing clinical practice, administration, research and education (CARE)—*Nursing Informatics: Where Caring and Technology Meet*!

The editors are especially indebted to Judith V. Douglas for her exquisite editorial and technical support, without whom this book could not have met its planned publication deadline. Her steadfast diligence and cheerful dedication have made this book the quality you see before you! Sincere thanks also go to Dr. Edward N. Brandt, Jr., Chancellor of the University of Maryland at Baltimore for his active support of informatics for the professional schools.

Our sincere thanks also go to Joann Sommers, who worked diligently on the preparation of the reference materials; Sandra Rogers, who coordinated the logistics of the information gathering and dissemination, and scheduled all necessary meetings; Amy Feng, Laura Nelson, Don Frese, Mary Ann Williams, and Inga Moten for their library searches of the reference material; Laura Nelson, Krysia Paré, and Sandy Giuliani, who helped proofread the individual chapters; and Marilyn Burnett, who labored diligently to transcribe tapes and assist wherever needed.

The editors also want to give special acknowledgment and express appreciation for the assistance of James Leoni, who created much of the graphics material; Linda Waring, who provided technical expertise; Yvonne Cager and the Operations Staff of the Information Resources Management Division, who assisted with the draft printings of the manuscript; Dr. James Craig, Dick Elliott, and Marie Toomes, who assisted in the photo production; and Mary Donhauser, who created some of the artwork.

Mr. Cyril Feng assisted the authors in taking full advantage of his highly regarded, fully automated Health Sciences Library. Dr. Thomas

M. Jenkins spent endless hours with the authors structuring the unique matrix overview of this book. He wishes to credit Jan Loper, President, Information Integraters, Inc. of Naples, Florida for the structural design of the format.

We owe special thanks to Noel Daly, the energetic executive officer of the Irish Nursing Board, whose support made this book part of the Third International Symposium on Nursing Use of Computers and Information Science in Dublin, June 1988.

Of special note is the senior editor's admiration for Ms. Sarah Holroyd, retired professor of music at the University of Kentucky who is completing her nursing degree now to devote the rest of her life to the nursing profession. A stronger love for the protection and preservation of mankind is unlikely to be found.

Also, our admiration and acknowledgment go to Mary Musick Lindberg, who represents the thousands of dedicated volunteer nurses who give their time, energy, and nursing expertise to those in need—silently and lovingly.

This extraordinary capacity for caring is shared by the senior editor's special friend, SaraKay Smullens. In her personal life, with her friends and family, Mrs. Smullens expresses her philosophy of self-respect and love for others. As a psychotherapist and an author, she stresses the importance of relationships. In networking with our colleagues for this book, we have put her philosophy into practice. As we finish this undertaking, we wish to thank those most important networks—our families.

Contents

Section 1—Nursing Informatics

Unit 1—Mastering Change

Section 1 —Nursing Informatics

Unit 2—Integrating Computing and Nursing

Section 1 —Nursing Informatics

Unit 3—New Roles for Nurses

Section 2 —Where Caring and Technology Meet

Unit 1—Clinical Practice

Section 2 —Where Caring and Technology Meet

Unit 2—Administrative Systems

Section 2 —Where Caring and Technology Meet

Unit 3—Research Frontiers

Section 2 —Where Caring and Technology Meet

Unit 4—Educational Innovations

Introduction

Susan J. Grobe

> The technological base of health care is changing constantly.
>
> (Hegyvary, 1987)

Nurses have a long and proud tradition of adopting technology into their professional practice. Stethoscopes, first used for measuring blood pressure, were gradually adopted by nurses for auscultation of lung and heart sounds. Today, electronic devices are increasingly being used to monitor respiratory and cardiac functions. This rapid adoption of technology is improving patient care, but it is also affecting care in ways not initially anticipated by nurses or other professionals.

Facing legislative and regulatory issues and experiencing increased specialization in nursing practice, the profession has been slow to acknowledge the increased responsibilities that accompany technological innovations. Newly required specialty skills tend to filter slowly across the fragmented practice field and into the professional education setting. The result is often a specialized arena for which both general practitioners and new graduates of the profession are inadequately prepared.

Yet change and increased adoption of technological innovations offer nursing strategies for responding to the external forces which threaten the profession—strategies particularly important in today's health care arena, where increasing economic pressures often conflict with nursing's caring philosophy.

Regardless of their national boundaries, nursing professionals must maintain quality of care and at the same time meet demands for cost containment, cost effectiveness, and increased professional accountability. Yet few nursing administrators have all the information they need about the critical issues affecting nursing practice and care delivery.

Specific data are required to document quality of care and cost control. These data must be gathered in a variety of settings, from the acute care institution to the realm of extended care, and on specialized and costly interventions that may not yet be reported in commonly available nursing literature. As technology continues to develop at a rapid pace, the capabilities conferred by computing place increased demands on nursing. Generating data for one particular purpose often results in more data being desired for related purposes; data definitions lead to increased sensitivity to the need for standardization.

While the demands for essential information outdistance efforts to identify and generate basic data, the urgency of the economic situation in health care requires nursing to use computer technology to make wise and informed decisions. Nurse researchers and nurse educators face the same dilemma.

The adoption of technological innovations requires responsiveness to change, and change can have unexpected consequences, both for the individual and for the profession. Once begun, changes occur in increasingly shorter time cycles. Unanticipated questions suddenly assume significance; and information handling skills, relatively unrecognized in the education of health professionals, take on new importance.

Thus, we have arrived at what the editors depict as the critical junction "where caring and technology meet." *Nursing Informatics* has patient care as its central focus, with associated clinical, administrative, research, and education components. The components are not unique to this book; however, the representation of these components as encircled by nursing informatics for this book is an important conceptualization. The book is divided into two sections. Section I delineates the field of nursing informatics, with specific reference to mastering change, integrating computing and nursing, and defining new roles for nurses. Section II, Where Caring and Technology Meet, describes computer uses in clinical practice, administration, research, and education. Here the contributors balance the promise of the technology for care with evidence drawn from their knowledge and experience.

Both sections bring us back to the question of what nursing informatics has to offer the nursing profession. Scattered throughout are references to nurses involved in nursing informatics and their influence on national and international nursing and multidisciplinary organizations.

However, I believe the essence of the question of what nursing informatics can contribute to nursing depends in great measure on the

- Importance of the research questions that are posed by nurse informaticians

- Soundness of the informatics research that is conducted

- Innovativeness of the nursing support systems that are created

- Rigor with which these systems are used and evaluated

- Excellence with which professional nurses are prepared and educated

- Adequacy with which nursing's professional organizations take leadership in guiding the profession through the changes associated with health care policy and the adoption of these technological innovations.

Fortunately, thoughtful deliberations on these key considerations by professional nurses and the nursing profession are one step closer because the editors had the insight to collaborate with colleagues on this extremely useful book.

Reference Cited

Hegyvary ST, Duxbury ML, Hall RH, et al: *Evolution of Nursing Professional Organizations: Alternative Modes for the Future.* Kansas City, Missouri: American Academy of Nursing, 1987.

Nursing Informatics

Unit 1

Mastering Change

Chapter 1
How technology transforms society

Chapter 2
How tools transform work

Chapter 3
How managers facilitate transformation

Chapter 4
How to get appropriate help in an age of transformation

Unit 2

Integrating Computing and Nursing

Chapter 5
Design principles of intelligent computing systems

Chapter 6
How people interact with computers

Chapter 7
Linking different computers and different users

Chapter 8
Environmental impacts of computing systems

Unit 3

New Roles for Nurses

Chapter 9
Justification for Nursing Informatics as a specialty

Chapter 10
How the market place and the bank impact Nursing

Chapter 11
What it takes to succeed in 9 different jobs

Chapter 12
Skills needed to be a Nursing systems analyst

Chapter 13
How Informatics will change the Nursing job

This contents array presents the architecture of the book in reader-friendly terms. Use it to get a feel for the thrust of the units and chapters and to quickly select what you want to study in more depth.

Where Caring & Technology Meet

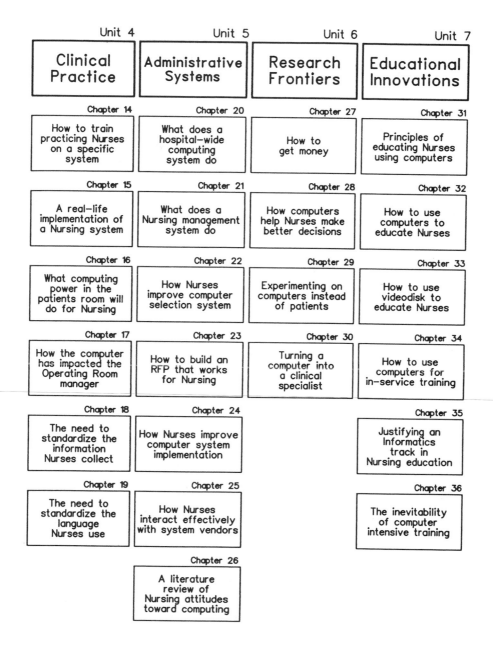

Unit 4	Unit 5	Unit 6	Unit 7
Clinical Practice	**Administrative Systems**	**Research Frontiers**	**Educational Innovations**

Chapter 14	Chapter 20	Chapter 27	Chapter 31
How to train practicing Nurses on a specific system	What does a hospital-wide computing system do	How to get money	Principles of educating Nurses using computers

Chapter 15	Chapter 21	Chapter 28	Chapter 32
A real-life implementation of a Nursing system	What does a Nursing management system do	How computers help Nurses make better decisions	How to use computers to educate Nurses

Chapter 16	Chapter 22	Chapter 29	Chapter 33
What computing power in the patients room will do for Nursing	How Nurses improve computer selection system	Experimenting on computers instead of patients	How to use videodisk to educate Nurses

Chapter 17	Chapter 23	Chapter 30	Chapter 34
How the computer has impacted the Operating Room manager	How to build an RFP that works for Nursing	Turning a computer into a clinical specialist	How to use computers for in-service training

Chapter 18	Chapter 24		Chapter 35
The need to standardize the information Nurses collect	How Nurses improve computer system implementation		Justifying an Informatics track in Nursing education

Chapter 19	Chapter 25		Chapter 36
The need to standardize the language Nurses use	How Nurses interact effectively with system vendors		The inevitability of computer intensive training

Chapter 26
A literature review of Nursing attitudes toward computing

Section 1—Nursing Informatics
Unit 1—Mastering Change

Unit Introduction

In our **CARE** concept, this unit addresses the **E** of Educational Innovations. Hannah introduces this section with an introduction of informatics pointing to education and training on a global level. Thomas addresses the current status of instructional computing in nursing education. Next follows Craig's discussion of the innovative uses of laser disk technology in nursing education. The fourth chapter by Hannah and Osis describes staff development activities. Heller and colleagues present the need for formal graduate education programs in nursing informatics and a plan for establishing such a program. In the last chapter, Hales focuses on continuing education with a list of minimum competencies for future nurse informaticians.

1—The Impact of Informatics on Nursing

Denis Protti

Introduction

What are the major issues surrounding this complex subject? Will the nursing profession change dramatically over the next 20 years and if so in what ways? Rather than presume to have definitive answers, this chapter will raise questions, questions that readers will eventually have to answer for themselves.

The chapter is structured so as to develop the following premises:

- Informatics is part of the larger domain of "technology."

- The impact that informatics will have on nursing can be seen by observing the impact technology is having on our society. Although technologies such as hydroponics, genetic engineering, and nuclear fission are important in the overall scheme of things, they are not discussed in this chapter.

- The nursing profession as we now know it will be impacted more by the attitudes and approaches to health care delivery than it will be by informatics.

In a chapter of this type, one must resist the temptation to "blue sky" unrealistically. Predictions of what the world will be like 100 years from now are easy; the predictor need not worry about being around to defend his/her views. The nearer to the present, the more difficult the task, because the political, social, economic, and emotional issues that influence change are much more apparent.

This chapter will attempt to identify the issues that are likely to affect nursing over the next 10 to 20 years. In doing so, it will restrict itself to discussing the issues as they pertain to hospital-based acute care nurses in western industrialized nations. Nurses in third world countries and those working in community health settings will also be affected by informatics but in slightly different ways. The extent to which one agrees with someone else's view of the future is very much influenced by one's own view of the past and present. The way in which each reader answers the questions raised will be governed by how the individual interprets and understands the issues and is challenged or threatened by the implications. One consolation is that all health professionals are having to wrestle with the same questions.

The Evolution of Information Technology

Informatics or, in less esoteric terms, information technology, is not a new phenomenon. It has been around since the beginning of time. It entails people communicating with each other, and recording their thoughts, ideas, and actions for others to read or hear.

In coming to understand information technology in a modern context, it is important to realize that the electronic computer is only one component in an elaborate and highly differentiated infrastructure. This infrastucture has grown through a succession of generations of computers, each of which represents a major change in technology. During the 8-year span of each computing generation (the first generation started in the late 1940s and the fifth in the early 1980s), revolutionary changes have taken place that correspond to those taking place over some 70 years or more in the aircraft industry. If we were to draw parallels to the rapid and massive advances in computing, with comparable development aircraft would fly 100 times faster, a $100,000 home would cost $20,000, and color televisions would cost $20.

The definition of generations in terms of electronic device technology captures some important aspects of computing technology such as cost decreases, size decrease, power increases, and so on. However, it fails to account for the qualitative changes that have given computing its distinct character in each generation. The change from mechanical to electronic devices has facilitated storing programs as data, using computers as general purpose tools, and developing programming languages. The transistor made possible reliable operation, routine electronic data processing, and interactive time-sharing. Integrated circuits reduced costs to the level at which computers became commonplace and made possible the personal computer dedicated to the single user.

Each generation represents a revolution in technology with a qualitatively different impact. Each generation subsumes the capabilities of that preceding it, providing markedly better facilities at significantly lower cost and adding new capabilities not possessed by the previous generations. One of the innovative new capabilities has been in the area of knowledge-based systems. The products stemming from breakthroughs in this area are expert systems that simulate some of the processes of the human mind—knowledge representation and inference—allowing expertise to be encoded for a computer and made widely available. This has generated a new industry based on creating systems that make the practical working knowledge of a human expert in a specific subject area, such as medicine, widely available to those without direct access to the originator. Are there parallels in nursing?

Technology and Society

Society is experiencing its second major revolution in less than 200 years. The first was the Industrial Revolution of the nineteenth century, which saw the substitution of mechanical processes for human muscles. It changed the nature of work, although not the size of the work force, and with it society's view of human values. The spinning jenny may have done the work of a thousand women, but hundreds of thousands were eventually needed in the mills. The automobile may have put the horse out of business, but Henry Ford saw to it that many more mechanics were needed than blacksmiths, many more oil industry personnel than haymakers.

Although it had a significant impact on the nature of work, the Industrial Revolution did provide untold opportunities for the individual to hold a job at some level. Even if the job was classified as unskilled labor, the person still had an identity as a breadwinner, and could feel a sense of worth from that. If that industrial job was classified as skilled labor, the person had not only the benefits of the unskilled laborer, but in addition a higher job status. As a rule, every major technologic advance destroys the civilization that existed at the time of its introduction into everyday life. The steam engine pushed us out of the fields and into the cities, and the automobile moved us out of the cities and into the suburbs. The movies gathered us in huge crowds in darkened halls; television returned us to our own darkened living rooms. The compass and chronometer made intercontinental travel possible, the airplane makes it trivial, and advances in communications technology may make it unnecessary.

The second major revolution is the so-called electronic or information revolution in which electronic circuits are being substituted for human mental skills. The electronic revolution is not only replacing the mental processes of the unskilled laborer—it is creating a genuine human value dilemma for technologists, managers, and professionals.

Technology is changing almost everyone's job. What is both exciting and frightening is that the rate of change in the next 20 years is probably going to be greater than the rate of change in any previous 20-year period in history. The fundamental economic activities of our society—agriculture and the multitude of extractive, manufacturing, and service industries—continue, but they are increasingly influenced by a new decision-making process. Vastly more information (on markets, costs, techniques, and other options) is being made available to decision makers because of the information technology now available. And this information is being eagerly sought, because more informed decisions, be they made in politics, in operating sawmills, in hospitals, or in waging war, are likely to produce better results.

The electronic revolution has made robotics a reality. The development and use of intelligent robots who perform delicate tasks that once were done by thinking human beings is increasingly commonplace in manufacturing sectors of society. Robotics are beginning to be introduced into health care. How long before they become commonplace?

While the industrial age found its symbol in the factory, the symbol of the information age might be the computer, which can hold all the information in the Library of Congress in a machine the size of a small refrigerator. Or its proper symbol may be a robot, a machine capable of supplementing age-old manual labor and liberating human beings from the most arduous and repetitive tasks. Or perhaps its symbol is the direct-broadcast satellite, which can send television programs directly into homes around the globe. Telephone companies the world over are joining forces under the banner of the Integrated Services Digital Network (ISDN), which is described as the key to linking all the elements of the information age. ISDN is several things at one time, but it will allow every home and business to receive simultaneously voice, computing, and video signals on a telephone line.

A popular way of looking at information technology is in terms of its utility. The reasoning most frequently used to justify purchases of information technology goes as follows: Labor expenses are high and getting higher; computer expenses are low and getting lower; it then logically follows that one should always trade an expensive commodity, e.g., labor, for an inexpensive commodity, e.g., computers.

One of the resulting dilemmas is that "value" has become less personal and more social or group oriented. In a technologic society, the individual may feel remote from the ethical and moral decisions that are projected onto society itself. For individuals whose identities are embedded in their jobs, traditional culture provides no guidelines to help them value themselves after they have been more or less excluded from the productive parts of society. The government public welfare system may provide money for the mortgage and food, but will it maintain one's sense of value or worth as a human being?

The Evolution of the Health Care Industry

The future of the health care industry is not the same everywhere. In many parts of the world, the health care industry is struggling to satisfy the most basic and fundamental of needs. In other parts of the world, the rapid advances in medical science are putting strains on governments to provide the best possible care, given the limited resources available. In the United States, the future of the health care industry is quite clear: The future is competition. Competition is not new, nor is it unique to the Americans; competition has always existed in terms of institutional pride, quality of care, medical staff prestige, and reputation.

In the United States, however, competition will be redefined over the next two decades to include price and marketing as important factors. In 1985, a White House working group on health policy and economics wrote that the prospective payment system (PPS) then used for Medicare inpatient hospital services should be viewed as a transition from cost reimbursement to a more comprehensive payment system based on competitive principles. This follows other health care payors—employer trusts, commercial insurers, health maintenance organizations (HMOs), and preferred provider organizations (PPOs)—in developing payment methodologies that promote price competition. The increasing emphasis on competition has spurred the movement toward what is called alternate site medicine, that is, the delivery of health care outside the traditional (and costly) hospital setting.

Of particular interest is the role technology plays in this new movement. Diagnoses that were once run in the hospital or in large clinical labs are now being performed in doctors' offices in minutes and at a fraction of the cost charged by the big automated labs. More and more surgical procedures are now performed routinely in outpatient day surgery units and in private surgicenters. Technologic advances such as the lithotripper can replace complex and costly major surgery, along with its 10- to 12-day hospital stay, with a 1-day procedure that shatters rather than removes kidney stones. A growing number of treatments (kidney dialysis and continuous antibiotic therapy, for example) are being administered in the home. The list grows with each passing year.

Much of the new technology focuses on small tabletop chemical analyzers that permit private physicians to test patient fluids for infection and other common disorders cheaply and within minutes. In the United States, there are approximately 40,000 physician-owned laboratories. By 1990, this is expected to grow to 70,000. The analyzers used in these small offices generally run the most common, most easily interpreted analyses, and are priced so low that even the cost-conscious solo practitioner is considered an important part of the market. One such analyzer performs the seven different blood tests (including glucose, urea nitrogen, and cholesterol) that account for more than 80% of a physician's needs. Other small instruments aimed at the private physician (and perhaps at the patient?) are a programmable three-channel electrocardiograph and an automated instrument for assessing the efficiency of the respiratory system. An ambulatory uterine activity monitor tracks possible abnormal conditions, alerting expectant mothers to premature labor by measuring uterine pressure through a small sensor attached to the abdomen. Until recently, the only way to predict premature labor before it actually began was through regular cervical examinations by a physician.

Diagnosis is only a part of the total health care picture. Medical costs are also being reduced by treatments that many patients can perform at home. The market, which includes not only the drugs used in the treatment but also auxiliary equipment such as small programmable pumps, now consists primarily of special nutritional products and services (aimed at patients with abnormal digestive systems), kidney dialysis, and continuous intravenous drug administration. Within a few years, home therapies will almost certainly embrace intractable disorders such as Alzheimer's disease along with many forms of physical rehabilitation.

One company markets a home chemotherapy system for cancer patients, many of whom would normally have to receive anticancer drugs in a hospital or physician's office. Patients who are healthy enough to live at home can often use a continuously administered, prepackaged drug or combination of drugs. The drugs are contained in a small plastic pouch that is attached to a catheter. A portable programmable pump delivers the drugs at a slow constant rate. One of the advantages to this approach is that the steady infusion of such drugs often eliminates the side effects, such as nausea, that usually accompany large doses.

The benefits of such procedures, moreover, extend well beyond lower costs. Recovery or remission rates for many patients are dramatically improved in the familiar and comfortable home environment. A lens implant in the eyes of a 75-year-old woman, for example, allows her to continue to live independently in the home and community, which is meaningful to her. Her quality of life is infinitely better than it would be if she were forced to move to a home for the blind in a nearby town or city. Similarly, neonatal intensive care units are allowing life to be continued in hundreds of cases in which death would have been a certainty 25 years ago. Microcomputing technology is providing artificial voices for those who cannot speak, workstations for the sightless, communication for those paralyzed by stroke. Seniors, handicapped people, and others with high-risk medical conditions can find a new level of security when their hospitals use a computer and the telephone system to guarantee them almost instant response in an emergency. This list also grows with each passing year.

Closer to home for the hospital-based nurse are the effects on the laboratory. The technologic impact on this area of the health care industry has been most pronounced. In the domain of clinical microscopy alone, the work being performed has changed dramatically over the past 40 years. In the 1940s, the work entailed the thoughtful manipulation of tissue and reagents and was carried out exclusively by physicians. A decade or so later, the work was structured and defined. Once rules were established, the work could be carried out by trained technologists. By the 1970s, the rules, particularly as they applied to measurement, were engineered into cell-counting machines. The work of the technologist now became one of monitoring the equipment for quality control and managing the exceptions the machine could not handle. Now, with newer, more sophisticated machines, quality control and exception management have also been incorporated into the instrument. Are there parallels in nursing?

Questions to Be Answered

All individuals have their own views, their own perceptions of the world around them that result from their individual background, culture, education, and values. We do not perceive that technology will affect each of us in the same way. A recent survey of nursing students found that more than 95% of them believed that they would never speak to a computer or use an expert system. Yet voice-recognition technology has moved out of the research laboratory, and expert systems are routinely being used in financial investment circles.

In an age when the rapid pace of research has lowered the half-life of knowledge to less than 5 years, how will the initial education and continuing education of nurses be affected? How will the new ways of caring for the sick, many of which are not a part of the standard conventional medical model, affect nurses? What effect will decreasing lengths of stay, resulting in large part from technology, have no our hospitals and hence on nurses?

In some parts of the world, a surplus of physicians has been identified. Given that public policy does not address this real or perceived situation through reductions in medical school admissions, will physicians begin to function in areas that are currently the domain of other health care professionals?

Will we have technologically based wristwatches that provide continuous monitoring of our physical status and perhaps even have drug-dispensing capabilities automatically triggered by our physiologic and biochemical needs?

Are we witnessing not only the automation of clerical activities, but also the automation of thoughtful technical and clinical work? If so, what are the consequences? Will the responsibility for the production of reliable information rest more with rules incorporated in equipment and on established procedures than on a nurse's judgment?

Nurses of the Future

Nurses of the future will require the skills to handle the technology that is driving the future of health care delivery. To care for the patient population in the hospital as well as in outpatient, community, and home health care settings, nurses need training in informatics to adopt the new roles required of nursing. There is no doubt that by the year 2000 every nurse must be capable of using information systems.

Questions

1. Compare and contrast the Industrial Revolution to the Information Revolution.
2. Describe one way in which technology has changed the way work is done in the laboratory of a hospital.
3. What are the characteristics of each new generation of computer technology?
4. Give examples, from nonhealth sectors, of how work has changed as a result of computing and communications technology.
5. Describe how nursing will likely change over the next 10 years as a result of technology.

2—Integrating Nursing and Informatics

Marion J. Ball and Judith V. Douglas

Introduction

Integrating computers into nursing is a challenge. Before we embark on this new challenge, we need to realize that nothing in life is easy. Change always elicits some fear, because it holds the unknown and unfamiliar. But we prefer to look at the partially filled glass of water as half full rather than half empty. We are in for great excitement and opportunities in the nursing profession as we move toward the twenty-first century.

Consider briefly the forces that are beginning to impact nursing, both external and internal. We can then look at the new tools information technology is putting within our reach and see how those tools will help us to address those forces.

Forces Impacting Nursing

Today, evolving standards of practice increase nursing accountability. The malpractice crisis has resulted in added emphasis on complete nursing documentation. Changes in reimbursement methods are affecting nursing care delivery. Cost containment and consumerism place additional pressures on not only the individual nurse but also the entire nursing profession. The profession and its practitioners need to address, acknowledge, and prepare for the expansion and extension in nursing roles created by advances in biomedical technology.

These external forces are exacerbated by internal pressures affecting the nursing environment. Hospital operations remain task oriented; systems do not promote practitioner accountability; and paperwork requirements have proliferated. These factors we cannot escape; we have to confront them and master them.

How do we do so? What are the new alternatives, the new tools available to us in the late 1980s that allow us to address these forces? How can we grow in our profession and meet these challenges?

The change masters, the leaders who have networked together to produce this book, will address these questions, repeatedly spiraling back to the host of issues and opportunities surrounding the use of computers in nursing care. These authors include nurses involved in every aspect of the profession, from clinical practice to education, from research to administration. They also include other professionals who have learned invaluable lessons in health care from the nursing profession and have lent their own special areas of expertise to nursing.

Stages in Integration

Whatever the use to which we put new technology in health care—clinical, nursing, hospital information systems, or elsewhere—we all pass through three defined stages before we become more or less comfortable with using the new technology. These three stages are classic in the adoption of computing and information technology.

Replacement

The first of those three stages is called replacement. Simply put, it means that when we get a new tool into our hands, the only thing that we are capable of doing with it at that stage is to try and do what we have been doing in a manual fashion. Maybe we can do it a little bit faster, a little bit more efficiently; but in effect we are replacing a function that we have done manually by this new tool, the computer.

Over the last 20 years, we have been in this first stage as we have brought computers into health care. New computer systems have been nothing more than replacements of manual systems. For example, in admissions offices, we no longer use the typewriter to enter the admissions information on a seven-part form. We brought computers into the admissions office, and we typed information into a computer terminal. We had some advantages in that we could more easily disseminate the information or we could make changes more easily without having to use correction fluid to correct the form. We could use a little bit of the technology that made the task a little bit easier. But we were really only in the replacement stage—slowly moving into using a new tool.

Innovation

Once we became comfortable with it, we said to ourselves, "Look, we have a new tool now that's very powerful. We might be able to do something that we could not do when we didn't have this tool at our disposal." So we move from replacement into what is called the innovation stage. We have gone beyond what we could originally do manually to doing things with the computer that we could not do before. The new technology begins to be diffused throughout our profession. Computer systems become commonplace in large-scale hospital information systems as they have in radiology and clinical laboratories.

Transformation

It is true that other industries—airlines, travel, banking—are somewhat ahead of health care and are approaching the final stage. This stage, called transformation, lies beyond replacement and innovation, and involves completely revolutionizing the way business is done.

In the health care profession, the one area to have entered into this third stage is radiology. Radiology practices today are a transformation of those common as little as 10 years ago. Computerized axial tomography has given us the now-standard CAT scan. Even the way in which radiographs (or x-rays) are read and reported is not at all similar to what was done before new computerized capabilities were available. And, of course, every one of these instruments is based on a built-in computer.

When we look at the nursing profession and its practices, it is very exciting to realize that we are going through these phases and all of us are somewhere in this process. Most of us are still in the replacement stage, moving into innovation. Over the next 5 or 6 years there will be a revolution—not even an evolution—a *revolution* into a transformed profession.

Information Technology Tools

Surveys by the American Hospital Association as well as by software vendors have shown that the hospital information systems (HIS) now installed in many institutions do improve communications. These systems also have the potential, when used properly, to increase access to and accuracy of data. Both are increasing in importance as we must respond to demands for more information-based reports and analysis.

Hospital information systems also give us the ability to forecast, by providing data gathering and storage capacities. With them, we can determine with some precision where we have been and where we are now. Software packages allow us to go beyond the present and to forecast where we will be in the future. This is particularly important in this new era of nurse involvement with overall health care delivery.

With that as background, let us focus on the health care environment with which we are all familiar and on the kind of tools that are coming into nursing. No health care profession has more contact with the many aspects of patient care than does nursing. No other profession has more involvement with hospital information systems that touch all these aspects than does nursing. Unfortunately, until recently nursing as a profession was not sufficiently involved in the selection, the implementation, and in the decision making as to what systems were best for their institutions. As a result, many of the earlier systems in the marketplace and in the hospitals have not met nursing needs. Many of them have failed because of that deficiency.

But there is little yield in dwelling on past failures—or even on the capabilities available at this exact moment in time. As Homer Warner, one of the United States' leading medical informaticians, has commented many times, "Let's not spend all our time and resources measuring how long it takes or how much it costs to get there with today's buggy. But let's get on with the job of building tomorrow's automobile and planning where to go with it." He means, of course, that we do not need to replicate. We do not need to see how we traveled with the old horse and buggy. Our challenge is to see how we can use this new tool to innovate and to transform.

Technologic advances are now available that will allow this transformation to take place. Several years ago, one of the authors (MJB) used to introduce to her seminar audiences a small laptop computer weighing less than 4 pounds that was carried by engineers, airline people, and academicians on the move. Now it is finding its way, not in the same form, into the working world of health professionals. Nurses no longer need to stay tied to a very large computer at a nursing station. This microchip technology is allowing us to augment as we innovate and transform by enabling us to take handheld terminals to the patient's bedside. This makes it possible to have information "at hand" when and where it is needed—at the patient's bedside.

Truly portable, these handheld terminals are under development by a number of manufacturers. Experimental models include 64K portable pocket terminals that the nurse can take to the patient's bedside for entering vital signs and some routine charting information. This frees nurses from having to jot down or to remember the information until they can return to the nursing station to enter it. The tools go with the nurses who provide the care.

We also have nursing station-based functional systems, including among others the Technicon, IBM, Travenol, Data Care, and some of the IBM PC-based systems. These represent what is now the more prevalent way of interfacing with hospital information systems development. The keyboard and the terminal remain at the nursing station where data is entered and the charting completed. Order entries are performed at the terminal by those who are providing care for the patient, primarily by nurses and in some instances by physicians.

To augment these systems, look at yet another innovation; the larger terminal may be taken away from the nursing station and placed at the bedside of the patient (Health Data Systems). This and other new ideas are being tested now. We do not yet know whether these ideas will come into the mainstream, but many companies and many vendors are obviously in the business of trying to market all kinds of tools to health care professionals.

Nursing Informatics

The nurse and all other health care professionals clearly will have to learn how to use these new tools. The learning process and the use that follows are covered by the term "informatics." The term medical informatics has been used for some time, nearly 20 years, and covers all the health care fields. Coined from the French word "informatique," the term is moving to greater use and a higher level of definition in the other health care professions.

Informatics includes all aspects of the computer milieu, from the theoretical to the applied. It covers learning how to use the new tools and to build upon the capabilities provided by computers and other information technologies. The part of informatics designed for and relevant to nurses has been labeled nursing informatics. This new term and what it represents will clearly be part of all our professional vocabularies and practices. The term combines all aspects of nursing—clinical practice, administration, research, and education—just as computing holds the power to integrate all four aspects.

We could go so far as to say that nursing informatics has arrived, and that the baby is starting to walk. It is exciting to see a whole new profession coming into its own. By becoming involved in the innovative phases of using the tools at our disposal, we can further nursing care and practice.

Nursing informatics has introduced new challenges and opportunities along with new computer applications. For nurses, it has created a new cadre of roles and a new vision of the nursing profession. Vendors of hospital information systems employ nurses as consultants now, as nursing liaison advisors to the data processing division. Nurses are becoming programmers, system engineers, and systems analysts.

We may ask ourselves, "Well, isn't this just individuals changing their profession and leaving nursing?" Not quite, for it involves more. Systems analysts and engineers who come from nursing backgrounds practice their profession differently from those coming from an engineering or mathematics background. This has tremendous advantages for nurses remaining in the more traditional nursing fields. Software development is critical for nursing, in that it provides the logic for applications. That logic must take into account what the profession is practicing on a daily basis, and who understands the nursing process better than a nurse?

Industry has realized this and is freely hiring people with nursing degrees to be involved in software development. The technical aspects are important, because the software does in fact drive the hardware.

From our point of view, though, the needs of the users are of equal or greater importance. Developers who understand the nursing profession and its needs, from abstract concepts to small details, are invaluable. Thus the evolution of professions—the hybridization of nurse and computer expert—is critical to effecting the transformation we are anticipating.

New roles evolving for nursing include consulting. Hospitals are now beginning to hire nurse consultants to assist in the design and implementation phases as well as in the process of selecting computers. They are concerned not only with input into what the software should be, but also with how health care professionals communicate with one another and with computing professionals.

Change

One key question remains: How do we get this new technology accepted by our colleagues? No hospital information system or stand-alone surgical software system will be installed successfully, no tool used effectively, unless there is an enormous amount of preparation and training. A diffusion pathway must be laid to bring something in that will completely revolutionize the way in which all of us practice our profession. If this pathway is never built, the attempt at computerization will be a failure. We don't have to guess at this. We've seen it happen.

As a profession, we have participated in government-funded investigations on the effect of hospital information systems on health care delivery in nursing practice. We are progressing beyond the clinical environment and moving professionally into the establishment of a bona fide research component. We will be looking at nursing practice and nursing education, assessing the problems and issues surrounding information technology, from implementation to ergonomics.

One of the biggest concerns now is that we provide strong master's and doctoral programs as well as superb bachelor's degrees in our nursing schools. Nursing informatics needs to be incorporated into the curricula offered by our schools. Only then will the nursing profession be prepared for what is in store.

All areas will be freed up as we move into the era of high technology. Hands-on care, or high touch, will continue to be at the heart of the profession. Nurses in computer-aided patient care situations will become involved in administering some nontraditional therapies, such as hypnosis, therapeutic touch, acupuncture, biofeedback, or sonic vibration.

All these changes result in another professional responsibility. Nursing needs to reassess its career paths and its status and reward systems. At this moment, nurses have but one main track for advancement. Nurses move from their traditional place at the bedside and achieve status and financial reward by taking on supervisory and managerial tasks. We firmly believe that as computerization changes the profession, nursing will reappraise its value system and reward professionalism in a wide range of nursing duties not traditionally recognized. In sum, nursing will have greater diversity by virtue of employment opportunities in the health informatics field.

The Future

What do we see in the next 5 years? We will see more computer power, portable computers and handheld terminals at the bedside, voice input freeing our hands for patient care, videodisk technology giving us vast quantities of stored data and visual information. We will benefit from expert systems, decision support systems, modeling systems, and artificial intelligence (AI) programs.

The greatest benefits, however, will not come from the individual tools, as powerful and as effective as they prove to be. Nursing will reap the most from the information that these new technologies make available. Computing will be a powerful utility, fueling our health care information systems just as electricity fuels our operating room lights and respirators.

In electronic terms, computing is the medium, information the message. The medium is the equipment that provides the connectivity, enabling the microcomputer user to access other computers, other systems. These computers link the user with colleagues, institutions, libraries. The medium provides new tools, giving to the health care professional new capabilities for multiple functions—education, research, clinical care, and management of all these. As we move toward integrating these functions through the computing medium, we must respond again and again to critical issues discussed by the other contributors to this book.

This new medium of computing holds our future. It is our charge to use it well, to create the information-rich environment where patient care and all the many functions that support it are of the highest quality. As a profession, nursing can do no less.

Questions

1. What are some of the forces impacting nurses today?

2. List and define the three stages of diffusion of new technology.

3. What role is industry playing in acknowledging the new discipline of nursing informatics?

4. Take a brief look into the future and give a description as to what you might be doing in your job 10 years from today.

3—Organizational Change

Noel Daly

Introduction

Organizational change is a major concern of nurses in today's health care system. Nurse managers in hospitals hold the key to a critical mass in health care delivery—the nursing services that are its backbone. How nurse managers structure health care delivery and what organizational climate they establish for nursing practice combine to influence quality of patient care and hospital performance. There is increasing evidence that comprehensive organizational change is an effective way to cope with current and future demands for nursing care.

Definition of Change

Change is defined as "to transform or convert or to be transformed or converted" (McLeod, 1982). Translated into organizational terms, this means that the environment contains at any time many strong forces. One of these forces is the increased use of technology in providing complex patient care. Another force is the pressure to reduce the growth in health care finances. These two powerful forces that have emerged provide nurse managers with the opportunity to evaluate and restructure the organization of nursing. It is clear that in this type of changing environment the nurse manager must establish a very cost-effective organization. Also, the nurse manager must act to gain a sustained advantage for quality nursing care.

The Role of the Nurse Manager

The nurse manager should have qualities of courage, patience, and discipline. Defining philosophy, goals, and objectives is part of the preparation before tackling any task. Knowing what is wanted and having a clear purpose are critical to the ability to recognize and use opportunities that arise. Clear purpose also engenders planning and action to create the opportunities needed to attain goals. Meeting the challenge of change in any nursing organization is real, and has many implications. But meeting the challenge of change is easier if a nurse manager thinks in terms of what can be accomplished instead of the problems and issues at hand. A proactive stance is necessary to challenge assumptions, and will result in creative solutions rather than piecemeal ad hoc solutions for specific issues.

In the past, change was the dominion of innovators. Today all nurse managers are expected to have the vision to manage change. Change cannot be achieved without comprehensive organizational revitalization and restructuring. Thus, nurse managers must become strategists, or those who have maintained organizations in the past may not be able to function effectively in top management.

Strategic Management and the Organization

Strategy involves understanding clearly the elements of the situation, restructuring those elements in the most advantageous way, and finding the best possible solution to the problem at hand (Ohmae, 1982). Ohmae goes on to describe strategic thinking as a combination of rational analysis, based on the real nature of things, and an imaginative reintegration of various elements into new patterns. The thinking manager achieves superior performance by evaluating the strategic three "C's": the corporation, the competition, and the customers.

Organizations can be defined as having five components: the top management, the technostructure, the operating core (those who perform the work), the middle line, and the support staff (Mintzberg, 1981). It is not necessary for all organizations to have all the five components. Smaller organizations tend to have fewer than the large older organizations do. Large organizations are more likely to have planning, training, and liaison departments than smaller ones. In Mintzberg's view, effective organizations are consistent internally as well as consistent with the organization's size and age, the community it serves, and the industry within which it operates.

In order to approach change in an organization, the first step is to assess where nursing fits. Most organizations are individualistic; they also vary according to their mission and resources. All hospitals operate within the same health care system. The nurse manager knows that there are good and bad arrangements, and must decide how nursing resources can be effectively utilized. Developing a sense of the whole organization helps the nurse manager find effective approaches to change.

Currently there is emphasis on strategic management in organizations. Five different levels of strategic planning and organization can be identified: product, market planning, business unit planning, shared resource planning, shared concern planning, and corporate level planning (Gluck et al, 1980). On all five levels, teamwork is the rule rather than the exception in strategically managed companies. Nurse managers are in a good position to initiate change in the nursing department as it relates to the total organization. A contemporary way to provide the organization with the flexibility needed to deal with changing environments is through executive management.

The first step in commencing change is to assess the organization. What is the organization's capacity to supply services? What is its potential? The following set of questions provides one approach to determining organizational capacity.

What is the organization's mission?
How does the organization fill that mission?
What services are provided?
What resources are used?
How does the organizational structure affect resource utilization?
What are the outcomes of the organizational effort?

Referring to Mintzberg's organizational components it is clear that nursing fits into each component: the strategic apex where the organizational mission is decided, the technostructure where systems and formal planning are designed, the operating core where nursing practice takes place, the middle line where nurse managers are responsible for division and unit function, and the support staff needed to make the system work.

The Change Process

To decide where the nursing department is, and what direction it should take in future development, the nurse manager must first develop an approach to visionary thinking. Once the nurse manager has a clear intention of where the nursing department should be, the next step is to figure out how to get there through strategic planning. Moving in that direction involves change. The classic theory of the change process has three main phases: unfreeze, move, and refreeze (Argyle, 1967). To deal with the change the nurse manager must decide what needs thawing. As a change agent, the manager examines who is affected by the intended change and what that individual's level of involvement is. Lewin's Force Field analysis expresses the theory that a balance point is reached between opposing forces for change and forces for maintaining the status quo.

Analysis of these forces requires the identification of the dominant groups/coalitions in the organization, those in positions of power in the organization's social system. This system is formed by the personal characteristics of the people, their internal organizational relationships, and the objectives and strategies of the organization. Involving the dominant coalition in the change process will help gain acceptance for the desired change in the organization. Another aspect of analyzing forces for change is to determine the sources of stimuli, such as society, the political system, or economic factors. The nurse manager can look to patients, nurses, professional organizations, the hospital board, the chief executive, the medical staff, government rules and regulations, policies and standards, and other sources.

Proactive change can be accomplished through organizational development, or, more precisely, through deliberate and reasoned change to improve organizational effectiveness. Change needs to be introduced, established, reinforced, and spread throughout the organization to create a proactive stance in regard to change. Nurse managers often suggest that they not only have to deal with changing attitudes of top management to achieve any desired change in the nursing department, but more importantly with the attitudes of staff nurses. Many staff nurses resist change if they are comfortable with their roles and ways. Staff nurses can be as powerful in blocking change as can top management. Movement in the change process involves establishing relationships conducive to change.

The nurse manager working toward change establishes an organizational climate conducive to growth and development. Organizational climate is defined as the psychologic setting characteristic of an organization that can be deduced from the way the organization deals with its members and the environment. Behaviors of employees are affected by the organizational climate. It is difficult to change behavior; what the nurse manager does is to change the organizational climate and employees will then change their behaviors accordingly (Bennis, 1976).

In departments of nursing, one of the most powerful measures top management can take is to create a system of values and beliefs recognizing the contribution of nurses to patient care and demanding of them the responsibility to fulfill the expectation of high-quality nursing care.

Promoting acceptance of change is the optimist's way of writing about resistance to change. A change agent has to be an optimist, albeit a realistic one, who learns to convey concepts and ideas in a positive and rational approach. Diagnosing resistance to change identifies four common reasons why people resist change:

- not wanting to lose something they value
- misunderstanding change and its implications

- believing that the proposed change is not good for the organization

- having low tolerance for change (Kotter and Schleisinger, 1979).

Remedies include:

- devising a program for open communication and for education about the change

- providing accurate information to allow people to understand the need for change

- actually involving people in the development of change (Kotter and Schleisinger, 1979).

Commitment to the change is generated if people have a part in designing it. When change involves learning new skills, people need to be supported by listening to their concerns, providing time and resources to learn the new skills, and recognizing their accomplishments. Establishing trust between employees and managers is an important condition of successful change. Prior experience with change affects current attitudes because organizations, like people, have a memory (Ginzberg and Reilley, 1957).

The use of planning techniques when designing and implementing change that involves many people in various departments is advisable. Plans are most helpful if they outline:

- the stages of the design for change

- the person responsible for implementing each stage

- the timeline for the period within which the change has to be completed

- the expected outcome at the end of each stage.

The cost of change can be expressed in both human and financial terms. It is the duty of the change agent to consider these costs when designing and implementing change. The amount of advanced planning with critical input from key persons and technical experts in the organization will mean cost efficiency in the way the plans are developed. There are many types of costs that are included in change plans; these can be categorized as follows:

- the time input of individuals involved for discussing, planning, and implementing

- consultants and technical experts

- print materials

- the resources needed

- changes in facilities
- education
- evaluation.

It has been observed that "the better the employee the more likely that he or she will become quickly dissatisfied with an assignment in which there is little discretion to make important decisions" (Ginzberg and Reilley, 1957). Improved motivation and satisfaction result from being involved, and both can be factors in recruitment and retention of the most qualified persons.

The Nurse Manager and Change

Competent nurses will be attracted to competent organizations in which they can have input in decisions that improve their practice and keep them stimulated to learn more. The benefits of change can be realized in lower turnover and increased productivity. To be effective, the nurse manager has to manage the change in the context of the organization and to be responsive to a situation.

It is imperative that the nurse manager finds ways to remain current in the nursing profession. An organizational support system can provide the forum for discussing common problems, exploring the feasibility of new ideas, or relieving pressure. Relationships with counterparts in other hospitals can be an enriching experience, giving nurse managers the opportunity to learn from peers in exploring and shaping new ideas. Contacts are invaluable in keeping the professional informed. The development of networks benefits both the nurse manager and the recipients within the network, be they local, national, or international.

The nurse manager needs to learn about new developments from peers and to acquire ideas of what to change or how to change. Among the sources helpful in this learning process are literature describing new projects and programs, site visits to places known for innovation, and sessions about change at conferences, symposia, and meetings. Useful strategies in planning and developing concepts for the future include:

- anticipating forthcoming innovations as products of theory development and research
- using the techniques of forecasting and projection to identify demographic changes, evolving or developing technology, and health care trends.

Thinking in terms of the future, engaging in forecasting, and having an open mind—these activities will allow the nurse manager to develop a sense of control over uncertain and unknown future events with the potential to affect the delivery of nursing care in hospitals.

Great satisfaction can be derived from designing and implementing change. The change agents who set a direction and work toward it are the pacesetters, the nurse managers who recognize the opportunity for change and use it. They are the nurse managers with the vision to plan for the future, the vision that will keep the delivery of quality nursing care up-to-date.

Questions

1. Give a classic definition of change. Then follow up with your own definition of change.

2. List five qualities a nurse manager must possess to be successful. List five more that would be highly desirable in addition to the five above.

3. Using an organizational assessment approach, determine your organizational capacity by answering the five questions listed in this chapter.

4. What is Lewin's Force Field theory? Can you describe how it could be used in a situation in your work place?

5. What are at least two benefits of change in an organization?

References

Argyle M: *The Psychology of Interpersonal Behaviour*. Middlesex, England: Penguin Books Limited, 1967.
Bennis WG: *The Planning of Change*. 3d ed. New York: Holt, Rinehart and Winston, 1976.
Ginzberg E, Reilley EW: *Effecting Change in Large Organizations*. New York: Columbia University Press, 1957.
Gluck FW, Kaufman SP, Walleck AS: Strategic management for competitive advantage. *Harvard Business Review* 1980; 58:154–161.
Judson AS: *A Manager's Guide to Making Changes*. New York: Wiley, 1966.
Kotter JP, Schleisinger LA: Choosing strategies for change. *Harvard Business Review* 1979; 57:106–113.
McLeod WT, ed: *The New Collins Concise English Dictionary*. Glasgow: Collins, 1982.
Mintzberg H: Organizational design: fashion or fit? *Harvard Business Review* 1981; 59:103–115.
Ohmae K: *The Mind of the Strategist*. New York: McGraw-Hill, 1982.

4—How to Select a Nursing Informatics Consultant

Elizabeth E. Ball and Gary L. Hammon

When to Employ a Consultant

Hospitals, specifically nursing departments, face major decisions as they plan to meet their computing needs. It is often advisable to employ a consultant in order to obtain expert advice with regard to a well-defined situation or problem that is beyond the capabilities or experience of the hospital staff. At times, the hospital chief executive officer (CEO) and/or board of trustees could benefit from independent validation of a future course of action, specifically with respect to nursing informatics. Not only are sizable financial resources involved, but often also the future efficiency and effectiveness of the entire hospital and nursing staff.

In considering when nursing informatics consultants should be employed, it is relevant to note what they can and cannot do. Competent nursing informatics consultants are able to review the present system and anticipate future needs. They will usually suggest alternative solutions for various organizational and technical problems in the nursing systems area. Consultants can hardly be expected to solve fundamental management problems in the organization, and they cannot legitimately assist in fighting private battles between or within departments in the hospital. A good consultant very rarely makes definitive decisions, but usually identifies a set of viable alternatives. Because professional nursing informatics consultants do not derive their income from the sale of a product, the institution must be prepared to pay for qualified consultation.

To answer the question of when to employ a nursing informatics consultant, you need a well-defined goal with specific objectives. In defining the goal, consider whether the consultant is to justify the current operation of a department. The director of nursing systems may have management problems involving technical, personnel, or legal issues that require an expert opinion of a very special nature. If there are major equipment decisions, reorganizations, or financial commitments in need of review, the computer department may want a different type of consultant to assist in coming to the most satisfactory solution. Another major reason for employing yet another type of consultant would be to review the current hospital or clinic situation to develop a strategic plan projecting future needs.

What to Expect from a Consultant

One of the most difficult tasks for the hospital board, CEO, or senior nurse executive is to define the mix of education and experience that constitutes the qualifications of a good nursing informatics consultant to meet the particular needs. Any consultant under consideration should be evaluated using the following criteria:

- Relevant professional preparation
- Significant experience
- Recognition in the field
- Recommendations tailored to needs of the client
- Report delivered on time and within budget
- Ability to accomplish change
- Good communication skills
- Fees comparable to those of similar organizations.

Given the above characteristics, the consultant would be able to address the defined goal(s) as assigned by the board of trustees, CEO, or senior nurse executive.

How to Find a Good Nursing Informatics Consultant

Before looking for a nursing informatics consultant, the nurse manager must prepare a detailed definition of the problem(s) and the desired objective(s). The results of this definition step should be agreed on by top administration, reaffirming the characteristics of the major problem(s), the scope of the problem(s) to be tackled, and the objective(s) to be achieved. The individual who is hiring the consultant should precisely define the parameters of the engagement.

In obtaining the services of a qualified nursing informatics consultant, it is important to differentiate between the independent advice provided by a recognized consultant and the more limited opinions that vendors provide. Most representatives of both hardware and software companies are not able to provide objective advice about computerization; their job is to sell their product. Conversely, the independent advice provided by a qualified nursing informatics consultant is based on firsthand knowledge of the hospital setting (Carithers, 1977, pp. 43–46). Carithers further states that the consultant should have state-of-the-art knowledge of hospital systems and their components.

One of the best ways to be assured of competent nursing informatics consulting assistance is to check with colleagues who have used a consultant who fulfilled their expectations. Subsequently, the consultant's references can be and should be checked by the prospective employer.

Another approach is to work through the various national professional organizations, which are often quite willing to suggest several consultants who are in business for themselves or who are affiliated with a major university. A review of the literature to find authors of knowledgeable articles in the field provides another source.

Organizations that may be of help include, but are not limited to, the following:

American Nurses Association, Council on Computer Applications in Nursing
American Hospital Association
Hospital Financial Management Association
American Medical Association
American Association of Hospital Consultants
American Management Association
Institute of Management Consultants.

It is desirable to have a preliminary meeting with several nursing informatics consultants before selecting the one for the job. At this time, the prospective employer should discuss the financial arrangements and the duration of the consultation. It is important to have a written specification of the job to be undertaken, clearly describing the expected products, or deliverables, of the engagement, such as a written report, a flow diagram, or an oral presentation to the trustees. All this is essential in order to find the right person or firm for the job. In the overall consideration, the employer should be aware of what can and cannot be expected from a consultant.

How to Work with a Selected Consultant

Before the start of the engagement, senior nursing management should announce the planned study in order to avoid uninformed adverse reaction from nursing personnel. Rumors and worries among the nursing staff can hinder and sometimes sabotage the timely completion of the task.

The competent nursing informatics consultant will be able to review the present system and anticipate future needs, both suggesting alternative solutions for various problems and offering advice on integrating the system with other systems in the organization. The nursing informatics consultant should play the role of the advisor, providing insight into alternatives and their possible consequences.

To work as a team, the hospital and the nursing informatics consultant must be sure they are working on the same problem. Since the consultant is there to assist the nursing department and the institution, it is helpful, whenever possible, to anticipate politically loaded situations and to pave the way for introductions and smooth working conditions. Timing can be the key to a constructive and successful engagement.

Conclusion

The employment of a competent nursing informatics consultant should be considered as one of the wisest decisions that nursing management makes. In effect, nursing management is hiring one or more individuals who have spent a lifetime acquiring the education and experience to handle the nursing informatics problem(s) being faced by the institution. For what amounts to a minimal financial commitment, the organization will have purchased competent advice addressed specifically to its defined needs. "Money spent with a consultant should be regarded as an investment, not as an expense," says Felix Kaufman, President of the Institute of Management Consultants. "The return on a consulting investment can be very great," he adds, "if not directly measurable in dollar savings" (Kaufman, 1975, p. 14).

Although the final decision for any organizational or systems change must lie with the chief executive officer, consultants can serve as important resources, bringing valuable expertise to bear upon the decision-making process.

Questions

1. What is the rationale for considering the employment of a consultant?

2. Name possible sources for locating a consultant who can be expected to address your specific requirements.

3. What are the institution's responsibilities for hiring a consultant, determining the scope of effort, and defining the deliverables?

4. What is the role of the institution's management and staff when a consultant is employed?

5. Describe the approach to the use of consultants that should maximize the investment as well as ensure a successful experience for all concerned.

References Cited

Carithers RW: What to expect from an outside consultant and how to get it. *HCM Review* 1977; 2:43–46.
Kaufman F: The role of the consultant. *Viewpoint* 1975; 14.

Bibliography

Block P: *Flawless Consulting*. Austin: Learning Concepts, 1981.
Lippitt G: Criteria for selecting, evaluating, and developing consultants. *Training and Development Journal* 1981; 35:24–31.

Section 1—Nursing Informatics
Unit 2—Integrating Computing and Nursing

Unit Introduction

The first chapter in this unit, by O'Desky, carries the technology from the "anatomy" and "physiology" software era to that of the current issue of networking, which is discussed here in terms of the central nervous system. The second contribution by Gerdin Jelger and Peterson addresses issues surrounding the human–machine interface and looks at what can be done best by the nurse and what can be done best by the technology in support of the patient. Gabler continues with a description of integration of systems as applied in the hospital setting, with a special emphasis on distributed processing. The unit is completed by Peterson and Gerdin Jelger's chapter on evaluation. They emphasize the importance of both the formative and summative evaluation approach to hospital information systems assessment, related to the way it affects the total fiber of the institution.

1—A Neural View of Computing for Nurses

Robert I. O'Desky

Computing in Health Care

For many years the health care community was introduced to the capabilities of computers by a comparison to fields of study relating to the health care profession. Basic computer hardware was compared to the human anatomy, and the software that was executed on the computer hardware was classified as the computer's physiology (Ball and Hannah, 1984). This was a valid approach that explained many computer concepts, but computer science has evolved to such a point that such a simple comparison is no longer justified. Today we must relate to a far more complex system when attempting to explain the current implementation of computer applications in a health care environment. The human system that most closely parallels evolving health care networks is the nervous system.

The Neural View

The nervous system can be considered as a large complex network of sensory nodes that pass information back to the central area of intelligence through electronic pathways (Fig. 1-1).

A current computer system can be considered as a topological network of intelligent nodes that pass information back to a central storage area via electronic pathways (Fig. 1-2). The nervous system is described in terms of neurons, dendrites, and so on; computer terminology—already complicated—is combined with communications terminology to create a potpourri of alphabet that is enough to confuse anyone. It is too great a project to attempt to explain all the computer abbreviations to which everyone is exposed (Kelly-Bootle, 1981; Ralston and Reilly, 1983), but the computer network can be compared, in a straightforward way, to the nervous system.

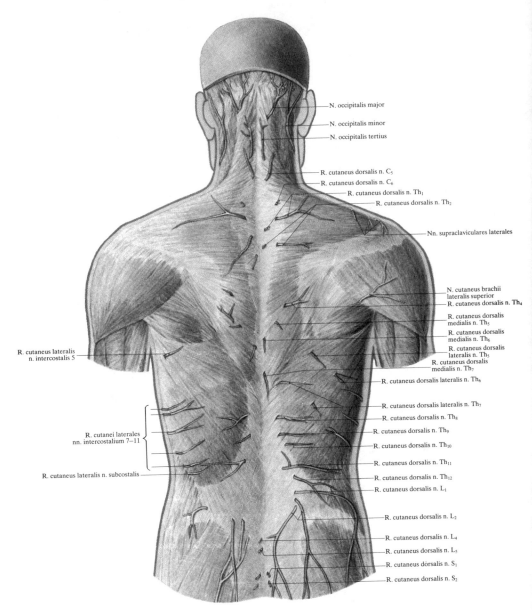

N. occipitalis major
N. occipitalis minor
N. occipitalis tertius

R. cutaneus dorsalis n. C_5
R. cutaneus dorsalis n. C_6
R. cutaneus dorsalis n. Th_1
R. cutaneus dorsalis n. Th_2

Nn. supraclaviculares laterales

N. cutaneus brachii lateralis superior
R. cutaneus dorsalis n. Th_4
R. cutaneus dorsalis medialis n. Th_5
R. cutaneus dorsalis medialis n. Th_6
R. cutaneus dorsalis lateralis n. Th_5
R. cutaneus dorsalis medialis n. Th_7
R. cutaneus dorsalis lateralis n. Th_6

R. cutaneus lateralis n. intercostalis 5

R. cutaneus dorsalis lateralis n. Th_7
R. cutaneus dorsalis n. Th_8
R. cutaneus dorsalis n. Th_9
R. cutaneus dorsalis n. Th_{10}
R. cutaneus dorsalis n. Th_{11}
R. cutaneus dorsalis n. Th_{12}
R. cutaneus dorsalis n. L_1

R. cutanei laterales nn. intercostalium 7–11

R. cutaneus lateralis n. subcostalis

R. cutaneus dorsalis n. L_2
R. cutaneus dorsalis n. L_4
R. cutaneus dorsalis n. L_5
R. cutaneus dorsalis n. S_1
R. cutaneus dorsalis n. S_2

Figure 1-1
The isomorphic view of the computer system.

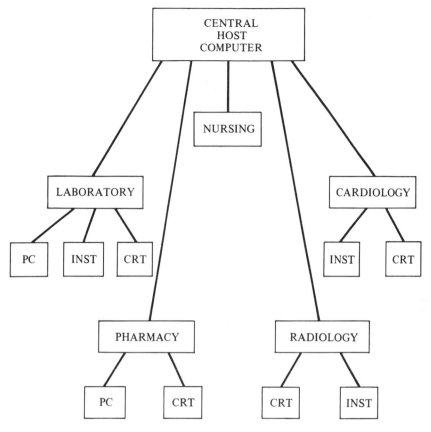

Figure 1-2
Schematic of central host computer.

Hardware

Just as our view of computer networks has evolved, the physical characteristics of computer hardware have developed greatly in the decade of the 1980s. Almost all computers were built along design criteria dictated by Von Neuman architecture. Basically, this architecture allows things to occur sequentially with only one task active at any point in time. The apparent ability of a computer to support many users simultaneously is actually an illusion created by the extremely high speeds of the computer. However, physical constraints such as the speed of electrons and the amount of heat generated by very dense computer chips have caused computer vendors to rethink their architecture. This has led to redundancy of computer components within a larger computer configuration and a capability to perform parallel processing. Many vendors are now taking this multicomputer-within-one-system approach.

Software

Other vendors have stayed with the proven hardware architectures and modified their approach to software networking. This concept has expanded from a simple idea of distributed processing to the current implementation of integrated data in a layered network (Huesing, 1986). This allows each department to maintain data necessary for its specialized functioning on its own system while sharing common data with other organizations. For example, the nursing staff is not concerned with the quality control samples run on a laboratory instrument and would not want access to that information. However, the results of a patient's laboratory tests should be available at the nursing station as soon as they have been validated and signed off by the laboratory. This is the kind of capability that a properly implemented layered network will deliver to the end users, who are typically the personnel providing direct patient care.

The Microcomputer

Another technologic innovation changing the face of health care computing is the introduction of the microcomputer into the system. This allows for computer intelligence to be located at any workstation for a reasonable cost. New approaches to applications software have resulted in significant development in data bases and inquiry languages, allowing the end user to access computer-stored information more conveniently. Thus, potential drug interaction problems can be pointed out before a drug is administered. As another example, no meal will be ordered for a patient if a lab test is ordered that requires the patient to fast. The benefits of this new generation of computers for health care are limited only by the ability of end users to describe their requirements to the computer people who are designated to implement this new class of applications. Nurses should be thinking about what they want the computer to do for them so that they can elucidate these requirements to the implementors.

The Impact of Technologic Innovation

The electronic technologic revolution—both a by-product of computer innovation and a direct contributor to enhanced computer capabilities—is one of the marvels of the past 40 years. How far computers have come since the early days can be measured by a number of attributes. Earlier computers required considerable space and air conditioning and were extremely expensive. Today, computer hardware is significantly less costly and, because of advances in electronic systems, is both smaller and faster. As a result, it is now possible to justify dedicating computers to applications that were not economically practical 4 or 5 years ago. Personal computers are now found at nursing stations where simple terminals were found in the past, providing an entirely new view of what functions can be accomplished at the nursing station.

The question arises whether these technologic innovations and enhancements can continue. In 1987, physics is putting a damper on what some scientists are attempting to accomplish in terms of computer hardware enhancements. The speed at which electrons flow has caused the size of electronic components to be decreased to a phenomenal degree. These smaller components generate more heat and are designed to run in a supercooled environment. However, it is difficult to keep a computer room at $0°$ absolute. Even the new superconductor research that has discovered zero electrical resistance at $40°$ absolute ($-233°$ centigrade) (Peterson, 1987; Weisburd, 1987; Fisher, 1987) does not offer much encouragement for any significant new advances in computer speeds.

Parallel Processing

Consequently, the computer manufacturers are moving in two different directions. The first direction is to put more central processing units (CPUs) in the system, resulting in a generation of parallel processors that can run significantly faster than the Von Neuman computers common today. If a system does not perform fast enough, adding a few more CPUs will increase the system's capabilities. This does, of course, have some significant drawbacks. The major one is that programmers do not understand how to structure their software so that it can run efficiently in a parallel environment. Another drawback is the lack of systems software required for parallel processing. This software, also known as operating systems, supplies to the computer basic functions that are very similar to the involuntary body functions of breathing and cardiac activity which the human brain provides to our bodies.

Obviously, this first direction is hampered by development and education problems that could be addressed and solved during the next decade. The redundancy provided by parallel processing capabilities is especially attractive in the health care environment, where systems must be operational 24 hours a day, 7 days a week, 52 weeks a year. However, this innovative architecture poses significant challenges, making it a long-term rather than a short-term solution.

Layered Processing

The second direction is available to us now. Currently, solutions—or, more precisely, sets of solutions—are available and implementable when the concept of layered processing is considered. Microcomputers are now powerful enough not only to solve particular problems, but also to become nodes in a comprehensive health care network.

Just as the senses serve as the transducers providing information to the nervous system, small but powerful minicomputer and microcomputer systems supply information to the health care network. An appropriate example would be a pharmacy system that runs on a minicomputer with a number of terminals. The system provides the pharmacy with information on inventory, billing, and everything else that facilitates its operation.

Nursing has no need for this information. What nursing needs is to be able to place an order and have the drug delivered and available when the patient is scheduled to take it. The nurse also needs access to the information provided by associated applications, such as inquiries into patient drug profiles and pending orders. The nurse does not want to be involved with how the information is exchanged within systems, but only wants the information to be available as it is required.

The technology to accomplish layered processing is available today, and many vendors are taking this approach to creating comprehensive health care systems. The layering effect can extend many levels deep; depth is a function of how much intelligence is required to accomplish a task at any node. As the intelligence requirement increases, end users should anticipate seeing more powerful mini- and microcomputer systems located at each health care workstation.

Data Storage

Another area in which technology is having a major effect is the area of data storage. New technologies such as optical storage modules will allow health care institutions to maintain comprehensive patient records for extended periods of time and make these records available on an inquiry basis. A complete 5-year-old anatomic pathology report can be available in a matter of seconds, rather than requiring a wait of days or weeks for recall. These new higher density storage media will allow for improved data retrieval and in turn lead to measurably bettter patient care.

The Impact of the Cognitive Process

During the early days of computing many people were afraid that computers would become smarter than people and take over the world. The general response was "Computers can't think and will never replace people." This usually pacified the skeptics, and computer development continued. However, a number of scientists decided that although computers could not create original thought, they could be programmed to appear as though they were acting and reasoning like humans.

Artificial Intelligence

This led to computer research in the area usually designated as artificial intelligence. The first researchers looked into games like checkers and chess in which logical deductions could be used to play a game at a competence level equivalent to a human player. Research into physicians' diagnostic-assistance programs was also done (Barr and Feigenbaum, 1981; Rumelhart and McClelland, 1986).

Expert Systems

Diagnostic-assistance programs belong to an area of artificial intelligence more precisely designated as expert systems. The major problem that occurs with the creation of an expert system is that no one individual appears to have all the required information available at one sitting. All too often the health care professional makes a diagnostic decision based on a comment that a professor or colleague made in the past. Yet the person making the diagnosis may not recall that expert information until a situation in which it is relevant presents itself.

Consequently, creation of expert systems is a time-consuming process, difficult for the layman to comprehend. Yet an expert system should not perplex anyone any more than a magician's illusion; once the illusion is exposed, it is no longer a mystery. Perhaps some manual dexterity is required in order to accomplish the illusion, but the procedure is typically rather straightforward. The same is true with expert systems. They may require some mental dexterity, but once the rules are well established, they perform the same logical process every time, resulting in the same final conclusion.

It would not be considered unusual if a nurse, at the start of a shift, received a message from the workstation computer that said:

> A barium enema is required for patient number 12345678 because of a radiology procedure early tomorrow morning. The evening meal for the patient has been canceled.

However, this would be the result of an expert system that reviewed the details of the radiology procedure ordered for the patient, deduced that the patient should be fasting, and instructed the dietary department not to provide a meal. The expert system would then inform the nursing station of what it had done.

The logic of this conclusion is not difficult to see, but a system that looks into a patient's many medical files—drug profile, dietary records, radiology records, and so on—to deduce what might affect the outcome of a particular laboratory test has many logical pathways and probabilities associated with each pathway. This type of logic may not be easy to follow and could appear as incomprehensible to either a nurse or a physician as any magician's illusion. However, systematizing this type of information is one technique for enhancing patient care.

Natural Language

The other area of artificial intelligence research that is particularly significant to nurses is natural language development. The classic method of allowing a nurse to communicate with the computer is to provide a series of menus that lead down a routing to accomplish a particular function. These can often become complicated and very confusing to the user. The area of natural language development attempts to allow the user an English language-type inquiry into the available information. For example, to find out what male patient Jones's drug orders were, rather than going through a number of screens to ascertain patient information and access pharmacy records, the nurse would merely enter:

LIST DRUG ORDERS FOR MR. JONES IN 3 WEST

The system would then come back with the appropriate information.

Some observers feel that this type of flexible natural language interface is much easier for a health care professional to use than the classic menu scenario. Driving these very sophisticated systems are new generations of relational data bases that integrate not only significant patient information, but also pertinent generalized medical information. Improved hardware and software technology will allow health care professionals to access information more easily and to use that information more effectively. This will not only make the jobs of health care providers more satisfying, but also make enhanced health care available.

The Infocentric View of Hospital Systems (O'Desky, 1986)

Everyone's view of hospital data requirements is prejudiced by how he/she wants to use the data. This author attempts to avoid those prejudices by considering the system as it appears to the hospital's customer, the patient. At the center of any information system are three generalized sets of information, all of which deal with the patient. These are (Fig. 1-3):

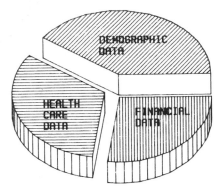

Figure 1-3
Core data.

1. Patient's demographic information

2. Patient's medical information

3. Patient's financial information.

If these sets of data elements are placed in the center of a set of concentric circles, then each of the concentric circles represents a new layer of patient involvement (Fig. 1-4). Departments like admitting, emergency, nursing, and surgery have direct patient contact. Laboratory, pathology, and pharmacy are ancillary areas whose contact with the patient is typically limited to sample or test acquisition. Patients are aware of these ancillary areas, but in general do not recognize how these departments affect their care. At the outer extremes of the concentric circles are the departments that keep the hospital functioning. Patients have little awareness of the hospital's administrative payroll department, but that financial department is definitely required to keep the hospital running.

Layered Processing in Nursing

If we consider each of the applications represented in the diagram, it is obvious that many of the application areas can be layered in order to provide optimum utility to the appropriate department. The data acquired by each of the ancillary areas must be accessible to the nursing station in order to provide the best patient care possible. The next generation of hospital information systems (HIS) will provide a number of innovative approaches to supply this information. New inquiry devices will provide nursing departments with new bedside capabilities for acquiring vital signs and other significant patient information. This could resolve many of the information exchange problems that can

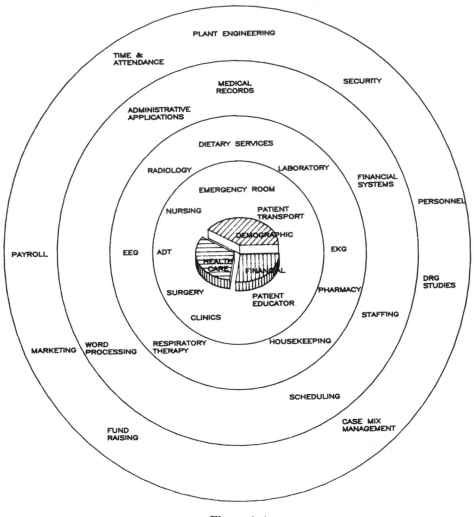

Figure 1-4
Infocentric view.

occur with shift changes. Handheld terminals with new technology data storage capabilities will provide nurses with information that was never before practical to obtain. This new ambulatory medical record will be augmented by new bedside technology to yield a more comprehensive patient profile to both the nurse and physician.

The key ingredient is, of course, data. The business world is just now realizing that data constitute a very valuable corporate resource. The health care community has always recognized this, but is just now beginning to take advantage of the data retrieval capabilities that computers can offer. Innovative computer technologies are going to offer many opportunities for improved work satisfaction and enhanced patient care. It is up to the health care community to maximize the benefits offered by this newly emerging environment.

The Future of Computing in Nursing

The nurse's view of valuable patient information is changing. Computers have modified the format of data storage from paper maintained in a patient record folder or sheet carrier to electronic data maintained on a computer supporting the nurse's station. Technology has just begun its inevitable intrusion into the functioning of the nurse's station. The resulting redefinition of how data is gathered, maintained, and displayed will have a significant impact on how nurses do their jobs in the future.

As we become more aware of how valuable an asset is up-to-date information in the treatment of a patient, the computer systems will provide easier methods to access the information. Hardware devices and artificial intelligent software techniques will be developed to facilitate the nurse's use of this valuable resource. The ultimate result will be improved quality of patient care from increased use of the enhanced information systems. Improvements, enhancements, and innovations in the whole area of computers and data processing are occurring at a dizzying rate. Even the most avid of readers can barely keep abreast of all of the new technology being implemented in the health care area.

However, the nursing community is not required to be in the most current technology mode. Nurses must be able to accommodate the systems available to them, and must be able to relate to the system providers the information and techniques that will assist them in doing their jobs more effectively. Data processing buzz-word generation is not a requirement for being able to use computer systems in a manner that benefits the nurse's job performance. For the health care professional, the use of computers is not an end unto itself, but only one of a collection of modern technologic tools that ultimately results in improved patient care.

Questions

1. Figure 1-4 shows the Infocentric View of hospital computer applications. What data should each of the represented systems make available at a nursing station? Are there any data maintained in the outermost circle that could be significant to the nurse who is attending patients? What subsystems provide significant data to nursing administration or management?

2. A large number of input/output devices are currently available to nurses. What device characteristics are most desirable for a nurse? Is manual dexterity an acceptable prerequisite for a nurse who is to use an input/output device? Is a keyboard an acceptable type of input/output device? How large a display is required for convenient use by a nurse?

3. What type of expert system would be most beneficial to a nurse? Would an expert system to assist drug administration be practical? How would a specialized calculator function provided at a computer input/output device be utilized? What type of calculator would you like to have available to you?

4. Do you have access to a microcomputer either at your job location or at home? What are the main applications that you use on the microcomputer system? Does the availability of computer graphics make the applications easier to use?

5. If you had two computers working on the same order entry application, how would you subdivide the job so that it could be accomplished in a shorter period of time? For example, one computer could be taking a drug order while the other computer was getting the patient's drug profile and checking for potential interactions. What would be the functions if you had three computers working in parallel? Four computers? Is there a practical maximum number of computers that could function in parallel?

6. Figure 1-1 is a representation of the human nervous system, and Fig. 1-2 is a representation of a potential computer network. Can you find comparisons between the pathways from the brain to outer extremities and the pathways between the computer systems? Is there something in the nervous system that compares to a computer modem (the device that allows the computer to talk to a telephone line)?

References Cited

Ball MJ, Hannah KJ: *Using Computers in Nursing*. Reston: Reston Publishing, 1984.

Barr A, Feigenbaum E: *The Handbook of Artificial Intelligence* (3 vols.). Stanford: Heiristech Press, 1981.

Fisher A: Super conductor frenzy. *Popular Science* 1987; 231:54, 58, 77.

Heusing SA: Layered processing—a new dimension? *Healthcare Computing & Communications* 1986; 3:40–42.

Kelly-Bootle S: *The Devil's DP Dictionary*. New York: McGraw-Hill, 1981.

O'Desky RI: An infocentric view of the hospital information system. *Healthcare Computing & Communications* 1986; 3:44–46.

Peterson I: New heights in superconductivity. *Science News* 1987; 131:23.

Ralston A, Reilly ED Jr: *Encyclopedia of Computer Science and Engineering.* 2d ed. New York: Van Nostrand Reinhold, 1983.

Rumelhart DE, McClelland JL, PDP Research Group: *Parallel Distributed Processing: Explorations in the Microstructures of Cognition* (2 vols.). Cambridge: MIT Press, 1986.

Weisburd S: Superconductive barriers surpassed. *Science News* 1987; 131:116.

2—The Human–Computer Interface

Ulla Gerdin Jelger and Hans Peterson

Health Care Professionals and the Computer

Health care relies on computer support in a large number of areas. Yet, information technology has not been integrated into health care as completely as possible or to the extent expected. In many instances, health care professionals exhibit concern and even skepticism about computer systems.

Nurses

Not unexpectedly, the profession of nursing has grave and valid concerns. Nurses are responsible for a number of tasks in a number of areas. Because of the considerably greater complexity of its work, nursing responds differently to computing than do other health care professions.

In the community setting, nurses frequently are called on to book a time for the patient for a visit to the physician, check information in the medical record, order analyses, and make notes at the same time they are talking to a patient on the telephone. If a computer system contains all these functions but does not provide the necessary support, coping with the computer can be a burden, especially for nurses, who are often also responsible for the manual handling of certain information.

In defining the relationship between computer and nurse, we must ask a number of questions:

- How does the nurse access and gain entry to the system?
- How is the confidentiality of the patient information arranged?
- How is the integrity of the nurse addressed?
- How is the patient identified in the system?
- How is the patient registered?

- How many screens does the nurse have to view before reaching the screen where the information being sought is presented?

- How many commands are necessary to move from a scheduling request to reading the patient record, and on to documenting an event?

- How does the nurse access clinical laboratory information?

- How many buttons does the nurse have to press to enter an order and verify (or transmit) the order?

- How does the nurse switch to the next patient?

The answers to these questions may alert us to some of the reasons why computer systems may create more problems for nursing than they solve. Nurses are already busy with multiple functions as they provide care to the patient. If they must also contend with multiple keystrokes to perform and record routine tasks, they cannot appreciate the fact that their input will make the statistics generated by another individual or another unit easier to produce and more correct. For those nurses, the routine is badly designed.

Patient Record Transcriptionists

Staff in other categories are experiencing similar problems. Because their tasks are not as complex as nursing tasks, they have not yet expressed their concerns as vocally as nurses have. The main work function for the patient records secretary is to type medical histories and discharge summaries. Whoever serves as transcriptionist, computer systems function better than manual systems for the input of patient records. The transcriptionist confronts difficulties similar to those of the nurse in handling reporting by multiple physicians on the same patient.

Physicians

The physician (and also the nurse) may feel unsafe with the patient record in the computer. Nobody questions that the information is accurate and that all information is there, but many professionals have a lingering feeling that they do not really know all that is in the computerized patient record.

This same patient record is the work material, the foundation for most decisions, from diagnosis to treatment and beyond. Here all information pertaining to the patient should be documented. The paper, the form, the volume, the colors, the structure, the content, the underlining—all give signals to the experienced reader. And the paper patient record has another advantage over the electronic record: the user can simply turn the pages and look through them.

Although the computer patient record has great advantages, including the capability to list, manipulate, and retrieve information, the changeover is difficult. We must observe and analyze conditions carefully in order to take advantage of the technique. Only then can we use computers comfortably and effectively.

Effects of Computerization

The American researcher Harold Leavitt in 1968 described the connection between the organization, standard business procedures, staff, and technology in what is called the Leavitt model (Leavitt, 1968). This model demonstrates the effect that changing any one of these factors can have on the remaining ones. In practical terms, this means that when a new computer system is implemented, we must expect and plan for changes affecting the other factors. By so doing, we can use the opportunity to optimize the quality and quantity of work produced and to raise the level of job satisfaction. The model highlights the real links between what affects the job satisfaction, the possibility of doing good work, and effective use of the computer systems.

Physical and Psychologic Environments

The physical environment has been studied. In several countries, laws and regulations apply to the working environment, both the physical and the psychologic. These laws are also applicable to computer workstations.

A good workstation should be:

- Placed so that reflections from windows and light fixtures do not disturb the user
- Provided with a screen with low electromagnetic and electrostatic radiation
- Situated in a room where wallcolors and textiles are not disturbing and do not give reflections
- Provided with a table and chair that have adjustable work position heights
- Sited in a room with nonstatic floor covering
- Housed with temperature and humidity controls
- Movable, with a separate keyboard and a screen that can be moved in different directions and angles
- Configured for text with a screen having a white background and black characters
- Quiet, with a sound level from the terminal and the printer not exceeding 40 decibels.

Even the most carefully designed environment has its limitations. In Sweden, the total working time at a terminal is recommended to be less than 4 hours a day and divided into two shifts. In the United States, limited exposure of workers to CRT displays has been recommended by occupational safety spokespersons. These recommendations would make job rotation necessary. Yet, as more and more work is computerized, the opportunities to change between computerized and manual routines decrease.

The psychologic work environment is not as easy to describe or to structure as the physical:

- Tasks must provide a sense of completion, i.e., should not be fragmented among multiple workers

- Work content must be meaningful and related to a clear goal

- Interpersonal relationships with coworkers are essential; isolation must be avoided

- Confidentiality and integrity issues must be carefully defined

- Responsibility and authority must be clearly delineated

- Changes in the psychologic environment must be done with a gentle touch and involve the workers themselves.

The Interface

The human being and the computer process information differently. The computer can store, retrieve, sort, analyze, and present large amounts of information, and never get tired! On the other hand, the human can think associatively, process several things simultaneously, choose between different solutions, and make decisions.

At this time, we understand more about how the computer and the human "think" than we do about how humans interface with the computer. However, researchers have attempted to describe this relationship and to define the skills that humans evidence in interfacing with information technology.

The Image

Psychologic studies indicate that the human being can recognize up to 1 million different images but can remember only about 7 numbers in series. Therefore, the memory of the human being is dependent on images; one difficulty with computerized medical records is that they lack the images needed to replace the impression given by their paper versions.

The manual system provides images of the organization and the routines in the form of the papers that are circulated. The computer system of today does not give any image of the system, its content, volume, structure, and the connection. The user feels deserted and without foothold. To gain confidence in a computerized system, the user must possess an image of the complete system and its functions. The same holds true if the user is to remember codes and commands for a computer system. They must be coupled with an image to be remembered.

Natural Language

Given the way computers process information, the development of computer languages has been enormous. It is not enough, however, to fulfill the needs of the human mind for variations and nuances.

As human beings work with the computer, the command to the computer becomes a common word in the language between workers in a particular workplace. Combinations of letters and digits replace whole words and sometimes even sentences. This means that the language of the workplace is changed, not as a function of the profession and roles within it, but as a function of the limitations of the computer, which cannot accept other than short commands. Thus, the work language begins to consist of short forms unfamiliar to those outside the workplace. The long-term effect is that it becomes difficult for professionals, in this case nurses, to exchange experiences and information from one workplace to another.

Coding

Patient records, which are structured, are amenable to computerization because they readily accept coding; it is easy to computerize a structured patient record. The computer can be programmed to translate the structured code, entered for calculations, into free text for reading, thus avoiding the double entry of information. Such translation follows a pattern, ending with the formation of complete sentences. The resulting text is consistent in appearance from one patient record to another. There is, however, a price to pay: The personal language is no longer there. Nuances are lost.

Questions

1. What do you think is the most pressing of all questions as we look at the many issues relating to the human–machine interface? Give reasons for your choice.

2. What are some of the physical requirements for good workstations?

3. What are some of the psychologic requirements for a good working environment?

4. Why is there a need for "natural language" in developing health care retrieval systems?

Reference Cited

Leavitt HJ: *Managerial Psychology: An Introduction to Individuals, Pairs, and Groups in Organizations*. 2d ed. Chicago: University of Chicago Press, 1968.

3—Informatics and Integration

James M. Gabler

The Challenge

Given the tremendous advances in medical science, the challenge for nursing is to integrate many specialized resources in the care of patients. Although nurses are trained to make decisions, the degree of their access to the necessary information is often an obstacle. Combined with the human need to be reminded, ready access to medical information in a timely manner is a major concern. Medical informatics must transparently integrate information from multiple sources in a manner that allows nurses to focus on the care being given rather than on how the information is obtained. Opportunities have never been greater for those willing to rethink and redefine what these problems are and how they can be resolved.

The Problem

One generally finds hospitals using a central processor with a single vendor's turnkey software or software developed in house. These systems are chosen as optimal for the institution and then used for many departmental functions. One naturally assumes that the system is "integrated" because most functions are on the same system. Although ready access to many data bases in a single system greatly simplifies communication of collected data, it is also possible to make multiple systems appear equally integrated while gaining significant additional benefits.

Before exploring the multisystem approach, one must understand the weaknesses in the single-system approach. First, most existing designs no longer meet competitive requirements. A system must have specific design goals around which compromises are made throughout the development and the maintenance/enhancement stages. Hospital information systems have generally been designed around financial goals, that is, having nurses enter orders at the nursing unit in order to capture charges in more timely and complete fashion. Although these adaptations have added valuable functions, the basic design is still event focused, not value focused.

As a result, existing systems primarily address financial/administrative requirements. Charge events are captured, stored, and historically accessed, but event values are viewable for short periods at most. Prospective payment, however, has accelerated the need for a departmental/clinical emphasis in order to control costs and to ensure quality care. Single systems, designed to optimize the whole institution, bias data collection processes toward their primary end result, generally revenue. This requires too many compromises from individual departments to accurately capture cost/quality details, e.g., submitting an all-inclusive charge and letting an accounting formula prorate cost and revenue to multiple departments based on historical (rather than actual) contributions. A multilevel design that focuses on departmental needs and then summarizes for institutional needs would be preferable.

A second weakness of the single-system approach is its inability to specialize. This is critical because three attributes—complexity, heterogeneity, and interdependence—characterize hospital information processing (Simborg et al, 1983). Individual hospital departments are more complex than their counterparts in other industries. For example, the hospital's accounts receivable department differs from that in other businesses because few of the hospital's "customers" pay their own bills. The resulting mix of insurance company payments, partial payments, and reporting requirements generates a uniquely complex environment. Also, a hospital scheduling system must allow for unpredictable factors (e.g., when a bed will be vacated) that are not an issue with other schedulers, such as those for airline reservations where seats have a fixed duration of occupancy.

Heterogeneity results from the significantly different computer processing requirements of each department. For example, the primary needs in the laboratory, radiology department, and pharmacy are process control, text processing, and dynamic data base update, respectively. Such variety often results in conflicting optimization strategies. Interdependence recognizes that a given patient will involve all or many hospital departments on a given stay or visit.

A single-system approach thus forces a compromise on processing characteristics, which generalizes the resulting product. In addition, these systems frequently come from a single vendor and have strengths in some areas and weaknesses in others. Although the centralized approach addresses the complexity and heterogeneity characteristics poorly, it does have the advantage, because of centralized storage, of addressing the interdependence characteristic more easily. Stand-alone systems, in contrast, address the complexity and heterogeneity characteristics extremely well because of their specialized and individual heritage. The interdependence issue, on the other hand, is poorly addressed in these systems because of the technical problems involved in connecting multiple stand-alone systems (Albright and Gabler, 1986). However, multiple systems are clearly preferable in that they address the variety of processing needs.

To summarize, a single system simplifies institutional coordination but reduces modular departmental independence. Two analogies illustrate that modular structures can be coordinated. First, the single-celled amoeba is not an appropriate design model for the more complex human body, which includes many specialized cells grouped in modules, such as heart, hand, brain, etc. Yet the human body is generally well coordinated in view of its "modular specialization." Second, when the scope and span of activities exceed one person's ability, organizational structures are established to manage (coordinate) a group of people for a common purpose. Clearly, modular systems can be coordinated, but an organizational/communication structure is necessary.

The Systems Approach

Computerization has gone through at least three design approaches. During the 1960s, the focus was on process-oriented approaches. During the 1970s and early 1980s, the focus was on data base-oriented approaches. Now the focus is shifting to a flow-oriented systems approach that concentrates on the movement of data (i.e., information exchange) rather than its algorithmic manipulation (process) or its storage organization (data base) (Sullivan and Smart, 1987). The systems approach is used to develop an organizational/communication structure for exchanging information and coordinating multiple systems.

Figure 3-1 illustrates the financial information flow in hospital systems. If this were implemented as a single centralized system, each functional ellipse in the diagram would share a single census file. An entry by registration/admission–discharge–transfer (Reg/ADT) is immediately available to the other functions, and charge events are immediately available for billing (Patient/Accounting); but all of the functions are locked into the single system's hardware/software environment. Conversely, if this were implemented as multiple departmental systems, each functional ellipse in the diagram could be a separate system module on separate hardware and software. An entry by Reg/ADT would flow to each of the other functions, and charge events would flow to patient accounting.

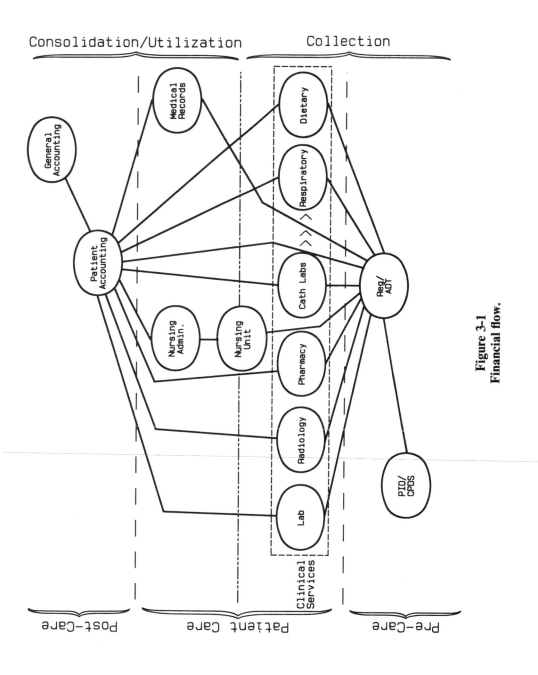

Figure 3-1
Financial flow.

If this exchange is standardized by specific protocols, an open architecture is defined that allows each module to be added, replaced, or removed independently of the other functions and their hardware/software environments. Although each function could be a separate, quasi-stand-alone system, some functions like patient identification (PID), Reg/ADT, and patient accounting can be a single system in some implementations (with loss of some flexibility). Departmental differences strongly favor separate systems for most of the other functions. Rather than consolidating all data in one data base, this systems approach allows relevant working data to be stored in each functional module while focusing on the small percentage of summary data that actually needs to flow between systems.

Since the systems approach requires some redundant data storage, special steps must be taken to address the synchronization issue. First, only one system can be the official source of each information element; e.g., Reg/ADT is the official source for bed control information. Second, the redundant data should be minimized to tag data, that is, sufficient identification data to allow subsequent regrouping (coordination) of independently generated information. For example, the medical record number, name, date of birth, sex, billing identification, location, etc. are needed in each functional module, but insurance, guarantor, billing information, etc. are only needed by patient accounting. Thus only a small amount of data needs to be copied to the other systems.

Third, timeliness affects the synchronization strategy. If synchronization is only necessary at certain times, information can be transferred periodically in files or batches of data. An example of this would be nightly billing in which charge events can be grouped in ancillary systems (lab, radiology, etc.) and sent to patient accounting. This method is technically simple, manageable, and easily recovered. However, some synchronization must take place immediately, such as patient admits, discharges, transfers, etc. A more sophisticated process must be established to insure timely information transfer, but a close examination of how information is actually used reveals that only key tag information must be immediately disseminated. With tag information synchronized, batch transfers handle most of the remaining flow requirements.

The synchronization process necessary for the Financial Flow (Fig. 3-1) allows other systems to be added that use the same collection modules (i.e., lab, radiology, pharmacy, etc.). Figure 3-2, Communication Flow, illustrates the ability to send ancillary orders and view ancillary results. Just as bed control (Reg/ADT) was the official census source, the ancillary is the official request/result source. Figure 3-3, Management Flow, illustrates the ability to consolidate collected data for multiple purposes. Patient accounting consolidates charge events for billing purposes, and the management reporting/archival system

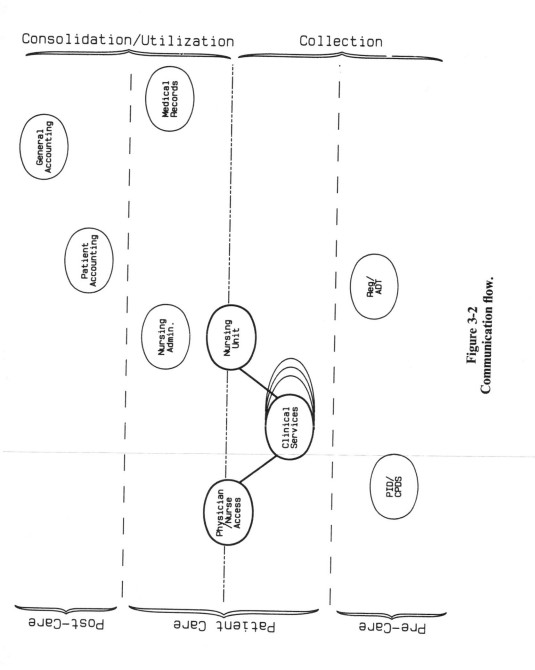

Figure 3-2
Communication flow.

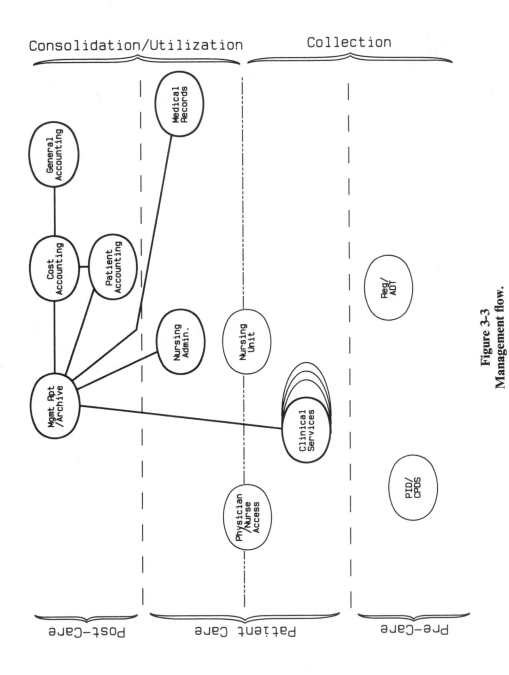

Figure 3-3
Management flow.

consolidates performed events for costing purposes independent of billing manipulations. The reporting capabilities of the management reporting system allow actual work performed to be compared to expected norms for concurrent review analysis, to various grouping for case mix analysis, to collection/charging methodologies for adjustments, etc.

Figure 3-4, Medical Flow, illustrates another data consolidation system that brings together clinical data for trend displays, clinical analysis, intervention indicators, medical decision support, etc. This has been a major missing component of most hospital information systems, but is easily added with the modular open architecture described here. Other nursing modules could be scheduling/staffing and a nursing data base. The latter would be similar to the other clinical service systems (Fig. 3-2), would maintain acuity factors, patient care data, nursing notes, care plans, procedure manuals, etc., and would be accessible via similar "request/result" (update/view) processes. The clinical data base is sometimes called the computerized medical record, and could be used for intervention reminders during the care of a patient. This also requires that bedside data collection be addressed so that medication administration can be cross checked, vital signs can be automatically captured, and other nursing care information can be quickly and easily collected. Bedside terminals and/or handheld (portable) computers can then be used to facilitate the collection process. Since this flexible structure allows collected data to be reused, medical informatics can more productively focus on how data is used rather than how data is collected. Much data collection is already automated, but without a coordinated communication scheme, manual reentry inhibits full usage of existing data.

The Benefits

Obviously, there must be quantifiable benefits to justify the systems approach rather than the traditional centralized database approaches. These benefits can be grouped into three categories: management control, management flexibility, and economics (Albright and Gabler, 1986). Management control is limited in previous approaches by the degree of computer expertise necessary. Because the systems approach allows functional systems to be defined at or below the department level, responsibility for both utilization and operation can naturally follow existing accountability structures. Individual systems are more easily grasped and more accurately evaluated and monitored for costs and benefits without computer expertise.

Because some general understanding is required to make good management decisions about technical recommendations, reducing

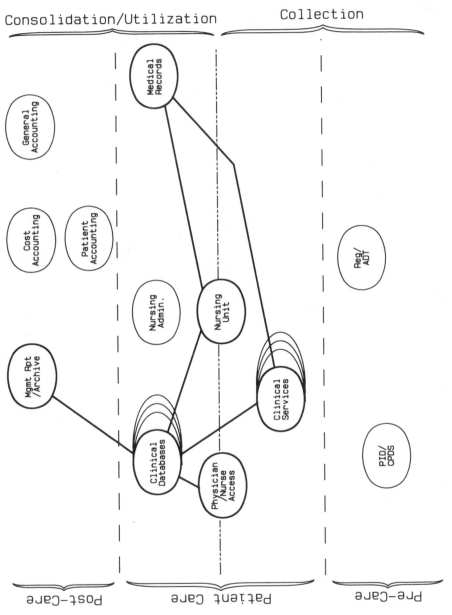

Figure 3-4
Medical flow.

computerization to identifiable modules allows management to make decisions without understanding all the technical issues involved. One does not have to understand copy machine technology in order to manage a copier—it is simply an issue of asking "Does it work?" "What features are needed?" "How much do they cost?" "Are they worth it?" and so forth. Management control also benefits from lower initial and incremental costs and from increased morale associated with the "ownership" of a system. This last point is particularly crucial, because user motivation has a much greater influence on success or failure than a system's objective superiority to other systems.

Management flexibility is a second major benefit. This flexibility starts with the system selection process, since each system area is free to choose, at any time, whatever system best fits its needs without being constrained by previous hardware/software decisions. This flexibility continues with the freedom to establish and change implementation sequences (priorities). Initial priorities reflect the current weight of various factors, but those weights will change during the implementation process because of government requirements, board requirements, management needs, departmental readiness, etc. These priorities are not as limited in a sequential implementation process as in traditional approaches. This means management can quickly adjust to a dynamic environment with minimal impact on overall objectives. This becomes even more important with our rapidly evolving technology. Flexibility is also realized in the natural redundancy inherent in the design. Since each system is quasi-stand-alone, it retains most of its processing capabilities even though other systems may be unavailable. For example, if the lab is down, the radiology system is unaffected; however, if Reg/ADT is down or the network is down, an ancillary system can manually enter tag information and continue processing departmental workload. Thus there is no single point of complete failure, but partial failures can degrade some capabilities.

The third benefit is significant economic savings. The modular design lowers initial and incremental costs. Total costs are also less than traditional single-system approaches because of significant technologic developments in interfaces and in economies of scale (Grosch's law). Interfaces have historically been discouraged, not only because they were difficult (and expensive) to develop, but also because they were difficult (and expensive) to maintain over time. Their complexity increases exponentially as the number of components interfaced increases. For example, connecting two computers requires two interface programs—one in each machine to "talk" to the other. Adding a third computer requires 6 programs; four computers require 12 programs, etc. This is known as the "$N^2 - N$ problem" where N is the number of computers (Simborg, 1984). Although limiting the hardware and software can simplify the maintenance, seldom are more than two or three computers directly interfaced.

Local area networks (LANs) have significantly simplified development/maintenance issues and costs, since only one program per computer is necessary for a LAN interface. The LAN simply delivers a message prepared and addressed by one computer to its destination, similar to the post office delivering mail. It is critical to note that LANs simplify only the mechanics of interfacing; the requirement for and content of messages (data exchanged) is a separate issue and must be addressed by the overall design as described. This simplification reduces costs as well. Costs are further reduced as standards evolve for the LAN interfaces. A group of hospitals and vendors have already started work on a de facto standard for hospital interfaces similar to those described above. Their approach is based on the International Standards Organization's seven-layer Open Systems Interconnection (OSI) model, as is General Motors' MAP (Manufacturing Automation Protocol) for a manufacturing environment.

The economies of scale have also been altered by technologic developments. Economies of scale have led to volume combinations in many areas. Computer centralization is typically based on this assumption. If all computers are plotted on a single price performance curve, the price per power measure would appear to decrease as computer power increased (Grosch's law). However, "when computers are grouped according to their size and power, Grosch's law seems to hold within each group, but not between different groups" (Ein-Dor, 1985). These groups are "...microcomputers, minicomputers, small mainframes, large mainframes, and super computers..." (Ein-Dor, 1985). It is important to note that a microcomputer is clearly not equivalent to a minicomputer for batch processing or intensive computations; however, if the processing can be redefined to function well on a combination of computers in a lower price/performance group, the total cost will be less since multiple units in the lower groups can be purchased for the same or less cost as one unit in a higher group. Savings result when large central processor requirements decrease even though the cumulative processing power increases. Thus, it can be economical to decentralize processing into multiple modules.

Summary

The challenge for medical informatics is to rethink and redefine how problems can be addressed in view of technologic advances. Problems tend to be defined in terms of the types of tools available to solve the problems. Although one can be creative in applying tools to problems, real innovation results from redefining the problems as technology produces significantly new types of tools. To make an analogy, at one time in history division was almost impossible to perform; but when

Arabic numbers replaced Roman numerals, division was greatly simplified. Most computerization today is based on a database approach that consolidates all data elements on a centralized processor. This is a natural result of interface difficulties and economies of scale (Grosch's law), which favor increasingly larger mainframes locked into a single-system design.

Now that local area networks (LANs) simplify interfacing and micro-/minicomputers have reversed the economies of multiple computers, a new approach can be taken that connects multiple computer systems. Rather than consolidating all data in one data base, the systems approach allows relevant working data to be stored in each functional module while focusing on the small percentage of summary data that actually needs to flow between systems. In essence, each system becomes a replaceable component of a larger composite system that one can more easily understand and manage without becoming a computer expert. This then becomes a flexible architectural structure that allows medical informatics to address the real patient care environment which has been poorly addressed with most existing systems.

Questions

1. What are the strengths and weaknesses of a single system for all hospital departments?

2. What are the strengths and weaknesses of a modular systems approach for all hospital departments?

3. What characterizes information flows?

4. What are the benefits of a modular systems approach?

5. How have technologic advances redefined problems and their solutions?

References Cited

Albright J, Gabler J: Distributed processing in a large hospital. *Software in Healthcare* 1986; 3:34–37.

Ein-Dor P: Grosche's law re-visited: CPU power and the cost of computation. *Communications of the ACM* 1985; 28:142–151.

Simborg D: The $N^2 - N$ problem. In: Lindberg DAB, Collen MF, eds. *Proceedings of the AAMSI Congress 1984*. Bethesda: AAMSI, 1984; 131–135.

Simborg D, Chadwick M, Whiting-O'Keefe Q, et al: Local area networks. *Computers and Biomedical Research* 1983; 16:247–259.

Sullivan C, Smart J: Planning for information networks. *Sloan Management Review* 1987; 28:39–44.

4—Evaluation: A Means to Better Results

Hans Peterson and Ulla Gerdin Jelger

Introduction

Implementation of computer support in health care means changes in work methods, work routines, work organization, distribution of responsibilities, content and environment of work, and degree of service to the patient. The cost of health care is also affected, as are the staff and the patient. Every computer installed in a hospital affects the entire organization. The work for many of the staff will be changed; some parts of it disappear; new activities are added. Depending on the way the computer support works, the daily work situation will be affected positively or negatively. Both direct and indirect users will be affected. At the point when a decision is made to introduce a system, the requirements are often only partially apparent. Routines and work may be incompletely identified, or data collection and output needs may be inadequately defined.

In spite of the fact that computer support has been used in the health care field for more than 20 years, every day we must choose new or different directions and solve problems in operations created by computer systems. During the 1970s, the motivation for development and the introduction of computer support was to increase the quality of care and the quality of information. In the 1980s, the motivation has changed. The cost of introducing a computer system cannot be covered in the budget without cuts in other costs. Thus, computer support is expected to increase productivity by helping to care for more patients without increasing staff or modifying facilities. These expectations influence the demands and prerequisites for evaluating the effects of computer systems implementation.

Attitudes toward computer support are different in different parts of the world. In North America and in parts of Europe, computer support in health care is not questioned. In Scandinavia, on the other hand, an endless discussion is going on with working parties, about how, where, and when computer support should be used and by whom. The Nurses'

Union has taken a strong role in questioning the consequences of computer systems for the working environment and professional roles. Before a computer system is introduced, it must be justified. Such a justification should always include

- Defining of tangible goals for the operations of a system

- Agreement on the expected effects of the introduction of computer systems among those whose work will be affected

- Analysis of and consensus on changes in organizational structure and educational program offerings required by system implementation.

For many health care professionals, the magnitude and number of unexpected effects connected with implementing a new way of working remain cause for concern. This is caused in no small part by evaluation efforts and their methodologies, which are responsible for

- Estimation and measurement of the effect of poorly defined expectations that often were never accepted by users

- Insistence on congruence between expected and actual effects.

Purpose of Evaluation

When computer-based workstations are introduced into the hospital setting, actual results should be compared with the expectations established and agreed to by all parties before implementation. The effectiveness of the organizational structure and the new systems should only be measured against clearly identified expectations.

Decision makers and hospital administrators may focus on financial implications and apply formal cost analysis methods. However, when determining whether a new computer system is preferable and which factors contributed to its success, other factors not related to cost are significant, such as service to the patient and the accuracy of information.

The purpose of the evaluation process is threefold:

1. To compare the results with the goals and the expected effects for

- the system

- the working conditions

- the service to the patients

- integrity and security of data

- finances.

2. To direct the work toward the expected result with the help of formative evaluation during the development and the introduction of the computer system.

3. To use the findings and outcomes of the evaluation process as an experience base for the next project.

The evaluation process is dependent on agreement regarding certain basic concepts. These include an understanding of what constitutes effective use of computer systems and what relationship should exist between expected, actual, and unexpected effects.

Effective Use

Over the years, higher and higher demands have been placed on computer systems. Expectations seemed to increase with every technologic innovation, every new software offering. Finally, we are learning that computerization is not the solution. It is simply a very useful tool that can help us do what we need to do. But before we can use computer systems effectively, we need to make extensive changes to the following:

- Methods and working routines
- Work organization and work distribution
- Distribution of work among different categories of staff
- The content of work.

This includes defining work routines on all levels and along all dimensions, including roles for professional staff. Additional considerations are the number of staff to be affected and the needs of staff for computer education and training. The success of these educational efforts is dependent on the level of motivation and engagement among the affected staff. To get the best results, all categories of staff within a certain part of the hospital must be involved.

In a large organization, it is difficult to know where the responsibility for these changes should lie. There are many interested parties. Because these are all new types of changes in the organization, good cooperation is necessary.

Effects

The expected effects are the summary of what we want to be changed and what we believe is going to happen when computer support is introduced. Just as all individuals have their own set of expectations, every category of staff should be given the opportunity to put demands on the computer system. The expected effects must be collected and coordinated. The expected effects describe both the effects that can be realized and those that cannot be realized. The expected effects are an essential part of the basis for the decision whether to implement.

Actual effects or real effects are those that can be measured and judged when the computer system is in operation and when changes in work have been finished.

The unexpected effects or the surprising effects constitute the difference between the expected and the real effects. They are a good measurement of how well we have succeeded in analyzing and understanding the expected effects. At the same time, they introduce new knowledge that has to be considered and used in the learning process for the next project.

Comparison: Basis for Evaluation

Evaluation necessitates comparison. The basis for comparison may be the work as it was done before or the level of computer support previously available. In the early 1970s, computer support was judged by asking whether it was better or worse than before. Today, formal evaluation is a part of the development and the change process. Growing financial constraints require that systems be justified as providing higher quality and greater productivity as well as fiscal benefits.

For evaluation to be successful, operational productivity must be well described in terms of expected effects. When precisely stated, expected effects cannot be misinterpreted, but clearly must be related to the actual work situation. For example, the expected effects for working conditions and for patient care could be measured by the following:

- Number of patient per unit and per nurse, per day, per month, and per year

- Items contained in the medical record, as reflected in their content, the record structure, or the number of pages

- Number of working hours and work breaks

- Nursing time for each patient; number of times patient record accessed

- Number of hours using a terminal

- Possibilities for job rotation

- Continuity in the contact with a patient

- Patient waiting time before a scheduled appointment
- Access to the patient record and the lab results at the time of the appointment.

Whatever the goals for a system may be, the sensitive areas of patient confidentiality and data security need to be described carefully. The descriptions can be generated through answering certain critical questions:

- Who shall have access to the patient record
- Who shall not have access to the patient record
- What should be documented and followed-up
- How should information be used.

Evaluation can take into account the operational goals of an institution, regardless of whether the system being implemented is large or small, custom-designed or commercially packaged or developed in-house. Evaluation can proceed regardless of questions of motives, methods of financing, or roles of the primary persons involved in the implementation.

Evaluating the effects of a computer system is often considered an unnecessary, bureaucratic exercise. The lack of support for evaluation contributes to this negative perception. True, there are no right or wrong methods established, but evaluation requires both fiscal and personnel resources and must be given priority as part of the implementation process itself.

The lack of accepted methods also means that the results can be questioned, especially by those whose expectations were not confirmed. Different constituencies within a health care institution focus on evaluating different aspects of an implementation. In brief, one's interests are a function of where one sits in the organization. The health care staff is concerned with service to the patient, professional roles, and working conditions. These areas are not easy to measure and cannot be expressed monetarily. Moreover, as is often the case, if the hospital staff lacks the knowledge, power, or means to direct the development and the evaluation, they will concentrate on effects other than those important to them. On the other hand, the decision makers, notably the hospital administrators, focus on operational matters, such as productivity and financial indices. These areas are easily described in economic terms.

It has been said before but bears repeating, "Implementing computer systems means change." In general, people do not like change, and it is difficult to convince them that change can bring about a better reality. However, different workplaces have different climates for change. Before introducing a computer support system and measuring its effects, it is important to take the temperature and determine what the working conditions are. Experience teaches us that computerization does not resolve organizational problems and flawed procedures. To the contrary, computerization often exacerbates them. A computer system can in fact transform negative conditions into what amounts to an organizational abscess.

Many problems are better addressed by types of solutions other than implementing a computer system. Organization of work, education of staff, management of the institution—all may be more effective than computerization. And even if the decision is to computerize, all those areas must be carefully assessed.

A recent study of the health care delivery system in Sweden concluded that its problems were those of work organization, in-service education for staff, and management. The only area that could not be resolved without computer support was access to the patient record. Computerization was the sole solution here because this record could not be in several different places (the ward, the outpatient department, the physician's office, and the examination room) at the same time.

Prerequisites to Evaluation

Before proceeding with computerization, certain prerequisites must be met. These will serve as guides in selection, implementation, and evaluation of a system. These activities should result in describing and/or defining the following as precisely as possible:

- Goals for the operation of the institution, expressed in tangible terms

- Expected effects

- Working conditions

- Operational functioning

- Information flow.

Areas of interest include patient care services, confidentiality and security safeguards, and financial implications. These should be expressed in quantifiable terms (preferably measures such as patient days) available and used by the institution for other purposes.

In addition, it is helpful to identify a representative sample of the individuals who will be responsible for the evaluation process. Both direct and indirect users must participate in evaluation. Their attitudes are particularly significant, as their work must be founded on the following principles:

- Positive and negative effects can only be defined by the users

- Both positive and negative effects must be described

- Detailed descriptions of existing and planned routines must be completed before the development work or before the start of the implementation

- The evaluation must be done in such a way that the users can participate.

Another prerequisite is that the evaluation process be included in the budget for the project. Through funding evaluation, the institution will improve the chances that the implementation is prepared for and directed in a manner that will give better results. In Sweden, 25% of the budget for some major projects is allocated for the evaluation.

The Evaluation Process

The evaluation process should start the same day that the decision is made to introduce a computer support system. The process then continues throughout the implementation, because its purpose is to direct the changes toward the goals and the expected effects that have been agreed upon. Those individuals responsible for the evaluation should work with the staff who will be the end users of the system, and who will be able to continuously monitor the project. This monitoring is essential to the evaluation of consequences and effects.

Whatever methodologies are agreed on, the evaluation process consists of four steps, as follow:

- Describing the goals

- Identifying the problems and specifying the desired changes (what one wants)

- Determining the expectations (what one believes will be the result)

- Analyzing the system once it is in operation (what happens).

The evaluation process invariably involves taking and analyzing measurements as well as arriving at qualified judgments of the results. However, since there is no single established method for evaluation, staff in each unit within the workplace should participate in determining which methods they and their colleagues find acceptable.

A problem can arise if all health care staff have to be given an opportunity to influence the work. In a small unit it is quite easy, but in a very large organization, it is impossible. Different methods of soliciting opinions can allow as many as possible to express their views about the demands on new computer systems and about the need for changes and the expected effects.

This participation is important because any project involving system development, and thus changed routines, creates expectations. Participation will help to make the expectations reliable. These expectations can be both positive and negative, depending in large part on the interest in a particular change.

To date, the most effective method has involved study circles, with a mixture of individual work, working parties, and discussions. With study circles, health care staff have gained knowledge of the project justification, goals, and activities, as well as insights into potential problems and alternative solutions. In order to have good results from study circles, as many as possible from all affected units within the institution should participate. Moreover, the participants should have discussions with colleagues who are not participating. The only disadvantage with study circles is that they are costly.

In Sweden, the choice has been made to modify the study circle approach. Working parties have been established, representing all different categories of staff. Members of the working parties are responsible for eliciting input and feedback from their colleagues. The working parties are supported by special staff, whose function includes educating members of the parties in the new areas of technology. There are no shortcuts to a more detailed knowledge of existing procedures. Although higher staff costs will result from the additional preparation, only collective knowledge can prepare effectively for computerization.

In the first step of the evaluation process, the working parties describe the following:

- Objectives

- Routines

  - All tasks step by step

  - The distribution of work (who is doing what)

  - The connections between different types of work

  - The volume of the information

  - The problems

  - What is functioning well; what contacts and relations are necessary and important

- Working conditions at every workstation

  - Tasks carried out

  - Numbers of persons working in the same room

- Kinds of equipment used
- Physical environment, specifically lighting and acoustics
- Changes needed for introducing a computer system
- Work organization
  - Distribution of the responsibilities
  - Distribution of tasks
  - Working hours
  - Number of staff and different categories.

When the description of each activity is complete, the problem area can be defined. A comprehensive view of the operations is essential because the expected effects must be seen in a total context.

The second step in the evaluation process involves analyzing the problems and their causes and assigning priority rankings to the different problems to be solved. One condition for success is an open and frank approach to solving problems caused by conflicts among the staff. This is especially important, since a computer system may exacerbate such conflicts. To solve problems, different alternatives must be explored. Usually a combination of computer support, changes in organization and management, and education/training programs gives the best possible solution.

The third step involves describing the expected effects in such a way so they form a foundation for the evaluation work that is understandable by all hospital staff. This includes the area of costs. They can easily be grouped in effects on the operations, effects on the working conditions, degree of service to the patient, and integrity. Projections of future costs are also made, based on available data judged relevant. These data include the following:

- Costs for staff: operations, development, introduction, maintenance, education
- Costs for hardware and software: computers, terminals, and printers, service and maintenance, communication, expendable supplies, programs and licenses, operations
- Reduced or eliminated costs: staff, typewriters, paper, archives.

Evaluation Outcomes

The difficulty in describing the expected effects of a computer system arises from the uncertainty of change. Questions of range and of probabilities associated with specific items are not easy to answer. A subset of expected effects, not realized in the short term, may in fact be achieved over the long term. Success may be affected by any number of reasons, from technical difficulties, problems with the change, or dependence on other workstations. Yet the evaluation of costs is based upon the effects realized in the short term. Effects potentially realizable in the long term cannot be accurately evaluated.

The proof of the quality of the initial work is the number of unexpected effects. These effects are not obvious until the system is in operation. Whether positive or negative, these effects create unplanned work in critical situations. Positive unexpected effects can compound and alter the end result, while negative effects can be disastrous. The only way to minimize the number of unexpected effects is to do the initial work better. Today the weak point is the limited knowledge concerning the change process itself. Evaluation will contribute to the knowledge base by defining conditions and analyzing expected and unexpected effects. As more insight is gained into the change process, the quality of description of the expected effects of implementing computer systems in health care will increase. Thus, evaluation will enhance the chances of effectively controlling the change process in future projects.

Evaluation methods now being developed, such as Sweden's working groups, will increase the quality of decisions when introducing a new computer system. The advantages and disadvantages of computer systems are being identified. At the same time, more and more nurses and physicians have had, or are taking, the opportunity to participate in projects and gain invaluable experience. These methods, notably those stressing preparatory work, can help to reduce the number of unexpected effects and to reach the best possible correspondence between expected and actual effects.

Known Effects of Computer Systems on Health Care

The justification for the evaluation of computer systems is simple. The knowledge gained from evaluation holds promise for the future. What is learned from the process can be used to create better computer systems and to integrate them more effectively into health care. From the evaluations done over the past 20 years, we have learned quite a lot. Some of the more important lessons learned follow.

More Users

All health care staff—physicians, nurses, auxiliary nurses, doctors' secretaries—will use terminals. This means that the rotation of work used in past years to avoid extended exposure to computer monitors will no longer be possible. All categories of staff will, for a large part of the working day, use terminals of different types in order to collect or enter information. This means that more and more staff will be dependent on the computer system. Accordingly, manual and computer systems must be not only reliable but also well coordinated.

Demands for Standardized Procedures

Hopefully, computer support will help to address the problems existing in the health care field today. To date, computer systems have been introduced in the attempt to solve a range of problems. The consequence has been duplication of work, since neither manual nor computer systems can resolve the difficulty. If either organization of work, the management, or the education component is not optimal, computerization cannot succeed. Planning conducted as part of the implementation and the concurrent evaluation process must clearly take this reality into account.

Experience has taught that introducing a computer system increases the demand on standardized procedures over the demand associated with manual systems. Manual systems are in fact more flexible; documentation can be done in different ways and take many forms. Paper and pencil can be brought around and used any time, and it does not matter what the letters and the figures look like, or how they are put down, or where on the paper they have been written. The flexibility is as great as the number of people who are going to do a specific task. The contrary is true with computer systems. Decisions must be made in advance specifying how input is to be done, in which order, and in which context. Flexibility in a computer system exists only to the limit it has been provided for and programmed for at the onset.

Less Dependence but More Informed Contacts

A well-known effect is that different categories of staff will become less dependent on each other. Today the medical record functions as the link between staff, joining them across specialties and professional categories as they enter data into and retrieve documentation from the medical record. In a computerized system, this dependency drastically changes. The nurse, the physician, or other health care worker can now access most needed information electronically rather than personally. The result is a marked decrease in the number of contacts between the various members of the health care team strictly for purposes of information updates. Significantly, studies have shown increased contact between physicians and nurses when they use the same information. Under manual systems, each profession maintained its own documentation. If based on shared minimal data sets and a common language, computer systems allow them to compare and read each other's information much more easily.

Broader Basis for Decisions

Computer support can provide all categories of staff with a better foundation for their decisions. As a result, there is greater opportunity to change the organization of work and to reassign the division of responsibility. In a manual system, the organization of work is frequently dependent on where and how staff has access to information to make the right decision. When a computer system makes information available as needed, these restrictions are lifted. Access, or lack of access, to information no longer dictates which category of staff or which individual should make decisions.

Shifts in Tasks

Whoever made the decisions in the past may not make them in the future. It might be better, easier, and less time consuming to reorganize the work and to reassign responsibilities. For example, with computer support, nurses enter orders for lab tests into the system rather than onto paper. Yet, if the system in laboratory does not print out those orders in a meaningful and useful way, lab staff may have to write them out. In that event, the task has not been eliminated or made easier to perform: It has only changed owner.

Acceptance by Staff

One very important prerequisite in implementing computer systems is the acceptance of the system by the staff who must use it. This acceptance is founded on the way the system functions and on what support the staff is given while the system is introduced and work routines are changed. The extent to which staff are invited to participate throughout the entire process clearly affects acceptance, as does the extent of information sharing and consensus building. Providing staff with opportunities for education and training also plays a part in creating the necessary perception of cooperation and participation.

Essential Characteristics of the Computer System

Certain characteristics of computer systems are especially important in the health care setting and can significantly affect acceptance of a system. First among these is reliability, which is absolutely essential given the 24-hour operation of hospitals. A system must function all the time, without fail. It must always be available to staff, whenever they need it. Unfortunately, all computer systems must have some scheduled downtime to perform preventive maintenance (including vacuuming the computer!) or to install enhancements (a new software package or added disk storage) or to test backup systems (a weekly procedure for alternate power sources in many hospitals). Any of these interruptions should be scheduled in cooperation with the hospital staff.

There must be well-accepted and well-documented operational procedures for the computer. Documentation must specify who is responsible for operations, who for backup routines, and who for maintenance. It is important that many of these tasks can be performed by hospital-trained staff, as they are on site should problems arise.

In many hospitals, the physical environment is inadequate. Computer installations, workstations, may present new problems. Small rooms may not house workstations and their associated printers. Wiring may be difficult in existing structures. Placing computers close to patients may require more terminals than are available and add a dehumanized element to rooms already filled with equipment.

The content and structure of a system play a key role in its acceptance by staff. If a system developed elsewhere is not sufficiently flexible to meet the needs of a unit or is not adequately adapted to the workstation within that unit, chances that the system will be accepted are seriously diminished.

Evaluation turns out to be the most important step to validate the circle of selection, implementation, and evaluation. Only after a system has been evaluated and successfully integrated can the project be defined a success.

At this point we are ready again to begin the process of constantly striving to find ways to improve our health care delivery system. If there is one lesson to be learned it is that evaluation is the ultimate in team effort. For evaluation to succeed, everyone must be involved in one way or another.

Examples of Other Questions to Ask in the Evaluation Process

How can I have access to the information?
How easy is it and how much do I have to enter to get the information I need?
How many steps in the evaluation process?
How can I enter the information?
Is there only one approach to evaluation?
How can I enter the information?
How much help can I get from the system?

Questions

1. What changes result from the implementation of computer support in health care?

2. What factors should be included in justification for the introduction of a computer system?

3. Identify the purpose(s) of evaluation.

4. Describe the three types of effects to be expected of computer implementation.

5. List the reasons commonly given for not evaluating systems installation.

6. Discuss the prerequisites to evaluation of systems.

7. Describe the evaluation process.

8. Discuss the known impact(s) of installation of a computer system in health care.

9. Identify the essential characteristics of computer systems for health care.

Section 1—Nursing Informatics
Unit 3—New Roles for Nurses

Unit Introduction

All chapters in this unit have taken a different slice out of the emerging new discipline of nursing informatics. This new discipline is leading to new roles for nurses. The first contribution by Ball and Hannah addresses the question of what is informatics and what does it mean for nursing. Jenkins narrows the discussion to address the economic and business trends in the health care market as he focuses on the emerging roles for nursing professionals as the entire health care delivery system changes. This chapter is followed by Hersher's detailed description of career paths for trained nurse informaticians and addresses the new environments and "cultures" in which we will see professional nurses function using both their nursing and informatics skills. In the next chapter, Jaekle, a nurse functioning in a new role, allows a glimpse into the actual activities of a nurse systems analyst. The unit concludes with a contribution by Orsolits, Davis, and Gross, who take a bold look into the future for this emerging discipline of nursing informatics of the twenty-first century.

1—What Is Informatics and What Does It Mean for Nursing?

Marion J. Ball and Kathryn J. Hannah

Introduction

Today, nurses around the world are rapidly increasing the extent to which they use computers and information sciences to assist them in the performance of their increasingly sophisticated and complex duties. Consequently, the field of nursing informatics is developing quickly.

Because of the evolution of nursing informatics, new roles for nursing are developing in industry, research, systems development, nursing education, nursing administration, and indeed at the bedside. One need not sacrifice an avocation for direct patient care in order to participate in the information revolution in nursing. In fact, the reason that many nurses have ventured into the field of nursing informatics is a common vision of information systems being used to enhance the practice of nursing and to benefit the patient by extending and improving the health care received by patients.

Developments in nursing informatics are beginning, and will continue, to have an impact on what and how nursing is practiced; further, this impact will be reflected in nursing education. In fact, the impact of nursing informatics ultimately will be so profound as to be a driving force for extensive change in the nature of nursing research and administration as well. The term nursing informatics can be operationally defined as referring to the use of information technologies in relation to any of the functions that are within the purview of nursing and are carried out by nurses in the performance of their duties (Hannah, 1985, p. 181). Therefore, any use of information technologies by nurses in relation to the care of patients, the administration of health care facilities, or the educational preparation of individuals to practice the discipline is considered nursing informatics.

For example, nursing informatics would include, but not be limited to

- the use of artificial intelligence or decision-making systems to support the use of the nursing process
- the use of a computer-based scheduling package to allocate staff in a hospital or health care organization
- the use of computers for patient education
- the use of computer-assisted learning in nursing education
- nursing use of a hospital information system
- research related to information nurses use in making patient care decisions and how those decisions are made.

In other words, advances in computing and communications are transforming health care in ways we could not predict 10 years ago. As the front line for delivering that care, nurses stand to benefit enormously from those changes and the new capabilities and opportunities they bring.

Professional meetings—and the literature to which they have contributed—have made increasing use of the term "informatics," from the French "informatique." The term first appeared in medicine, where computerization was most developed. Over the past 3 or 4 years, what was initially referred to as "medical informatics" has become more precisely defined. Today the literature applies the term to the full spectrum of the allied health sciences, yet at the same time singles out specific areas, such as "nursing informatics" and "dental informatics."

As all sciences, the field of informatics is continually undergoing self-analysis and redefinition in order to find its niche in our fast-changing world. A recent attempt at definition argues that

> *Medical informatics* is a developing discipline, a multidisciplinary field, which has grown out of the recognition that effective utilization of computers in health care will occur only when there emerges a critical mass of individuals who understand both the fundamentals of medicine and those of engineering and information science. By *medical*, we do not mean M.D., but all parts of the health-care arena: allied health; biological sciences; health-care facilities; health-services research; medical specialities; and nursing. (Stead, 1987, pp. 14–15)

Stead further explains that "In the medical setting, *informatics* is used in a broader context than *information science* to include all aspects of the computer milieu," which he then itemizes as the following:

- Algorithms
- Artificial intelligence
- Biometry
- Communications

- Data base methods

- Imaging and signal analysis

- Hardware design simulation

- Modeling and systems organization (Stead, 1987, p. 14).

Stead addresses the problem in interpreting the term "medical" narrowly. Many others share his concern and see a much broader orientation, with "health informatics" encompassing subsets such as in medicine, dentistry, nursing, and pharmacy. A move to this more global definition would clarify the place of "informatics" as we work to take advantage of information technology.

The growing acceptance of this concept is evidenced in the December 1986 issue of *The Western Journal of Medicine*, devoted wholly to medical informatics. In his introduction to the issue, the editor explains that

> Like many of my colleagues, I had spent a fair amount of time over the past few years trying to explain the meaning of "medical informatics." When it was decided to feature this subject in the December issue of the journal, this offered an unusual opportunity to *illustrate* what medical informatics is, and to put some of its best examples on display. It also seemed useful to draw attention to the important distinction between *information* (the commodity with which informatics deals) and the *computer* as a tool for use in processing this commodity. The computer continues to be an exciting object, it is increasingly present and it rarely fails to attract attention. Unfortunately, the commodity which is processed by the computer tends to be overlooked. (Blois, 1986, p. 776)

Blois concludes his discussion of medical informatics by arguing that

> what have now become necessary are better means of managing this information and locating it when needed. It is here that we have turned to computers and to information science for help. This is a major undertaking and a new adventure for medicine. Developments ... continue to break new ground so that we can look forward to an increase not only in knowledge itself but in the means of analyzing, organizing and disseminating it. (Blois, 1986, p. 777)

The Association of American Medical Colleges (AAMC) is addressing these concerns for medical education. At their Symposium on Medical Informatics, Lindberg (1986) proposed the "seven levels of understanding medical informatics" as a more detailed definition. This approach begins to specifically address the educational and curricular definition of informatics. Moving from the fundamental to more complex, those seven levels are

- Computer literacy
- Independent learning
- Minimal personal skills
- Knowledgeable consumer
- See new applications
- Build a system for one's application
- Tool building (Lindberg, 1986, p. 93).

The AAMC reports agreement that today's health care professional must be skilled in problem solving, concept formation, data processing, and in the ability to analyze, summarize, make judgments, and form valid conclusions. The study of informatics, the AAMC argues, enables students and professionals alike to sharpen and enhance these skills. Among the contributions of informatics are the capabilities for

- managing the information base available to treat patients

- treating patients more efficiently and cost effectively by reference to a broad range of experiences documented in national data bases

- providing more time for physicians to spend on the important personal aspects of patient care through delegation of some information handling and processing tasks to computers

- improving the educational process through the incorporation of information technology and decision-making science and through the utilization of computer-mediated instruction

- broadening and rationalizing the clinical experience in medical education (Steering Committee, 1986, p. 3).

Recently, the Nursing Working Group of the International Medical Informatics Association established an education task force. This task force convened in Sweden in June 1987 for the purpose of competency statements regarding nursing informatics knowledge required by nurse administrators, nurse educators, nurse clinicians, nurse researchers, and nurse informaticians (Peterson et al, 1987). These competency statements are expected to be used in the formulation of educational curricula and job descriptions.

In the field of informatics, notably in the areas of dental, medical, pharmacy, and nursing informatics, we are seeing a substantial growth in the use of computers as a basic tool and integrated into the disciplines that make up these professional fields. We will see a succession of a new generation of informaticians develop. The National Library of Medicine has for years funded training programs in medical informatics, and it is our prediction that the same will occur in dental, nursing, and pharmacy informatics.

There is no doubt that informatics as a new discipline has a bright future as the professional schools utilizing informatics in the specialty areas of nursing informatics, dental informatics, medical informatics, and pharmacy informatics become further involved. As we move into even more sophisticated uses of computers in health care, the field of informatics will thrive.

New Roles for Nurses

Developments in nursing informatics are beginning to have and will continue to have an impact on what and how nursing is practiced. In fact, the impact of nursing informatics ultimately will be so profound as to be a driving force for extensive change in the nature of nursing practice.

A side effect of the changes in health care and the evolution of nursing informatics has been the growth of new roles for nursing, as discussed elsewhere in this volume. Such roles are developing in industry, research, systems development, nursing education, and nursing administration. Nurses, most notably those with bachelor's and master's degrees, are participating in the selection and implementation of systems for use at the bedside. Nurses also articulate the information needs of health care professionals and of clients in clinical practice settings to the system designers and engineers. A new phenomenon is the hiring of the nurse consultant by hospitals to assist in the design and implementation of computer systems. The input of nurses into system selection and design is growing exponentially, as health care facilities use computers to interpret electrocardiograms, monitor patients, and prevent drug interactions by cross-referencing drug incompatibilities and warning appropriate staff.

For the Clinical Nurse

Nurses with a vocation for direct patient care need not sacrifice their calling in order to participate in the information revolution in nursing. In fact, the reason that many nurses have ventured into the field of nursing informatics is a common vision of using information systems to enhance the practice of nursing and to benefit the patient by extending and improving health care.

Informatics will free nurses to assume the responsibility for systematic planning of holistic and humanistic nursing care for patients and their families, for continual review and examination of nursing practice (quality assurance), for applying basic research to innovative solutions to patient care problems, and for devising creative new models for the delivery of nursing care.

The advances in the use of information technology will necessitate a more scientific and complex approach to the nursing care process. Consequently, nurses will require better educational preparation and a more inquiring and investigative approach to patient care. Nurses will also need to be more discriminating users of information.

No longer will nursing practice focus on the assessment and care planning phase. Rather, it will emphasize the implementation phase. Thus, nurses will require an expanded repertoire of intervention skills. These nursing intervention skills reflect the autonomous aspects of nursing practice. Based on the body of nursing knowledge and the nurse's professional judgment, autonomous nursing interventions are complementary to, not competitive with, physician-prescribed treatments.

In this context, clinical nurse specialist training at the master's degree level offers nurses the opportunity to use increased knowledge and clinical practice skills at the bedside. This intensification of the role of bedside nurse provides an alternate career path for nurses who prefer patient care to administration, research, or education.

In the delivery of health care, nurses have traditionally provided the interface between the client and the health care system. They are now fulfilling this function in new ways as they move into a technologically advanced environment. With nursing informatics as a guide, nurses will become increasingly more involved in the design, use, management, and evaluation of computer systems in health care agencies and institutions.

Today, nurses are identifying and developing new ways of using computers and information science as a tool to support the practice of nursing in the performance of their duties. At the same time, computers and information science are facilitating a more sophisticated and expanded level of nursing practice. There is an interactive and synergistic effect between nursing informatics and nursing practice. The boundaries of nursing informatics are thus contiguous with those of nursing, and like them, dynamic and constantly changing.

Questions

1. Define in your own words what you understand nursing informatics to be.

2. Give the name of four or five organizations and/or monographs in which the area of informatics is being addressed as an evolving discipline.

3. What impact will informatics have on nursing as a field?

4. Where in the practice of nursing will we see "caring and technology meet"?

References Cited

Blois MS, ed: What is medical informatics? *Western Journal of Medicine* 1986; 145:776–777 (special issue).

Hannah KJ: Current trends in nursing informatics: implications for curriculum planning. In: Hannah KJ, Guillemin EJ, Conklin DN, eds. *Nursing Uses of Computers and Information Science*. Amsterdam: North Holland, 1985; 181–187.

Lindberg DAB: Evolution of medical informatics. In: *Medical Education in the Information Age—Proceedings of the Symposium on Medical Informatics*. Washington, DC: Association of American Medical Colleges, 1986; 86–95.

Peterson H, Gerdin Jelger U, Grobe S, eds: *Competencies*. New York: National League for Nursing, 1987 (in press).

Stead WW: What is medical informatics? *M.D. Computing* 1987; 4:14–15.

Steering Committee: The evaluation of medical information science in medical education. In: *Medical Education in the Information Age—Proceedings of the Symposium on Medical Informatics*. Washington, DC: Association of American Medical Colleges, 1986; 2–61.

2—New Roles for Nursing Professionals

Thomas Jenkins

Introduction

This chapter looks at nursing from the perspective of economics and business. Trends in the health care marketplace are interpreted in terms of their impact on the structure of the nursing function and the overall structure of the health delivery system.

Trends in Health Care

The health delivery system in the United States is undergoing a fundamental transformation from a provider-driven monopoly to a customer-driven market. This transformation was initiated when Congress enacted prospective payment legislation. Diagnosis Related Groupings (DRGs), originally intended as a cost control mechanism, triggered a flood of derivative actions in the private sector. The thrust of these actions is to restore customer control of health decisions.

These are the key trends that will exercise major influence on the nursing profession:

- surplus hospital capacity

- diminishing flows of new professionals into the allied health and nursing professions

- a glut of MDs

- excess medical education capacity

- increasing gap between what is taught in nursing schools and what is needed in the marketplace

- increasing entrepreneurial involvement in providing nursing and nursing education resources

- insufficient and inefficient health information capacity

- increasing numbers of both independent and dependent seniors
- insufficient nursing home capacity
- insufficient noninstitutional health services capacity
- increasing customer demand for health services vis-à-vis disease management services
- decreasing ability of health professions to establish monopolies via legislation
- increasing ability of alternative health service professionals to compete with medical professions
- increasing requirement for health service professionals to be effective educators
- increasing requirement for health professionals to be effective marketers.

Breaking the Medical Monopoly

There are important lessons to be learned from the history of hospital-centered medical practice. Our discussion initially focuses on the medical profession because of its centrality in the growth of hospital-based health care practices: medical, nursing, and allied health care. We then explore transformational strategies for nursing in the hospital context and beyond the hospital.

In the period after World War II, the explosion of medical technology, facilities, and insurance programs created a windfall for MDs. The nursing profession has grown and diversified in parallel with the growth of medicine and hospitals. From the economic and business perspective, growth and diversification of the medical profession were the primary drivers in this time frame. Hospital-based medicine expanded its market during the 1950s and 1960s using standard business approaches to service. This should come as no surprise, because most hospital boards still have significant business representation.

Four basic principles for running a service business, which are effective whenever customers are better served by depersonalizing the service function, are listed below:

- Get the customer to come to you rather than for you (the service provider) to go to the customer
- Create a thoroughgoing dependence of the customer on the service provider
- Create payment mechanisms that eliminate the bill-collecting routine from the professional's practice

- Develop an assembly line approach to service, which, as much as possible, standardizes the interaction with the customer and reduces the probability that unique customer demands will be placed on the service provider.

Before DRGs were introduced, this business development strategy was effective. However, the systems developed to implement this approach to service create major problems and competitive disadvantages in today's health services climate, which increasingly demands personalized service. In order to establish viable professional practices, professionals must gain and maintain credibility in the eyes of the public at large. The fundamental sources of professional credibility are law, education, advertising, and media.

These sources of credibility have been used with great effect by the medical profession to create a public mindset favorable to medicine, especially to hospital-based medicine. The medical profession has worked assiduously to establish a legal climate favorable to itself and, conversely, unfavorable to its competitors. It became a model for other health care professionals in the use of lobbying strategies to forge legislated monopolies.

So long as the public accepts the premise that health care is defined as medicine—or as surgical and chemical intervention to control body processes—this is a viable strategy. Its viability decreases dramatically as the public questions the definition of medicine as health care.

Education became the mechanism by which the profession governed entry—medicine has created a truly magnificent educational system. Medical education grew at the same pace as medical practice but a few years ahead of it, and teaching hospitals became the bastion of medical research. Educational procedures, testing, and continuing education became the bulwark of the credentialing process, not only for medicine but for most other professions as well. The result of this emphasis on education is that the business of health care is organized primarily along academic lines. Movement by an individual practitioner among the functional components of a hospital is hindered by the academic requirements imposed by the credentialing process. In most businesses, this movement is a major source of new ideas and adaptation to changes in the environment. For the individual, it is the primary source of managerial development.

All businesses have a stake in the success of their customers. Therefore, businesses that support the medical profession advertise heavily to ensure its success. This is particularly true of drug companies, whose messages saturate prime-time television and all other advertising media.

Because advertising revenues are the lifeblood of media, it is not surprising to see the media reflecting this in their programming. Hence we see large numbers of movies, television programs, and news stories about hospitals, doctors, nurses, and patients. And, as demographics change, we can expect to see more and more media attention to health issues of aging.

As is true with all issues of power, the sources of medical power contain the seeds of its demise. The medical profession's legal monopoly has called forth a legal counterbalance: malpractice. As the society became more health conscious, it became obvious that medical education left a lot out—such as nutrition and such as wellness. And as medical research and practice sought to establish dominion over the body using surgery and drugs, the importance of the mind and spirit to a healthy body became more obvious, thanks to people like Norman Cousins. Alternatives to allopathic medicine—homeopathy, acupuncture, chiropractic, body work, body–mind–spirit work—successfully emphasized aspects of health that medicine ignored or deplored. And when payors began to realize that the benefit-to-cost ratios of health promotion were extraordinarily superior to those of disease management, the honeymoon was over. No longer could MDs believably claim to be the sole arbiters of matters of life. Legally, however, they still have sole arbiter power over matters of death. Somebody has to.

The same advertising and media power that supported the medical profession's monopoly on the way up now works against it on the way down. Malpractice suits attract wide media coverage. Advertisers urge consumers to ask questions and coach them on the kinds of questions to ask. Television programs and novels depict ordinary people challenging doctors, with effect! Adults as well as children learn how to deal with life by imitating what they see on television.

Lessons for Nursing

It is critical to remember the fundamental nature of the transformation occurring in health care: from a provider monopoly to a customer-centered, market-driven, health-oriented marketplace. For nursing, the question becomes "How can we as professionals gain from this transformation?"

We first examine strategies for nursing that maintain the status quo. The first is the legal/educational credentialing strategy. Attention to this issue by major nursing organizations will not present a problem to the profession unless it is given more priority than it deserves. Representatives of the profession need to remember that the value of a degree has been diminishing with time, not increasing. Requiring a bachelor of science in nursing (BSN) for entry into the profession is therefore appropriate to maintain status. It will not create an increase in nursing power.

Legal efforts to certify independent nurse practitioners form the second status quo maintenance category. This has higher priority than the BSN thrust from a strategic perspective. To be successful, however, it needs to be strongly coupled with a customer-centered marketing approach and with development of essential managerial skills.

Transformational Strategies for Nursing

Strategy Number 1: Be Clear about Who the Customers Are

Nurses have functioned in the post-World War II era as the humanistic counterbalance to an increasingly technology-driven medical profession. This is an important role. However, it has diminished rather than advanced the interests of the nursing profession. Customers are the true source of power in business. When a professional group is perceived as actively counterbalancing one of its key customer groups (MDs are hospital and nursing customers, as are patients), it cannot help but lose credibility in the eyes of that customer. Effective nursing in today's environment means serving the needs of the customer. In a hospital environment that means serving the needs of both patients and physicians.

Strategy Number 2: Nursing Diversification

To date, nurses have specialized according to practice disciplines: medical/surgical, psychiatric, critical care, and so on. Within those disciplines, the profession has been generally egalitarian. While there has been a differentiation according to the type of license a nurse holds (LPN, RN, etc.), from the business perspective all are nurses. This accounts in large part for the dilemma that nursing organizations face when interacting with employee relations departments and hospital administration. There has been insufficient marketing differentiation among the various nursing skill categories. For the primary customers of the nursing organization, too frequently a nurse has been "just" a component of the total labor force, i.e., an assembly-line worker.

The developing shortage of credentialed nurses will lead to specialized titles, pay, and positions for hospital-based nurses. Hospitals will have to develop more attractive packages to remain competitive. However, the major opportunities for nurses are outside the hospital. Hospitals are a shrinking component of the total health care system.

Development of market-oriented, entrepreneurial businesses is the next major challenge for the nursing profession. The following are some areas of need that will be driving forces for independent market-driven businesses: physical rehabilitation, immune system rehabilitation and maintenance, health and wellness teaching and training, primary nursing, direct patient care, exercise therapy, home care, psychologic rehabilitation, remotivation therapy, geriatric nursing, physician assistance, pediatric and maternal services, nutritional services, movement therapy, imaging therapy, health informatics, health system advocacy, chemical dependency, unit management and operation by contract, and so on.

Strategy Number 3: Develop Managerial and Personal Skills

The skills of management, marketing, negotiation, clinical reasoning, problem solving, and decision making are central to independent practice, whether this practice is conducted inside or outside the hospital setting.

Nursing has been severely hampered in its development as a profession by its insularity regarding these skills. The insistence on nurses teaching nurses has created vocabularies and thought processes that isolate nursing from the mainstream of skill development in managerial areas. Few educational programs effectively develop these skills. The challenge to educators is to build programs that do develop them. Those programs that meet this challenge will thrive; those that do not will eventually die.

Literally thousands of resources developed for the business community have direct bearing on these skills. They take the form of live seminars, packaged seminars, self-study materials, audiotapes, videotapes, and books. Many are reasonably priced. Nurses who are able to transfer what they learn from these resources to a health care context will be amply rewarded for their efforts. Nurses who learn how to learn from people in other disciplines will be doubly enriched.

Nursing entrepreneurs who have developed these skills will increasingly create businesses to teach them to others. The combination of nursing background, professional credibility, and solid products will provide many with substantial incomes. Satisfaction of existing marketplace demands absolutely requires that these skills—management, marketing, clinical reasoning, problem solving, and decision making— become a standard component of every professional's practice. The marketplace of the future will place an enormous premium on these skills.

Strategy Number 4: Develop Computing Skills

The computer is to the mind what fire, the wheel, the internal combustion engine, and the airplane have been to civilization. It is a tool that transforms the way individuals, groups, and organizations think and interact with each other. It is a tool that nursing must master, a tool with which nursing must learn to innovate.

Let's look at some specific areas of opportunity. Several systems approaches to the hospital-based nursing function are either on the market or under development. To date, none has caught on. They have not caught on because nursing organizations are being asked to make a huge leap: from a labor-intensive paper system to a full-blown electronic system.

This violates all we know about how humans learn. We learn, individually and collectively, by associating the new with the known. Until we have integrated something new with what we have already mastered we are unable to handle it effectively. This means that we first must take a new tool and use it on a familiar task and in this way get a feel for it. Next, we begin to experiment with the tool. This experimentation leads to small innovations. The more we experiment, the better we are at innovating, and soon we're innovating in a major way. Eventually we transform the old familiar task.

You can create your own examples to prove this point. Consider any area of nursing or medicine—cardiac care, burn care, trauma care. Go back a decade and trace the innovative path that ends with today's state of the art. What does this mean for nursing and computers? We need more people applying known computing tools to more confined problem areas, more small experiments, in every nook and cranny of nursing. To do this, more nurses need to get hands-on experience with microcomputers earlier in their careers. More nurses need to acquire a home computer, so they can safely "play" with the tool.

Strategy Number 5: Develop Computing Applications

Nursing is the hub of information in the direct patient care setting. Nurses will become more proactive in developing computing applications that leverage this hub position, both in the hospital setting and outside it. Literally all information that nurses deal with on a routine basis has the potential for a computing application. The critical objective is to get on with the process of building something, using it, improving it, rebuilding it, and so on.

Applications holding particular promise in this market-driven transformation are those that help consumers deal effectively with health resources. Examples are meal and shopping planners for people with special dietary needs, programs that train self-care patients in specific skills, and recordkeeping programs for promoting health and fitness (exercise, weight, caloric intake, and so on).

Summary

The key trend transforming health care is the movement from a provider-driven disease management monopoly toward a customer-centered, market-driven health services industry. The old sources of professional power—credentialing, legal barriers to entry and practice, exclusive support from advertisers, and media—are themselves being transformed. Entrepreneurialism in nursing will be strongly fostered by this transformation.

Critical skills for practitioners include management, marketing, clinical reasoning, problem solving, and decision making. Essential tools for developing and employing these skills are the tools of health informatics: computers, software applications, and artificial intelligence. The essence of the transformation is learning ... and unlearning. It is not optional.

Questions

1. Discuss in a short paragraph how alternative health professionals are competing with traditional medically based practices.

2. Prepare a two-paragraph discussion on what "effective marketing" of nursing services means to you.

3. Discuss how hospitals have implemented the four basic principles for improving the efficiency of a service business.

4. Prepare a list of 10 books on marketing and management skills that you would like to read during the next 2 years. (Then, read them!) Prepare an abstract of one article from the *Harvard Business Review* that is relevant to nursing and/or health care.

5. Outline a small-scale computer project with which a nursing unit could experiment.

3—Careers for Nurses in Health Care Information Systems

Betsy S. Hersher

Introduction

For nurses, this is the ideal time to enter the field of health care information systems. Prospective payment has stressed not only the need for financial reporting, but also the importance of date collection and order communications systems. Systems are being developed to address nursing productivity issues as well as to provide acuity measures. Point-of-care, bedside terminal systems are surfacing and gaining the attention of the industry.

With a nursing shortage emerging, these systems will take on more importance. Nursing administration as well as chief executive and chief financial officer positions will become a targeted market. Departmental systems have taken as much of the spotlight as financial systems and alternative delivery systems are being developed to meet the needs of the changing health care environment. Nurses are needed to define and design, install, develop, manage, consult, and market these systems.

It is desirable to complete a bachelor's degree and continue on for a master's degree in business administration, computer science, or nursing administration for advancement in many of these areas.

As a reinforcement for this additional education, or possibly as a replacement for it, practicing nurses may find it helpful to act as user liaisons within the hospital where their work can serve as the transition into a new career in medical information systems. The experience gained can combine with their nursing expertise and with their additional education to carry them into this new field.

User Liaison for the Hospital

When a medical information system is installed in a hospital setting, it is necessary to coordinate the needs and staff of the institution with the capabilities of the system. Usually, a systems steering committee is formed. Participation on the steering committee is an excellent way to gain systems knowledge.

Nurses are often naturals as systems people because of their training and background. There is order and organization in nursing. Efficient and effective methods of patient care delivery are developed using a step-by-step, problem-solving approach. Automation of patient care systems effectively helps nurses to analyze and handle problems. The role of the nurse includes teaching, accurate and complete documenting, and motivation.

A place on the steering committee would allow for interaction with hospital-wide users, the vendors (the companies who develop and sell hospital information systems), consultants, and administrators. The role of the steering committee includes needs analysis, participation in the selection of the systems, definition of the systems, and coordination of installation of the systems. This is an excellent place to discover if you are interested in a career in systems. As a steering committee member you have an opportunity to conduct site visits and see a variety of systems, and may attend training classes given by your chosen vendor. Active participation on the steering committee makes you highly visible and the obvious first choice when your institution is looking for a coordinator.

An ability to learn, excellent communication skills, patience, and a comfort with leaving the bedside are needed skills. It is a natural transition for some nurses to leave bedside nursing and move into the development of patient care-related systems. The negative factor in a move such as this is that you must learn to be a facilitator, using resources but not necessarily controlling or having authority over them.

New Roles in Medical Information Systems

Coordinator for Health Care Institutions

In many hospitals the patient care systems are managed by nurses. The skills required for this job are a working knowledge of systems and excellent communication and management skills. The ability to hire and supervise technical people is a plus. This position involves installing the systems and interfacing with the vendors, the users, and management. It is an excellent stepping-stone to a position with vendors, as a consultant, or as vice president of information management.

Installer of Medical Information Systems for a Vendor

The need for qualified candidates to install various components of medical information, order entry, communication, productivity, acuity, and staffing systems is growing. An installation person is often on the marketing team during and after the sale of a software package. (Software is the term used for the programs and operating managements that make the system run. They help the user define his needs and explain documentation.) The main task of the installer is to train the users and help them over the rough spots during and after conversion to the new system. Many of the skills outlined above are operative in this job. Additionally, the installer must be a negotiator and liaison, acting as the bridge between the user and the software vendor.

Working for the software vendor adds a new dimension. While an advocate of the user's position and needs, your job is to have the system installed according to the design parameters. The vendor is paid as the various modules are installed. You can imagine that this position can sometimes be that of a juggler.

These positions often require 50% or more traveling time, a solid understanding of how hospitals work, excellent communication and presentation skills, and an understanding of systems. A move into an installation role with a vendor can lead to a number of career possibilities.

Product Manager

One of the most exciting professional moves has become available in the last few years. The responsibilities of product management/production definition are loosely defined and can change from vendor to vendor. The duties often overlap into marketing. This is a position that is beginning to be developed on the hospital side.

A person in product management is responsible for constantly updating the current product and keeping abreast of all new developments in the field. Product managers must be cognizant of the current and future needs of the clients and determine whether these needs can be or should be incorporated into the product. The people determining the product direction are the watchdogs of the product and the industry.

The characteristic role of product manager is the same in any industry. They must interface with marketing staff, client, technical staff, and management to produce a usable and marketable product in a timely manner at the best price. They must satisfy the needs of one client without compromising the needs of others or the capabilities of the technical staff. This position generally begins as a staff role requiring excellent communication and negotiation skills. You need to possess or acquire internal and external marketing expertise. Both vendors and health care organizations are under pressure to define their current and future needs accurately, and this is a key role. Success in this position can lead to high-level strategic planning positions with expanding responsibilities and compensation.

Market Support Person

Market support is defined differently in various organizations. The classic definition involves technical sales support to the salespeople and additional explanations to the client. With so many patient care and ancillary systems in development, nurses are needed to assist in closing the sale.

To be a good marketer, it is important to listen well to the needs of your clients. Finding the reasons why your software products answer the needs of the clients is a key element. Market support personnel must possess excellent written and oral communication skills and understand the marketing cycle. They must be able to identify the decision makers. On some occasions, it is necessary to act as a negotiator between the clients and the salesperson.

The salesperson's role is to sell the product and close the sale. The market support person adds the technical information, often demonstrates the product, and attempts to ensure that the client is not oversold or undersold. They play a key role before, during, and after the sale.

During the sale cycle, market support staff will interface with the product management team, the technical staff of the hospital, the vendor, and salespeople. In many vendor situations, market support departments will answer requests for proposals and be involved in contract negotiations.

In a software vendor situation, the move from market support to sales rarely occurs because of the additional skills required. The notable exceptions are the patient care, ancillary, and alternative delivery systems. Additionally, medical personnel often move into sales for highly technical products such as biomedical equipment.

The move into sales from marketing should not be taken lightly. It is a rare individual who makes the transition successfully. The skills required are negotiation, sometimes selling more than is there, patience, and the ability to close a sale. A successful transition can be quite rewarding.

Consultant

Nurses are in great demand today in most of the large consulting firms. The ideal candidate for a consulting firm has a master's degree, possesses excellent written and oral communication skills, and has a good knowledge of systems. Consultants should be analytical problem solvers, independent, creative, and assertive. Additionally, an outgoing marketing personality is a plus and would ensure growth.

Nurses make excellent consultants if they have the right personality. It is often necessary to make instant decisions based on analysis of fact. Generally speaking, nurses tend to have strong personalities, to know how to take charge and how to establish their professional credibility. These are all traits that a consultant needs to possess.

Consulting is a high-pressure field. Assignments are not usually carried out in project teams of more than two people. Projects can range from needs analysis and selection of vendors to strategic planning, cost-benefit studies, and systems audits.

Consulting offers excellent personal growth potential. You must operate independently and successfully, learn to lead projects, and be able to handle a variety of products. Consulting forces you to stretch your ability. You also take on the role of liaison and expert. Some of the negatives are a heavy travel schedule and opportunity for project management but little opportunity to manage large numbers. In many instances, consultants make recommendations but do not remain to implement them. If you are accustomed to follow through, it can be difficult to walk away before the entire task is completed. A career in consulting requires a drive and ambition to seek high levels of achievement. Consulting firms hire carefully and look for candidates who will be partner material.

Sales Representative

Nurses make excellent salespeople because of their keen ability to motivate, negotiate, and be seen as credible. An additional factor in their credibility is the need to thoroughly understand a process, such as illness, and observe many signs at once. If this skill is translated into sales, the nurse should be able to present the product from a sound base of understanding rather than a "smoke-and-mirrors" approach.

Because of training and experience, the nurse has the need to bring something to closure. A key requirement in sales is the skill of closure. A career in sales can be very rewarding financially and lead to sales management or operational management in a vendor environment. The downside is that it is a high-risk, high-frustration environment that requires a strong tolerance for rejection. Being tenacious is a real plus.

Management Engineer

Operations review and management engineering would be an exciting area to explore. A degree in industrial engineering or health systems is generally required. Management engineers work closely with the information systems department evaluating new application requirements, needs analysis, and benefits derived from computerizing a system. They are often involved in productivity studies with heavy emphasis in nursing. Nurses are particularly suited for this profession, and there are very few nurse/management engineers. With productivity and staffing computer systems joining the marketplace, this would be an ideal career opportunity to explore.

System Analyst/Programmer

Nurses may opt to work in a hospital's computer services department as a system analyst or programmer. A bachelor's degree is usually required as well as a working knowledge of that hospital's computer system. This person may or may not work exclusively with nursing applications.

New Product Development

Nurses will be in high demand in the development of some new applications, including:

Decision support systems
Clinical ancillary systems
Managed care
Nurse staffing
Productivity measures
Acuity systems
Bedside and handheld terminals.

Summary

It is important to continually upgrade your skills and goals, examine career options, and be flexible. This is an ideal point in the growth of health care information systems for nurses to consider before becoming actively involved. The future of our industry will be total health care systems expanding far beyond hospitals. There is and will be a greater need to provide information for decision making in the vast areas of alternative delivery, preventative medicine, industrial and occupational medicine, and the adult long-term care market. Large, non-health-care corporations and business coalitions will have a strong influence on our industry. Terminals will be set up in the workplace for early detection of disease and to provide wellness programs.

Because of severe financial pressures, we will finally be forced to use our technology for medical research and to provide access to national data bases to provide better health care and allow for prevention, early detection, and a faster cure for some diseases. The nurse consultant will play a major role in this area. This evolution will happen only over time. As many mergers take place among the major health care vendors, we can only wonder what this means to our industry. As larger consolidated corporations sort their priorities, entrepreneurs will have the ideal opportunity to use their creative ability to provide products and services to the industry. The survivors will be those firms and institutions providing the best and most flexible service at a competitive price.

What is important in this market is the people. They must be global thinkers with an understanding of the present and future of the health care market. They must be managers who are flexible and able to use resources and technology creatively. In both a profit and nonprofit environment, these leaders will be required to be risk takers and decision makers, and to operate in a proactive manner. They will need to be entrepreneurial and be open to joint venturing.

The health care systems industry is more open to clinical specialists than ever before. This is an ideal time to consider a career as a systems specialist.

Questions

1. Given the material on careers for nurses in information systems, plus your background and skills, design a position description that describes a career move for you.

2. What have been the changes in the hospital industry that would lead to nurses playing a more predominant role in health care systems?

3. What are the new application areas and technical advances that nurses should be aware of? Name at least 10.

4. Why would nurses do well in sales and marketing?

5. Given the information in the text, describe at least three additional roles for nurses in information systems.

Bibliography

Hersher BS: Symposium on computers in nursing. In: Pocklington D, Baron JL, eds. *Nursing Clinics of North America*. Philadelphia: WB Saunders, 1985; 585–594.

4—The Role of Nurse as Systems Analyst

Beth Jaekle

Introduction

During recent years, specialized roles for professional nurses have emerged at an exciting pace. These positions offer new challenges and opportunities for growth. One such new role is that of nurse as systems analyst in hospital data processing departments.

JOB DESCRIPTION

THE MOSES H. CONE MEMORIAL HOSPITAL

TITLE: Application Support Analyst

DEPARTMENT: Management Systems

Job Summary: The Application Support Analyst acts as facilitator, negotiator, advisor, trainer, analyst, and catalyst for change during the evaluation, selection, implementation, and ongoing support of nursing administration/clinically-based computer systems. The primary focus is on monitoring interdepartmental and intradepartmental information flows.

Reports To: The Application Support Analyst reports directly to the Data Processing Director.

Major Duties and Responsibilities

1. Analyzes interdepartmental and intradepartmental information flows before, during, and after computer implementations in order to assure system integrity.

2. Acts as facilitator during meetings with nursing and other ancillary departments in order to identify specific system requirements and solutions to interdepartmental problems.

3. Trains nurses, ancillary departments, and management systems colleagues on the functionality of nursing administration/clinically-based computer systems.

4. Acts as problem definer, problem solver, and negotiator while working under the pressure of complex variables including multiple departments, multiple vendors, multiple procedures, multiple personalities, and unproven technology.

5. Participates in detailed testing of nursing administration/clinical computer systems.

6. Assesses departmental system needs and measures needs against available systems in software market.

7. Plans and presents software demonstrations and assists in preparing panel discussions and presentations at national health care conferences.

8. Coordinates site visits for visiting hospitals and vendors.

A nurse in this position establishes and maintains communication and mutual understanding between nursing and data processing professionals by combining the expertise of both disciplines. The result is the development, implementation, and ongoing support of automated nursing systems that are technically sound as well as functionally appropriate for the nurses who will use them.

A systems analyst gathers and analyzes data, studies problems, identifies needs, and determines how computerization can most effectively facilitate the smooth flow of information. A nurse wishing to assume this role has a very good foundation on which to build. Nursing education develops may skills that are similar to those used during systems analysis. These include assessment, planning, evaluation, and problem-solving skills. The tools are extremely important; however, the role requires that they be refocused, refined, and expanded.

A systems analyst also evaluates both intradepartmental and interdepartmental information flows. For this reason, a nurse in this position must establish a global view of the hospital and maintain an up-to-date understanding of nursing administration and clinical practice. Computer skills must also be acquired. Computer capabilities as well as technical limitations should be understood. With this expanded knowledge base, a nurse assuming the role of systems analyst can successfully contribute to the development and implementation of computer applications that enhance productivity in previously nonautomated work environments. In today's world of cost containment and budget restrictions, this is extremely important.

As computer applications in health care continue to expand, a systems analyst with a nursing background will prove increasingly beneficial. This person can add a much-needed dimension to hospital data processing departments. As health care computing becomes more complex, it is only logical to seek input from an individual who is able to combine both clinical and computer skills. Such input can only enhance the operational smoothness of hospital information systems.

Questions

1. What skills acquired through nursing education and practice can be refined and expanded by a nurse assuming the role of systems analyst?

2. Why is it important for a nurse in a systems position to maintain a global view of the hospital and an up-to-date understanding of nursing administration and clinical practice?

3. Why is it beneficial for hospital data processing departments to employ nurses?

5—Nursing Informatics and the Future: The Twenty-First Century

Marcia Orsolits, Carolyne K. Davis, and Mark S. Gross

A Nursing Perspective

The use of computers in nursing practice, administration, education, and research is becoming increasingly important. The need for nurses with the knowledge and skills to provide leadership in the design, application, and management of information technology in health care is also growing.

Several critical issues will need to be considered by the health care industry as it moves into the twenty-first century and into the era of informatics. These issues will center around two prime areas of technologic innovation. First, as bedside computer systems are installed in hospitals and have the potential to link to computerized home monitoring systems, a new wave of information will be available. Organizational management decisions will reflect a reliance on this new continuity of care data to maintain both cost of care and quality of care. Accountability for individual actions will be more easily tracked in the future. Nurses will become more vital in their role in the quality of care when the computer is able to discern whose responsibility it was to perform each aspect of care.

Second, nursing is seeking to evaluate its traditional methods of payment within the room-and-board category and moving to establish a separate payment directly to nursing based on actual services rendered. Information from nursing input will be vital to establishing accountability for correct payments.

With these two moves—direct payment of nursing services as a separate component within the hospital bill and direct accountability for continuity of care—nursing's future in the organizational management team will be enhanced by the individual nurse's command of informatics. Thus, nursing as a profession will need to address concerns related to documentation practices, standardization of information, and shifts in nursing's power base in the health care organization.

Documentation

A subtle yet critical issue facing the health care industry is the documentation practice of professionals. As we attempt to enter the age of fully automated health care we must consider diagnostics and treatment, patient record generation and maintenance, as well as organizational management. Traditionally, we have focused on the task of automating what is currently documented in patient records and management reports. There has been little attention given to addressing the appropriateness, effectiveness, and efficiency of the content recorded by physicians, nurses, and other care-givers. Impacting this content are the philosophies and attitudes surrounding the paperwork demands of today's complex health care delivery system. We would suggest that professional practice documentation is one of the key factors contributing to the less-than-anticipated progress of automation in health care when compared to other industries in the United States.

Professional education and socialization processes emphasize the timeliness and appropriateness of information and seldom address efficiency issues. Timeliness refers to the information being available to key users when it is required for decision making. Appropriateness refers to the factual accuracy of the information: Is it correct in terms of "trueness," and are there necessary and sufficient amounts? Efficiency refers to the use of minimum resources (people, time, and materials) to provide the information. As new practitioners enter the real world of health care delivery, often the pressures of time and multiple demands result in a drastic alteration in documentation behavior. Students generally have time to document all their observations, actions, and conclusions. There is little value placed on setting information priorities, succinct recording, and relevance of information. However, when time is scarce, the new practitioner may consider documentation less important than either direct care or administrative duties, and may enter information that is not clear or complete.

Standardization

Only recently are we seeing a willingness of professional nurses to standardize nursing care plans and nursing notes. The high value placed upon "professional judgment," "patient individuality," and "practice uniqueness" had somehow been translated into a concern about and mistrust of standardizing anything that nurses do. Standardization will be necessary for automation and comparability within and among health care organizations.

Power Base

The introduction of an objective and highly efficient mechanism, in this case the computer, can be a traumatic experience. There is a potential for creating new expectations and levels of accountability among patient care providers. More importantly, there is a potential for nursing to experience a redefinition of their power base in the organization. Information is power, and head nurses have managed and controlled a large amount of information in their role as orders manager. Over the past 5 years we have seen head nurses and staff renegotiate roles as a result of automated nurse staffing and scheduling functions. The power to influence sensitive management decisions regarding staffing levels and work schedules was not easily relinquished by nursing. The automation of patient care information may well result in the realignment of roles and responsibilities between head nurses and staff.

Practice Patterns in the Future

Health Care versus Hospital Care

The industry will shift its focus from hospital-based acute care to broad-based health care. The mobility of our society, a growing emphasis on prevention and wellness, and a resistance to institutional care will move us to a wide variety of delivery sites and scenarios. Technology will allow the automation of an entire patient care record on a credit card-sized tool. We will complete employee physicals from the work site with a network of diagnostic and physician linkages for simultaneous reading and interpretation. Consumers (patients, insurance companies, and employers) will shop for health care with the latest consumer guide available on personal computer networks for access at home or office. Self-care software will be purchased at the local drugstore or video shop!

Patient Care versus Nursing Care

Paradoxically, in an age of ever increasing specialization, we may see a return to a centralization of patient care functions. Few health care organizations will be able to support five or six separate and distinct administrative departments to provide one service—patient care. For example, nursing, physical therapy, occupational therapy, dietary, respiratory therapy, and social service may need to be consolidated into nursing in order to provide more efficient, coordinated, patient-centered care. Health care organizations that survive and seek to excel (to be profitable!) will necessarily become structurally flat (decentralized management) and lean (centralized care delivery).

Case Management versus Orders Management

A key issue in the future world of comprehensive information system environments will be the ability of traditional health care organizations (hospitals) to change and nursing's ability to adapt, define, and accept new roles in these organizations. As order entry and patient care functions become automated, substantial changes occur regarding the role of the professional nurse. As the manager of orders, the head nurse has provided the critical central control, disbursement, and follow-up of physicians' orders. When information was lost, the head nurse sought, found, or recreated the needed data. When implementation was slow or nonexistent, the head nurse "did the job for someone else" (dietary, lab, social services). The sense of satisfaction that things did get done and patient care needs were met was tempered by the burden of negotiating, cajoling, and often pleading with a variety of independent departments participating in an orchestration of "I don't know," "never saw it," "we're too busy." Similarly, the primary nurse focused on the delivery and coordination of care for a defined set of patients. This role was usually limited to a period of hospitalization and defined by the boundaries of a nursing unit.

In contrast, future role expectations will focus on nursing's role in case management. The responsibility of coordinating and at times directly providing patient care during an episode of illness, as differentiated from a hospitalization, will offer unlimited boundaries for nursing practice. Information will also need to transcend the traditional boundaries. Home visits will be supported by and supplemented with computer visits between the nurse who is case manager and the patients and their families, perhaps even to the individual patient's work site.

An aging population with multiple health and treatment needs will further stress the delivery system for creative solutions. The retired couple that spends 6 to 9 months in a southern climate will be in touch with and perhaps treated by a computer link to a northern health care system. Their health care record will be readily accessible to them and their care-givers.

New Roles for Nurses

As executives in a major health care consulting firm (and one of us is a former nurse administrator and educator), we have noted a wide variance in the knowledge and skills of nurses in the area of information technology.

Informatics in Nursing Curricula

We believe that several levels will soon need to be addressed in nursing education programs. These often reflect differences in kind rather than differences in the degree of knowledge and skill. For example, computer literacy, comfort, and skills as daily users will be most important for the staff and first-level managers in nursing. While informatics focuses on designing systems to meet management and clinical information needs for nursing administration, the executive levels of nursing need to prepare the organization for automation and for evaluation of system effectiveness.

There are now plans underway for graduate-level education in nursing informatics, such as at the University of Maryland, that are very much in keeping with these future role expectations for professional nursing. The content of such programs will benefit from a planned integration of organization, management, and information science theories. Initially, this content is most appropriate for the graduate level. Thesis options will offer opportunities to work with undergraduate students and practicing nurses in selected informatics research. Longer range plans will need to integrate informatics science into the baccalaureate levels as well.

Career Opportunities

The career opportunities for nurses in informatics are multifaceted. In the hospital setting, nurses are being assigned as project directors for nursing management system installation and implementation. As hospitals become totally automated and add patient care systems, the knowledge and skills of nurse project directors will be broader based. The success of hospital information systems will rely on organization-wide readiness, participation, and evaluation.

However, career opportunities for nurses will extend into many other nontraditional fields. Education in nursing informatics and experience in the application of information technology to nursing will offer new powers and new horizons to nursing professionals.

Career Opportunities for Nurses with Clinical, Management, and Informatics Skills

In Nontraditional Settings

- Third-party payors (insurances, fiscal intermediaries) and professional review organizations
- Alternative delivery systems (home health and health maintenance and preferred provider organizations)
- Management consulting firms
- Health information systems vendors.

In Nontraditional Roles

- Chief information officer
- Research and development analyst

- System analyst for implementation and management
- System marketer and installation expert
- Consultant in the design and selection of systems.

Questions

1. What should we be giving attention to as we document professional practice?
2. Why is standardization recommended in the area of nursing care planning?
3. Describe the shifts we are seeing in health care delivery.
4. From your work experience, what basic skill in the field of informatics could help you today?
5. Looking at the set of career opportunities, which would you most likely adopt if you should move into a new role? Give reason and justification.

Bibliography

Brodt A, Stronge JH: Nurses' attitudes toward computerization in a midwestern community hospital. *Computers in Nursing* 1986; 4:82–86.

Dowling AF Jr: Nursing information systems. *Journal of Medical Systems* 1985; 9:1–3.

Dowling AF Jr: Consideration for data set development: planning for future needs and the nature of the information. *Proceedings of the Nursing Minimum Data Set Conference 1985.*

Dowling AF Jr: Successful strategies for HCIS planning. *Software in Healthcare* 1987; 5(2):13–14.

Miller JA: The hidden dimension in information systems technology. *Computers in Health Care* 1987; 8(4):16–18.

Sox HC Jr: Decision analysis: a basic clinical skill? *New England Journal of Medicine* 1987; 316:271–272.

Section 2—Where Caring and Technology Meet

Unit 1—Clinical Practice

Unit Introduction

The first unit of Section II discusses the **C** of the **CARE** acronym—Clinical Practice. Warnock-Matheron and Plummer begin by exploring the factors to be considered in the implementation of nursing information systems. Tranbarger provides a case study to illustrate one institution's approach to adoption of nursing information systems. Hughes describes pioneering efforts related to data capture at the point of care. Berg and Larson consider a particular type of clinical application—operating room information systems. In the final two chapters, Werley describes progress in the development of a minimum data set for nursing in the United States, and McCormick explores the need for a uniform nursing language system encompassing nursing diagnosis and a nursing minimum data set.

1—Introducing Nursing Information Systems in the Clinical Setting

Ann Warnock-Matheron and Cheryl Plummer

Introducing Nursing Information Systems (NIS)

The current trend toward computerized systems in hospitals has a major impact on nurses. Therefore, nurses need to be aware of and participate actively in the selection, implementation, and evaluation of systems. Nursing systems managers must be cognizant of the changes in procedures, functions, and roles that will result, and must develop change management approaches that will promote nursing user acceptance of the system.

For introduction of a nursing information system to be successful, three components must be addressed. These are

1. management of the changes required

2. implementation of the system

3. training of the users of the system.

The introduction of a nursing information systems requires that attention be paid to the hospital culture and to the human factors. Successful management of change results in user acceptance of the system. Poorly managed change will generate resistance. When this occurs, attempts to circumvent changes will undermine the effectiveness of the system and the organization will fail to attain the full benefits of computerization.

Nursing acceptance of the new computer system can be facilitated by preparing nursing personnel for automation and soliciting their participation in the implementation process. This will enable them to cope with the changes in their work environment, to adapt to procedural changes, and to utilize the new tool, the computer system.

Impact on Organizational Change

The introduction of computer systems into the hospital changes the environment. These changes have been identified as:

1. More formalized and structured job functions, thereby reducing flexibility and autonomy

2. Newly created roles and a greater number of specialized occupations

3. Clarification of roles and departmental functions

4. Increased status differentiation (stratification) of occupations and organizational units (Farlee, 1978).

Each of these changes may be viewed by individuals and organizational units as threatening, and this can contribute to increased dissatisfaction and lower job satisfaction.

In order to gain the organization's acceptance of the computer system, Farlee recommends that:

1. Formalization be kept to a minimum

2. All occupational groups and departments be brought into the decision-making process when selecting a system and when specifying system modifications

3. Stratification be minimized

4. Good communication be maintained

5. Adherence to agreed-on plans and schedules be employed.

Human Factor Considerations

The successful implementation of the nursing information system (NIS) can be facilitated by anticipating the potential reactions of nurses to automation. If the reasons for these reactions are identified and understood, effective strategies that will foster acceptance and support for the system from the nursing users can be developed.

One strategy is to focus on the factors that make change rewarding rather than on the resistance to change. The balance between positive and negative reinforcement determines how the nurse will react to change. When rewards are perceived to outnumber drawbacks, acceptance will occur. Resistance occurs when the negatives appear greater than the rewards, and is expressed as a desire to maintain the status quo.

One study indicated that "the individual will operate on the basis of his perceptions even though they may be erroneous or colored by a variety of factors, such as poor communication or internal psychological mechanisms" (Youker, 1983, p. 37). Others have reported how hospital staff perceive computerization (Hodgdon, 1979; Ball and Hannah, 1984). Punishments can exist in the form of negative perceptions regarding the system's effects on organizational procedures or professional responsibilities. Negative perceptions may also result from a failure to respond in a complete or timely fashion to concerns about computerization or, interestingly, from unrealized expectations. The manner in which such issues as security, status, and social satisfaction are handled can tip the balance toward reward or punishment.

Strategies to Enhance Adaptation

Adaptation is viewing change as rewarding rather than punishing. By observing how the nurse perceives the impending changes, we can influence the reaction toward the nursing information system. Based on the writings of several change theorists, three key strategies to facilitate staff adaptation to change can be identified (Kirkpatrick, 1985).

Empathy. Empathy is used to determine the probable perceptions of nurses of the proposed changes. A program to decrease negative perceptions and increase the positive ones will enhance the probability of a successful implementation.

Communication. Communication is defined as the ability to "create understanding." By fostering understanding, the changes may be perceived to be more positive. Communication of a change should include all of those who need to know as well as all of those who want to know.

Participation. Participation requires that the manager of the change ensures that those concerned with and affected by the change are involved. "Participation increases the potential intrinsic rewards and results in ownership and commitment" (Youker, 1983, p. 39). True participation means that the users can influence the direction of the project and the change manager must be prepared to respond to the concerns of the user.

Nursing systems managers can promote nursing user acceptance by

- Ensuring adequate preparation of the nursing users
- Encouraging involvement of nurses in system testing
- Soliciting feedback from nurses and responding to concerns
- Communicating with nursing staff during implementation
- Providing support during the implementation period.

Few hospital computer systems have been installed without the staff experiencing fears and frustrations. By understanding the nature of user reaction to change, communicating, educating, and training, nursing system managers are able to minimize the period required to reach a high level of nurse-user acceptance.

System Implementation

The successful implementation of a nursing information system requires the participation of all affected individuals and organizational units. To integrate all these people into the project, a project team should be established. The project team will be composed of those responsible for developing or installing the system and user representatives. The users play an integral role in guiding the functional design and supporting the implementation. Unless the project is carefully structured, the diversity of views represented will result in a counterproductive environment.

The Implementation Plan

The implementation of the nursing information system must compete for resources with other ongoing projects and normal work activities. A master plan for the implementation, therefore, allows for

- Scheduling of resources
- Setting priorities
- Avoiding costly delays and duplication of effort
- Identifying of personnel required.

Definition of Roles and Responsibilities

A clear division of roles and responsibilities is necessary to

- Promote an effective and productive work environment
- Prevent costly duplication of effort
- Facilitate communication among team members.

When everyone knows what has to be done (implementation plan), who is responsible (definition of roles and responsibilities), and when to do it (implementation plan), the chances for a successful implementation are greatly enhanced.

Management of the Implementation Plan

For the implementation to progress, a means for allocating resources, making decisions, and reviewing progress must be established. Normally, these functions are the prerogative of a steering committee composed of the upper management of all the affected organizational units. The steering committee is chaired by a user with decision-making authority. User participation in the decision-making process enables the committee to influence development according to their needs and priorities. Among the functions of the steering committee are

- Allocation of resources
- Setting of priorities
- Review of progress
- Approval of any significant change system content
- Approval of any major change in the development timetable.

System Conversion

There are four basic approaches to system conversion.

1. Direct or Crash Conversion. This occurs when the old system is stopped and is immediately replaced by the new system. This method of conversion places the greatest stress on individuals and the organization because the change is abrupt.

2. Parallel Conversion. This occurs when the automated and manual system operate simultaneously for a period of time. The primary disadvantage of this approach is that the user workload is doubled. Provision should be made to have additional staff available during the conversion period in this approach.

3. Phased Conversion. In phased conversion, parts of the system are made available to users at discrete intervals. A major disadvantage is that the new system can be used for specific functions only and that other functions must be performed using the existing procedures.

4. Pilot Conversion. In this method, the system is initially made available to only a small part of the organization. At intervals, other units of the organization will receive access to the system. The disadvantages of this approach are the inability to move staff freely between organization units and potential communication problems when the functions that the pilot group performs must interact with those of groups not on the new system.

The four basic conversion approaches can be combined in various ways; for example, a crash conversion for a pilot group, phased parallel conversion, or a phased conversion for a pilot group. Each of the conversion approaches has inherent problems. These problems can be minimized by giving careful consideration to the effect of the conversion method on the organization and producing a plan to address potential problems.

The plan must be able to identify time frames, personnel to be involved during the conversion period, specification of how problems are to be documented, and strategies for assisting users when problems are encountered. Successful implementation is also dependent on notifying affected personnel about the conversion plan and providing clarification if necessary. Help desks manned by nursing system personnel and other designated system users can provide verbal assistance by means of a telephone and direct terminal access to function being performed by users.

Training

Definition of the Target Group and Needs Analysis

Nurses as a group appear to be resistant to computerization. A review of research literature related to nurses' attitudes to computers and automation indicates that the degree of resistance varies in relation with education, length of employment at a given hospital, and work experience. Therefore, it is essential that the attitudes of the nursing staff be assessed before any implementation. By measuring nurses' attitudes, target groups may be identified that require more intensive orientation and education.

It is reasonable to assume that the target population will be adult learners who may have predetermined opinions and/or anxieties about computer training. They are mature individuals with a variety of life experiences and responsibilities.

Adult learners have been described as

- "goal oriented

- persistent

- highly motivated

- geared to success

- committed to family, work, and/or other responsibilities

- limited in time allocated to educational activity

- best able to meet educational goals using their individualized learning style

- learning best when there is direct application of theoretical concepts and skills to the work situation" (Cobin and Lewis, 1983, p. 271).

Several factors contribute to the complexity of the task of orientating staff. The nursing staff who need to be trained in the use of the new system may consist of administrative coordinators, nursing unit supervisors, head nurses, staff nurses, and unit clerks. Presenting information simultaneously to people of widely varied backgrounds and educational levels can be considered a major challenge (Zielstorff, 1976). It is fair to anticipate that some of this group will oppose the incorporation of computers into the health care environment. Nurses are a very traditional group who tend to view any change with a certain amount of skepticism (Ball and Hannah, 1984).

In addition, it is necessary to identify common apprehensions of these nurse learners. It would be threatening to nurses if they believed that a patient's welfare might be endangered if they did not adequately understand the technology. Nurses would also be fairly resistant if they viewed the computer as a source of change or threat to long-established nursing practices and procedures (Ball and Hannah, 1984). If the "machine" is viewed as a barrier in the relationship between nurse and patient, resistance will develop. The expression and/or repression of these anxieties will impact training.

Purpose

Preparing the nursing staff for automation is crucial in establishing staff user acceptance and minimizing resistance. This can best be accomplished by designing a training program that will:

1. Provide nurses with a basic understanding of computer systems

2. Inform staff of the benefits expected

3. Define the roles and responsibilities of nursing personnel during and after implementation

4. Orient staff to the use of the system.

Questions arise whether a training program should attempt to influence nursing staff attitudes about the computer system in addition to presenting the information required to effectively use the system (Zielstorff, 1976). Zielstorff indicates that if the affective components of an introduction to automated systems are ignored, an important adjunct to orientation is bypassed.

The attitude of nursing personnel toward the system and, ultimately, their morale are often a function of the quality of the training provided. Many systems professionals attribute the success or failure of the system to the degree of user acceptance achieved.

Objectives

Objectives for the training sessions should be developed. Defining objectives is essential not only for specifying the material to be presented, but also for evaluating the effectiveness of the course. "Each objective should be clearly stated, limited in scope, and measurable, so that the learner can gauge the degree to which he or she has assimilated the material, and so that the planners of the program can evaluate its effectiveness" (Zielstorff, 1976, p. 15).

Training objectives should include:

1. Familiarizing the nursing learner with the use of the hardware
2. Familiarizing the nursing staff with the functions of the nursing information system
3. Providing nurse learners with basic information about computer systems, how they operate, what the benefits are to nursing, and the progress of the project to date
4. Promoting a positive attitude among the nurse learners toward computerization within the hospital environment
5. Generating feedback from the nursing staff in defining the system functions.

In the development of the training program, consideration must be given to the needs of the organization, the clients to be served, and the needs and interests of the learner. The resolution of issues such as comprehensiveness of the training program and efficient performance of the "graduate" of the program are inherent in the developmental process.

The training program should acknowledge the differences in knowledge, attitudes, and skills of the learner. By addressing these differences, providing factual information, and allowing the learner to express and interact in a stimulating environment, a training program does much more than teach nurses "how to compute." A training program provides the basis from which the learner may begin to grapple with the revolution of technology in the hospital setting, and thus promotes a more sophisticated level of nursing practice.

Instructional Approaches

"To ensure for accountability and measurable results, training programs are often structured using a systems approach" (Darkenwald and Merriam, 1984, p. 66). The various components of a program or organization are analyzed and consolidated to achieve a specific goal or product.

Humanistic philosophical principles have also been incorporated into the development of training programs. The emphasis on personal growth and development is recognized as being "important to the overall effectiveness of the organization" (Darkenwald and Merriam 1984, p. 67). This emphasis influences the role of the teacher and learner within the instructional process. Research on the learning process relevant to adult education can be derived from the theories of behaviorists, Gestaltists, and cognitive theorists.

Recent research indicates that the novice and the expert learn differently. The novice deals with the information in small parts and does not have an overall framework within which to reference new information. Therefore, the novice learns best when goals or subgoals are identified and frequent feedback is given after each action or decision. On the other hand, experts can readily recall information and use problem-solving procedures (Larkin et al, 1980).

In relation to establishing or changing of attitudes, one study found that the learner must identify with a respected model who performs the desired kind of behavior (Bandura, 1969). An earlier study defined three dimensions for the role of the teacher: the helper who furnishes a model for the learner, the expert who knows more about that which is being studied than the learner, and the therapist who removes attitudinal blocks to learning (Benne, 1957). Training facilitators obviously need to appreciate the importance of their role and be aware that for some they may be acting in the capacity of a role model.

A variety of methods can be utilized in presenting the hands-on training component of the program. These include live or videotaped demonstrations, followed by return practice by the learner that is guided by the facilitator. Presentation of material in a modular fashion allows the learner to control the rate of learning. Each module provides the learner with the information needed to successfully complete the function. This method of training allows for higher facilitator-to-learner ratios. In order to ease initial anxieties, all hands-on training exercises should be performed on fictitious patients. This allows the nurse learner to be more relaxed and provides the freedom to err without concern for patient safety. There is also no fear that the learner will corrupt real patient data during training.

The training program should be designed to integrate the elements of the instructional methods discussed. This represents an attempt to meet the learner's needs while taking into consideration the resources within the hospital setting.

Preparation of Organizational Resources

To meet one of the primary objectives, i.e., the nursing learner becoming competent in performance of the various functions of the system, hands-on experience is required. Hands-on experience can best be provided in a training room that is located away from the patient care areas so that nurse learners are not interrupted by the demands of patient care.

Training rooms should be equipped with the same hardware that learners will be required to use in patient care areas. Each learner should have an individual workstation and sufficient space for printed material and accessories. Arrangement of the workstations in a semi-circle allows the facilitator to monitor several learners simultaneously.

Training Program

Once the training facilities are complete, preparation of the trainers can proceed. Each facilitator should complete a basic training course and be provided with additional supervised time on the computer system. Group sessions permit discussions on how to structure a session, the application of adult learning principles, and methods of dealing with a variety of situations that may arise. Each facilitator should be evaluated by the training coordinator.

Content

Nursing learners need to become competent in the use of the equipment and the performance of functions on the system. Nursing staff must be provided with information relating to the use of the nursing information system and its benefits to nursing practice so that the learners become cognizant of issues related to the computerization of patient data. Myths and misconceptions about the system can be dispelled through the presentation of facts in the orientation sessions (Zielstorff, 1976).

The information-sharing component of the training program can occur during the orientation of the nursing staff. At this time, computer terminology is being defined and issues related to computerization such as ergonomics, confidentiality, and security of patient data are discussed.

Tools

The material provided to learners should include a training manual detailing the steps required to perform necessary tasks and functions on the system. It is important that the learners become familiar with this manual during orientation so that they will be able to use it efficiently on the nursing unit. Self-evaluation and facilitator evaluation tools are valuable in generating input for the refinement of the training program. Additional training tools such as audio and video cassettes or computer-assisted instruction modules can be used to instruct learners on keyboard operation and troubleshooting sequences.

Scheduling

The timing of the training sessions requires careful consideration. The number of staff to be trained, the physical facilities available for training, the number of trainers, and the overall staffing situation within the hospital are factors that affect the number of personnel that can be trained at any given time. Whatever the training rate, time should be blocked out immediately before implementation to allow review by the nurse learners who require or request it.

Access to the system is given when the learner has successfully completed the training program. For each training objective, minimal competency levels must be determined. Each learner must be able to achieve these levels before receiving system access. Each institution should determine what additional remedial activities will be provided should a nurse not meet the minimum standard.

In addition to the overall consideration given to the development of institution-specific confidentiality and security policies and procedures, attention needs to be focused on reinstating access to those individual nurses absent during implementation of new functions and systems.

Postimplementation Audit

At completion of implementation, an internal postimplementation audit is undertaken to evaluate the following.

Training

The objective is to determine the effectiveness of the training program and whether users have encountered problems because of inadequate training.

System Functionality

The overall functionality of the system is rated on whether user requirements have been met. This will also determine what enhancements or upgrades to the system are required.

Implementation Process

The audit process views the success or failure of the implementation primarily as a learning exercise for future implementations. The lessons learned may be applied to the implementation of enhancements or extensions of the system. Questions that should be answered include:

Were the budget and timetable estimates realistic?
What were the causes of missed deadlines and budget overruns?
What obstacles were encountered?
Does the system perform up to expectations?

User Satisfaction

User satisfaction is of primary importance. If the users are dissatisfied, they will not use the system. Factors affecting satisfaction levels include the following:

What problems are users encountering?
How are or will these problems be resolved?
What suggestions for improvements have users made?
Do the users find the system easy to use, and if not, what can be done to make it so?

Problems in these areas, appropriately identified and documented, can be addressed by appropriate personnel after the review. It should also be remembered that the evaluation of these four areas is an ongoing process, and that little items of frustration will have a long-term impact on the attitude of users to the system.

Significance

The implementation of nursing information systems holds great promise for nursing practice. With these systems, nursing as a profession will benefit from the recent advances in information technology. Computerization will move beyond the fiscal concerns of traditional hospital information systems and into the true center of health care: the well-being of the patient.

Questions

1. Identify and describe the three elements essential to successful implementation of a nursing information system.

2. Discuss the impact on the organization of the implementation of a nursing information system.

3. For each of the seven negative perceptions of nursing information systems listed in the chapter, write a brief paragraph describing corrective actions you would take.

4. Define the stages of system implementation.

5. Compare and contrast the four basic approaches to system conversion.

6. Relate the principles of adult learning to the instructional approaches for training nurses to use the system.

7. Discuss the major elements to be considered in developing the training program.

8. What is a postimplementation audit and what are its major foci?

References Cited

Ball M, Hannah K: *Using Computers in Nursing*. Reston: Reston Publishing, 1984.

Bandura A: *Principles of Behavior Modification*. New York: Holt, Rinehart & Winston, 1969.

Benne K: Some philosophic issues in adult education. *Adult Education* 1957; 7:67–82.

Cobin J, Lewis J: Solution to a dilemma: computer technology facilitates non-traditional post-basic nursing education. In: Scholes M, Bryant Y, Barber B, eds. *The Impact of Computers on Nursing: An International Review*. Amsterdam: North Holland, 1983; 269–276.

Darkenwald GG, Merriam SB: *Adult Education: Foundations of Practice*. New York: Harper & Row, 1982.

Farlee C: The computer as a focus of organizational change in the hospital. *Journal of Nursing Administration* 1978; 8:20–26.

Hodgdon JD: ADP management problems and implementation strategies relating to user resistance to change. In: Dunn RA, ed. *Proceedings of the Third Annual Symposium on Computer Applications in Medical Care*. New York: IEEE Computer Society, 1979; 843–849.

Kirkpatrick DL: *How to Manage Change Effectively*. San Francisco: Jossey-Bass, 1985.

Larkin J, McDermott J, Simon D, Simon H: Experts and novice performance in solving physics problems. *Science* 1980; 208:1335–1342.

Youker R: Implementing change in organizations (a manager's guide). *Project Management Quarterly* 1983; 14:34–40.

Zielstorff RD: Orientating personnel to automated systems. *Journal of Nursing Administration* 1976; 6:14–16.

2—Nursing Information Systems: A Case Study

Russell E. Tranbarger

The Setting

Located in Greensboro, North Carolina, a major urban center in the Piedmont region, the Moses H. Cone Memorial Hospital is a 547-bed, private, not-for-profit, community hospital and regional medical care center. On an annual basis, the hospital has an average daily occupancy of 92% and provides 150,000 patient-days of care.

The hospital serves as a level-two trauma center and a level-two neonatal intensive care center, provides a poison control center for the region, and is a center in the North Carolina area health education program (AHEC). The hospital provides exceptional services through its laboratory, radiology, radiation therapy, cardiology, oncology, and infection control services, and has the only inpatient hospice unit in North Carolina.

The hospital provides medical residency programs in family practice, internal medicine, and pediatrics. It also provides a 12-month nurse internship program and a 12-month post-master's residency in nursing administration.

Planning for an Information System

In 1980, Moses Cone embarked on a plan to purchase a hospital-wide information system. At that time, the institution determined that it would go beyond standard computerized hospital information systems, with their focus on financial data, and address the design and development of nursing software. The financial orientation continues even today in many institutions, as evidenced by a recent report stating that in most institutions the data processing director reports to the chief financial officer (Packer, 1987); moreover, nursing software remains in its infancy.

Involving Nursing

At Moses Cone, the strategy was to make nurses part of the decision process. Thus, a strong emphasis was placed on the clinical care component of information systems. The first step was to become familiar with the technology and its applications. The executive committee of the department of nursing sought out individuals with an interest in and/or experience with computerized systems. A few had worked in hospitals with such systems, and at least two had participated in the purchase or implementation of systems in other settings. A search of the literature revealed some articles on information systems, and these articles were distributed to key individuals.

Vendors were invited to demonstrate their hardware and its applications at the hospital. The nursing group devised a system for evaluating each demonstration for its nursing applications and for comparing ease of use as well as essential features. As much as possible, each member of the group sought time to use the system personally during the demonstration.

The hospital had contracted with consultants to assist in the process. All department heads and top-level managers were invited to at least two separate seminars, led by the consultants, on the technology, its uses, and its value. Each member of the nursing group became better educated through these efforts. Interestingly, there was some apprehension that nursing had gained a better level of knowledge than other department heads or managers.

Opting for a Local-Area Network System

For a variety of reasons, the original request for proposal was withdrawn and a new director of management systems was employed. The institution reached a different decision at this point and decided to implement a local-area network (LAN) system instead of a hospital-wide information system. Several reasons guided this change in direction: The technology seemed developed sufficiently to ensure success; no single system on the market did everything that was believed essential; inevitably, one product had a better pharmacy system and a less satisfactory laboratory system, and so on.

At Moses Cone, for instance, the laboratory had been computerized for several years. Experts in and supporters of computerized technology, the laboratory staff were most emphatic about what they would or would not accept. Perhaps a driving reason for this belief was the institution's strong commitment to decentralization. The LAN solution was not only compatible with decentralized management practices, but it also seemed invented to support and strengthen the hospital's decentralized system of decision making. Thus, the LAN solution enhanced nursing's ability to drive the decisions toward a solution beneficial to patient care applications in ways not always possible with hospital-wide applications.

STAT LAN was selected as the appropriate system for Moses Cone and arrangements were properly negotiated. The original nursing executive committee became the nucleus of the group convened to develop and implement the system for nursing.

Planning the System

The group dusted off the articles from the first efforts and added articles on networking to them. The group also added two unit secretaries and two head nurses (unit managers) to the task force. Discussions led to a consensus of features required, those desired, and those that would be nice to have but not necessary. Nursing identified those current consuming or problematic time-functions that computer applications might aid in solving.

For example, with a large number of daily transfers within the hospital, time was lost locating a specific patient for physician, visitor, or ancillary department. The ability to ascertain current location of each patient was judged essential. Also identified was the need to know the appointments for each patient for each day so that nurses could schedule nursing care around visits to such departments as radiology, physical therapy, or surgery. The nurse must also help the patient shepherd his strength and resources. Without knowing easily where the patient is to go, approximately when and for how long, this coordination and advocacy role is virtually impossible and frustrates the patient, the primary nurse, and all involved departments. Reliance on the telephone for timely communications of information was also an identified problem. Difficulties in getting through and then finding the person with the answer combined to make the telephone a time-waster and a source of frustration for all.

Establishing System Criteria

Always important, system criteria take on even greater importance when a new system is being developed and implemented. The most essential criterion was that the person at the unit level would process items according to a standardized method. Decentralization sometimes borders on anarchy, and the concept of LAN presents an opportunity for each departmental system to develop procedures that serve the single department well but may be totally different from any other department's procedures. The agony of nursing is that every department in the hospital interacts with nursing at the unit level in some manner. Consequently, the potential for the unit person needing to process each action differently depending on which department is the receiving one was both real and alarming. From the beginning, the Moses Cone development group insisted that the software convert all departmental applications into a common procedural entity.

The second criterion was one of efficiency. The system must be keystroke conservative, requiring the fewest possible keystrokes to accomplish the task. The next criterion was more philosophic in nature: The unit system was not to be considered the nursing application. The unit system was simply the *processing* of physician prescriptions, admission/transfer/discharge data, and other elements related to the support services nursing provides to other departments. Although these elements are not essentially nursing services, nursing personnel must coordinate and retain some control over them.

Initiating Software Development

The next step in the process was to initiate software development. To accomplish this goal a group of individuals including the unit secretary, a head nurse, a middle manager, the vice president for nursing, and representatives of hospital administration went to the STAT LAN corporate headquarters. This group met for 2 days with various members of the staff to design the software.

Group members always require some time to become comfortable with each other before the real work begins. This group developed slowly and carefully and shared ideas with growing confidence. By the end of the second day, the conference room was papered with flipchart pages identifying requirements, enhancements, timetables, persons responsible for the specific task, and so on. Considerable time was spent in explaining nursing functions to the computer people and for them to explain the reality of software to the nurses. Like most interdisciplinary groups, they had some miscommunication, some suspicion, and some doubting Thomases.

A nursing task force was formally appointed to coordinate the implementation of the local area network system. A report was presented to the task force on the initial efforts of software design that began at Simborg Systems corporate headquarters.

The task force began exploring how it would function and manage the process. After some fitful beginnings, the group devised its strategies. The group was expanded to include more unit-based individuals, including staff nurses; nursing staff development was represented along with support services and management systems people.

Interdepartmental Involvement

Since decentralization was a driving force in this instance, the group began to explore the ramifications of departmental selection of systems and their independent implementation of each system. Experience had taught that individual departments often forget that nursing must assist in their functions. For example, nursing transmits physician prescriptions to the pharmacy and administers the medication after its arrival on the patient unit. Nursing transmits the radiology request, prepares the patient for the procedure, and often transports the patient to the department. Each department may devise a method for achieving these functions without asking what consequences these decisions have for nursing.

Dyad System

To better manage the interdepartmental process, the group instituted a dyad system. This system established dyads by assigning a nurse from the executive group to each user department. It was the nurse's responsibility to establish a relationship with the leader of that department's computer efforts before any implementation. Subsequently, the dyad was to explore the interdepartmental implications of each department's efforts and to decide the method and process that would maximize benefits to each and minimize disruption to each. Each dyad was then asked to present its efforts to the task force and to provide for further discussion and refinement through this process. This negotiated process perfected decisions, kept departments informed of progress, and aided each department in understanding how nursing interacts with all departments and how the hospital fits together. These insights, in fact, have filtered into other functions, benefiting nursing as well as the user departments.

Cyclical Review Process

The software, developed by programmers at corporate headquarters, was delivered to the hospital's management systems department. It was reviewed for bugs and then handed over to the task force. Hardware was installed in the staff development office, and individuals then worked with the software. In addition to familiarizing the staff with the system, this process demonstrated what training materials were necessary. A meeting was then held for hospital and Simborg Systems staff to discuss problems, required changes, and needed enhancements. This cycle of development, review, critique, and change was repeated many times.

Meetings were also held between the hospital, the software developer, and the vendors for various department systems. Interconnecting the various systems through the network proved to be difficult at times but possible. Eventually the first patient care unit was ready to pilot the system and Moses Cone went on line. This provided a new round of cycles of enhancement, revision, and occasional disappointment as the network took shape. Each new addition to the network, whether a unit, a process, or a new system, caused a new round of problem solving and revision.

Interaction between Nursing and Dietary Department

The benefits of the dyad system and the cyclical review process were demonstrated by the interaction between nursing and the dietary department. Dietary had requested and been denied approval for a computerized application in the previous fiscal year, and consequently was both familiar with computerization and somewhat resistant to the LAN concept. Nursing was responsible for reviewing, creating, and resubmitting individual patient menus for each meal; this required considerable nursing time. In addition, the hospital averaged about 50 transfers daily so patients were often somewhere other than where their meal was delivered.

Both departments grew to share one goal: to use the LAN system to manage better. The STAT LAN staff developed dietary software early and added it to the system, allowing dietary to receive admission/transfer/discharge information on a terminal in their department. It also supports the timely transmission of diet orders without the disruption of the telephone call from the patient care unit personnel to the dietary department. This unexpected benefit engendered respect for the system that might have been slow in coming otherwise.

Similarly, the cyclical review process established plans for building on the initial skeletal framework, moving to incorporate all the features identified as necessary ones and, finally, some of the desirable options. These enhancements will occur over the next 2 to 3 years.

Implementation

When the software was sufficiently developed to use, the first unit was brought up. What the staff did and did not know about the system became apparent, as well as what worked well and what did not work at all. Order entry, results reporting, and electronic mail for the laboratory were already being used on each nursing unit. Accordingly, these same functions along with admission/transfer/discharge functions were the initial network applications. As soon as one unit was fully operational and reasonably effective, a second unit was brought on line. Essentially the same process was followed until all project units were up and running.

Project units were selected on the basis of two criteria: first, to provide for the testing of as many application/situations as possible; second, to limit travel time from user unit to user unit for those assisting in the phased implementation plan. When all project units were up, the task force developed a schedule for bringing the other patient units up. One week was required for each three units. About every 2 weeks, a 1-week hiatus was called to allow software development to catch up and departments to recoup their energies.

Units that came on line early began to request removal of the laboratory terminals before physician training on the new system was accomplished. Similar requests evidenced how very quickly the staff had mastered the system and were pushing onward.

A time schedule was then developed for units such as the operating suite, emergency services, postanesthesia care unit, and medical day care, which did not admit patients but held them on a temporary basis. Again the software had to be developed and tested since these units were a temporary location for the patient but also needed to be able to order and obtain results, etc. The same process of development, testing, and revision occurred.

Evaluating and Enhancing the System

At the time of this writing, the head nurse for each unit on the network was scheduled to appear before the task force and evaluate the system, its effective use, and existing problems from their unit perspective. These evaluation meetings were planned to provide a solid information base for suggested software enhancements. Because every unit has a distinct patient population as well as a slightly different nursing population, these unit perspectives produce unique insights.

The next step in the process is to add other ancillary departments with separate computer systems to the network. Each new department will be linked with all nursing terminals at once, but the same process of testing, refinement, and revision will occur before another new system is added.

Several cycles of enhancements are planned. Among the first to be added will be a function called exploding orders. This function transmits all orders associated with a single patient event on the transmission of the first order. For example, when a physician orders a barium enema radiologic exam, the nurse must order the procedure in radiology, order a bowel preparation from pharmacy, and change the diet orders in dietary. The exploding order function will automatically complete the entire transaction when the barium enema is ordered. Additional enhancements will include patient schedules, nursing care plans, policies, and procedures for individual units as well as for the entire hospital, and printed discharge instructions.

The next phase of the process consists of a new use for the network concept that focused on a purely nursing application. Nursing has used NPAQ by Medicus, Inc. to classify patients according to acuity as well as for quality assurance and some other applications. Presently this requires that nursing classify each patient by marking an electronically readable patient acuity rating form on the unit and sending the form to the nursing office. The forms are fed through a reader into the computer, which calculates workload, census, and so forth, and then projects the staffing required for the next 24 hours. One of the early goals at Moses Cone was to add the Medicus computer to the LAN and eliminate the sending of papers from unit to nursing office and data from the nursing office back to each unit. Meetings were held between the software developer and the Medicus staff to achieve this result.

Future Nursing Systems

The vision of the nursing task force at Moses Cone is to develop a computerized nursing system, providing decision-support functions for nurses as they provide patient care. These functions, also known as expert systems or artificial intelligence, have the potential to improve patient care as it is delivered.

In order to explore this potential and to begin the developmental process, a meeting of computer vendors and nurses along with information systems staff was convened. This meeting brought Moses Cone considerably beyond the original goal of designing software for the LAN network. The potential applications discussed are perhaps years away, yet reflect the consensus of an educated and properly managed group of interdepartmental staff working to achieve shared goals.

This group firmly believes that the development of systems will enable hospitals to contend with the shortage of professional nurses now making itself felt and projected to remain a factor for at least the next 10 years. In that shortage, new systems will help to overcome the critical distinction between the neophyte nurse and the experienced nurse: the ability to collect and analyze data and to draw inferences predictive of patient outcomes. Systems hold the promise of helping the beginning nurse go beyond identifying respiratory distress to predicting impending respiratory arrest. Systems will provide the beginning nurse with the ability of the experienced nurse to associate subtle changes in the patient's affect, respiratory rhythm, and laboratory values, and thus to abort the respiratory arrest before it occurs.

Other patient care features might include a microchip embedded in the patient's identification bracelet, readable through a handheld computer for the purposes of identifying the patient and providing information on and documenting medication and dosage, patient data, or treatment. Handheld terminals with artificial intelligence functions could assist nurses in assessing patient outcomes through identifying trends in vital signs, laboratory values, or any combination of data.

These systems would enhance nurse productivity and allay the growing nursing shortage. They also would improve patient safety and risk management. By addressing nurse staffing imbalances, individual errors, and related incidents, such systems would help to decrease the significant numbers of hospital-acquired complications that now occur.

The Moses Cone Experience

Designing software for computer applications holds great promise for nursing practice. It is a skill few nurses today believe they have. Yet once they lose their fear of the untested and untried, they will discover, as they have at Moses Cone, that they have the knowledge and skill to accomplish the task. They are eminently qualified to translate their professional expertise in nursing into technologic processes. Once again, they have found ways to direct the actions of others toward the goals of nursing. They can lead the way and achieve minor miracles, enhancing patient care by automatic nursing functions.

At Moses Cone, their secret to success has been the development of trust and effective communication among a team of nurses, managers, and computer systems staff. True, groups can sometimes be difficult to manage, but at Moses Cone they have been exciting, venturesome, and extraordinarily effective in achieving their assigned mission.

Computer technology is clearly a significant part of nursing's future! An oft-quoted Chinese proverb states that a journey of a thousand miles begins with the first step. Nurses at Moses Cone have taken that first step in designing nursing software. The remaining journey is an exciting series of little steps mingled with joy, frustration, and challenge.

Questions

1. What factors need to be considered when selecting a computerized information system?

2. How can an institution prepare for computerized information system implementation?

3. What must be accomplished following implementation of a computerized information system?

4. What skills are necessary for an individual to design nursing software?

5. How does a local area network (LAN) system differ from an integrated hospital information system?

6. What advantages and disadvantages are associated with the local area network (LAN) system? With the integrated hospital information system?

Reference Cited

Packer CL: Information management. *Hospitals* 1987; 61:92.

3—Bedside Information Systems: State of the Art

Shirley Hughes

Patient Information in Today's Health Care Environment

Patient information documentation and review requirements have taken on some very new aspects in the current acute care setting. The nursing professional has always needed to document care given and to review patient information to make care decisions; but in the current environment, those same requirements have taken on qualities of urgency and intensity. With today's hospital environment of more acutely ill patients and (often) fewer staff, it is imperative that health care professionals have more and better informational tools to assist them in caring for the patient.

This is especially important at the point of care. Nurses must have immediate access to patient information to make instantaneous decisions regarding care. They must be able to document care provided and assessments of patient conditions completely, efficiently, and in a timely manner. The recent introduction of automated information systems at the bedside affords nurses the ability to do so.

Nursing Information Needs

Bedside Data

Collecting and recording data about the health status of the patient and its accessibility and communication to other health care professionals is an important aspect of the practice of nursing. This recording function, however, can be a very time-consuming task. Nursing professionals spend a significant amount of time on paperwork. More and more hospitals are beginning to explore the potential of automating this recording function at the source, the patient bedside:

- to minimize the time required

- to eliminate redundancies when charting information

- to improve the timeliness of the documentation effort.

Documentation routinely done at the bedside can and should be automated at the bedside to maximize professional productivity. Data are commonly documented at the bedside and transcribed later at the nursing station, into the designated charting medium. Examples of this documentation duplication include the following:

- vital signs
- fluid balance
- admission history
- medication and blood administrations
- treatment and therapy administrations with results
- specimen collections.

Productivity and Quality of Care

Productivity is critically important today as hospitals attempt to contain costs without compromising quality. Bedside information systems can assist in that effort by eliminating the nonproductive time spent returning to the nursing station to check vital signs or the last administration of a pain medication before administering therapy.

Access to this information at the nursing station is not efficient or effective. Both productivity and quality of care will benefit when information is available to the care provider where the care is administered, i.e., at the patient's bedside. Proper administration of medications requires that the care provider have immediate access to records of what was ordered for which patients that specify dosage, scheduled and completed administrations, and potential drug or allergy interactions.

Quality of care and minimization of risk to the patient and the institution are of major concern. An excellent quality of care is expected by the patient and striven for by the nursing profession. However, medication errors can still occur. Treatments are sometimes overlooked or administered late. On occasion, test specimens are collected late or mislabeled. Mistakes are the exception, not the rule, but any occurrence is too many as far as the patient is concerned. Mistakes also diminish the quality of care provided and increase the cost of liability coverage. All of these mistakes severely compromise the hospital's ability to respond to cost containment measures. A bedside information system can provide this verification/warning of potential errors function before the error occurs, thus making a major impact on delivery of quality care.

Documentation can be more complete, more timely, and more accurate when captured at the source. A bedside information system that can assist the nursing professional to increase professional productivity and improve quality of care will result in maximizing resources and minimizing the health care delivery costs.

User friendliness and ease of data entry are especially important concepts when applied to bedside data entry. At the bedside, the main focus must remain the patient. A system requiring more documentation or time than a manual system will not enhance the time spent with the patient, only the time spent in the patient's room.

The most effective bedside information system presents a minimal amount of intrusion into the patient environment. The system should not present a problem or inconvenience for the patient or for the caregiver. In other words, the needs should dictate the form the solution takes.

Bedside Terminals

The bedside information needs are apparent, but the form the bedside information system solution should take is not as readily agreed on. There are several very different approaches in use in hospitals today. Because this is a fairly new aspect of hospital information systems, no one solution has yet been determined to be the solution of choice. Patient needs in such areas as critical care, obstetrics, or medical/surgical create very different care environments. It is possible that different vehicles will be required to meet the unique bedside information needs of each.

Stationary Terminals

Standard Terminals

A common first step toward bedside information solutions is to move the standard CRT or PC used at the nursing station to the bedside. This is the most expedient approach, for it provides the same full functionality that nursing is accustomed to at the nursing station to the bedside and involves minimal development effort and no additional user training.

There are, however, some disadvantages. The patient environment is invaded by a high-tech but not necessarily high-touch solution. There are often problems with placing a full-sized terminal into an already crowded area. Both space and location are significant. Since the terminal is a stationary device, the nurse must leave the patient to go to the terminal to look up or to chart information. The humming noise usually associated with CRTs and PCs may not be noticeable at a busy nursing station, but can be very irritating to a sick patient.

From a systems viewpoint, there is also the danger that the hospital information system (HIS), if not designed for bedside applications,

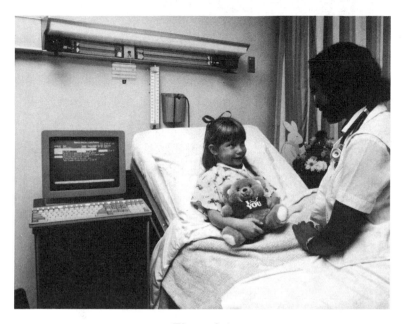

Figure 3-1
Stationary bedside computer terminal (Ulticare).
By permission of Health Data Sciences Corp.

cannot accommodate the addition of the large number of terminals. The system may experience unacceptable decreases in response time. In addition, if special wiring is required for each patient room, this can be an expensive alternative.

The commercially available Ulticare System offered by Health Data Sciences includes a software package designed specifically for the bedside application, but uses a standard fully functional CRT at the bedside. (Fig. 3-1). Nurses may sit or stand at the terminal, which is mounted on a hydraulic lift.

At the University Hospitals, University of Alabama at Birmingham, PCs are placed at the bedside in the critical care areas for charting and data review functions.

Specially Designed Terminals

A terminal specially designed for use at the bedside can satisfy physical space limitations and provide for quick and easy data entry. With special function keys and specially designed menu selection screens with minimal typing required, the task of documentation can be made very efficient. This will accomplish the goal of time savings and, if not too limiting in its functionality, maintain the completeness of the information. The disadvantage is that the terminal is a stationary device and thus not available at all times to the nurse caring for the patient.

The Medtake System by Micro Healthsystems, Inc. uses this hardware approach. The system uses a small footprint terminal with function keys and a numeric keypad replacing the complex keyboard of most CRTs. Menu-driven screens are used extensively.

Portable Bedside Terminals

Data Collection Storage Devices

The immediate advantage of a portable device is that the nurse can be with the patient at all times and still document care as it is provided. The disadvantage is that these data collection storage devices are not real-time interactive. Charting data is collected in the device but is not available to others on the health care team until it is downloaded to the mainframe (usually through a device located at the nursing station). Review of real-time patient information to support care decisions at the point of care is impossible with these devices.

The NCR Peanut was one of the first nursing terminals offered. It received a great deal of attention from nurses and had many excellent features. It was, however, eventually taken off the market after it was realized during actual installation and use by nurses that, among other things, a real-time interactive device was a major criterion for bedside information systems.

Portable Interactive Terminals

Portable interactive terminals can give the nursing professional the best of all possible worlds in bedside information solutions. They allow quick and easy data entry (often using bar coding as well as special function keys and menu selections), real-time documentation and retrieval of patient information, portability so that the nurse can be with the patient, and a design especially suited to the patient care environment. There may be disadvantages to this approach if the portable devices prove to be too heavy, cumbersome, or restrictive in function for the nurse to use them easily.

Systems Available

Examples of this approach include CliniCom's CliniCare, a portable handheld terminal with a built-in bar code reader, special function keys, and a back-lighted liquid crystal display for menu selection and screen display (Fig. 3-2). A wall-mounted full-screen monitor is also offered with CliniView. This facilitates display of larger amounts of data for review, graphic displays, and menus for assessment charting. The handheld terminal acts as the keyboard for the full-screen monitor. Thus, this is the only fully interactive and truly portable device currently in use.

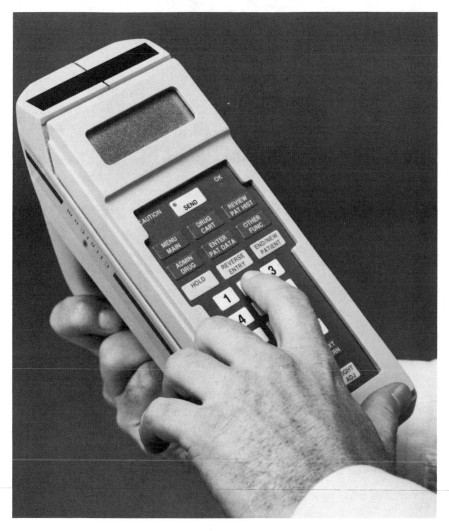

Figure 3-2
Portable (handheld) terminal (CliniCare).
By permission of CliniCom, Inc.

AT&T has announced a bedside information system development project in which a lightweight flat-screen terminal with a touch-sensitive screen is used for menu selections and for typing of additional patient data. This portable terminal plugs into a wall outlet in the patient room (Fig. 3-3). Vancouver General Hospital is also developing a portable terminal for use at the bedside. This device is slightly larger than a clipboard and consists of a miniature keyboard and a small graphics-based liquid crystal display screen.

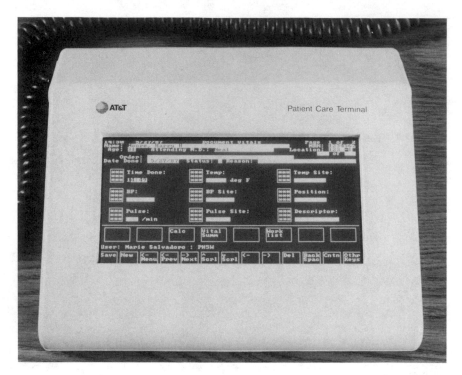

Figure 3-3
Portable bedside terminal (CareComm).
By permission of AT&T.

Bedside Terminals and Patient Care

One common approach to the bedside information system software solution has been to simply move the HIS functionality to the bedside. Although this approach does not take into consideration the uniqueness of point-of-care information needs, it does provide a familiar and fully functional system of whatever order entry, results retrieval, and documentation functions are available on the HIS. A centralized data base is a key advantage with this approach. Data are available to all members of the health care team from any terminal location in the hospital. Some of the features required at the point of care that may not be included in a system designed for the nursing station include security, confidentiality, quick data entry techniques, specific functions such as validation of therapies, and expeditious retrieval of critical patient information.

Systems designed specifically for the bedside can offer additional benefits to those found with the approach just described. These systems focus on the patient, quickly capturing information normally jotted down by the nurse on paper worksheets. Reminders of treatments and medications to be administered are provided to the nurse. Validation of these therapies and/or warnings of potential error conditions are highlighted. Shortcuts are provided to facilitate quick access to critical information. Although these systems are designed specifically for the bedside, typically they are tied into the HIS so that the need for data accessibility throughout the hospital is satisfied.

Both Ulticare and CliniCare are examples of specialized bedside information applications. However, they represent two very different approaches. Ulticare is a complete HIS, including order communication and results reporting, as well as nursing documentation, with the patient bedside as the focal point for data collection and review. CliniCare, on the other hand, provides the point-of-care information functionality as an enhancement to the hospital's existing order-communication and results-reporting information system.

The Medtake System has approached the bedside information needs from another perspective. This system provides the nursing documentation functions at the bedside and communicates this information to a PC located at the nursing station. Additional information can be added to the charting at the nursing station and chart documents can be printed. A link to the HIS is not required.

Bedside information processing is certainly not a new requirement, but a long-established one to which new technologies are now being applied. The major features included in the successful systems are those of fast and easy data entry, data accessibility, quality checks for accuracy of patient care, and, most importantly, nurse and patient friendliness. The computerized bedside information system is new to hospitals. Over the next few years, as the various approaches in use today are tested, the less effective approaches will be replaced. The more effective will grow and expand to provide the important quality and productivity improvements needed by nursing.

Questions

1. What benefits can a bedside information system provide specifically to the nurse?

2. What benefits can a bedside information system provide to the hospital in general?

3. List three important differences between a nursing station-based system and a bedside information system.

4. Compare the pros and cons of a standard CRT versus a specially designed bedside terminal.

5. What considerations do you feel are important for the patient environment when considering a bedside information system?

4—Operating Room Information Systems Software

Constance M. Berg and Darlene Larson

Computerization in the Operating Room Suite

History

In the late 1970s, very few hospitals enjoyed the support of computerization in the operating room (OR). The few that used such applications were those that put in-house programmers to work on developing scheduling programs and offering capabilities similar to those in outpatient appointment scheduling. Usually these functions were developed on mainframe computers.

Next came the personal computer, which supported the material management component for the entire hospital and thus the operating room inventory, or at least the portion of the operating room inventory managed with the entire hospital inventory.

In the early 1980s, vendors began appearing in the marketplace with software packages specific for the operating room department. At first, functions focused on scheduling and/or materials management, then preference cards and management reports. Functions rapidly expanded and are now as diverse as personnel experience/credentialing records and clinical data tracking. Hardware choices range from personal to mainframe computers. Data entry choices include bar code readers, light pens, voice-activated recording, keyboards, and automated notepads. While many systems are designed for data entry to occur at one central location or a limited number of centralized locations, terminals are beginning to appear in each operating room for direct data entry, thus facilitating expanded data collection. As a result, today the operating room manager has many software functions, hardware, and data input options from which to make a selection that best meets the department's needs.

Current Status

In the United States today, an estimated 7 to 10% of the operating rooms in the 5500 hospitals having more than 50 beds use some type of computer support. In 1987, 167 subscribers to an American newsletter, *OR Manager*, responded to an editorial survey on the use of computer services in the operating room suite. The results showed 103 operating room suites (62%) have some type of computer capability. The remaining 64 suites (38%) are not using any computer services. In the suites using computerization, 36% use stand-alone systems, 42% use the hospital mainframe, 13% use a combination of stand-alone and hospital mainframe, and the remaining 9% use remote services, or remote services in combination with the hospital mainframe or stand-alone system. The stand-alone systems are ranked the highest in user satisfaction (Schrader, 1987).

One research evaluation study of 18 OR systems reported "software capabilities can go beyond scheduling to fulfill hospital needs for cost tracking, clinical abstracting and other information requirements in support of the overall goals of cost containment and quality assurance." The same study stated 21 functions are available, but the number available in any one system was variable (Ball et al, 1986).

While many functions are available, the *OR Manager* survey reported "only 22% of those (hospitals) with stand alone systems were using their system for all the functions of scheduling, inventory, reports, materials management, and charging." However, it is important to know that all systems are not designed to provide the wide range of functions that some of the systems can provide. Therefore, some departments may be using all of the functions available on their particular systems, but the system itself does not have the capability to perform all of the functions another system can do.

It is not surprising that so few hospitals have or are using operating room systems, or that only portions of an installed software package are being used. Several reasons contribute to this fact.

- Systems for the operating room are in their infancy, as are many of the software companies. Vendor research and development are determining what clients want, and vendors simultaneously are trying to educate clients about their needs.

- Another significant factor limiting widespread use is that computer systems are a capital budget item, costing from $12,000 for a software package to over $500,000 for systems that also include the hardware. Usually this amount of expenditure requires preparation of a cost justification document by the operating room manager, who is frequently inexperienced in this task, specifically for acquisition of a departmental (versus clinical) computer system.

- Product evaluation can be difficult; frequently only some of the functions available in a system have actually been implemented in user sites. Because there are few fully implemented systems to see, buying software is like buying an almost intangible product.

- Equally if not more important, there is no way to know if a system can actually perform as claimed if it has never been fully implemented and/or implemented at the volume level with the number of terminals and/or sites a specific hospital may require.

- Many operating room managers need to be educated about the benefits of an operating room system, determining which system is best for their hospital, acquiring as well as implementing the system, and finally using the system to its maximum capability.

- Many hospital administrators and financial officers also require education about the benefits of an operating room system.

The Future

In the United States, the Joint Commission on Accreditation of Hospitals (JCAH) is now advocating more stringent standards of quality assurance for patient care. The resulting focus is on mechanisms to monitor and evaluate patient care in the operating room. As of 1987, there is no mandate to install computer systems for the operating room suite to effectively monitor care and accomplish generic screening for quality assurance outcome criteria standards. However, one wonders how patient care will be monitored unless computers are made available to professional nurses to capture data at its source. With manual systems, it is costly, difficult, and time consuming to detect errors in patient care. It is next to impossible to manually manipulate the type and amount of data needed to detect errors, facilitate research, monitor care, and make informed decisions to improve patient care practices.

Need for Computer Systems in the Operating Room

Cost Containment and Competitive Factors

Why are computer systems needed for operating room suites? Operating rooms face incredible challenges, especially in the United States, because of the changes in reimbursement for surgical services. Also, competition is omnipresent.

The operating room is a major cost and revenue center and one of the most expensive resources in the hospital. Thus, the OR manager is constantly challenged to contain costs, increase services, increase market share, increase the profit margin, and "ace out" the competition. Powerful and sophisticated software is available to provide the necessary information to assist the OR manager in meeting these goals. The computer with appropriate software is a tool for the operating room manager to identify and analyze costs, expenses, and trends while improving overall efficiency. Meanwhile, the entire operating room team wants to ensure that patient care will not be compromised as cost containment measures continue. As operating room managers are increasingly pressured by their administration for more information and recommendations, they are showing an increasing desire to learn how to acquire and install computer technology designed specifically for the operating room suite.

The biggest challenge for the operating room manager is convincing hospital administration that computers in the operating room suite can be beneficial for the hospital.

Impact on Nursing Care

Computer systems are designed to reduce the time and effort required to keep track of everything. With a terminal in each operating room, data is recorded once by the circulating nurse as the case is occurring. Without a terminal in each OR, some data is recorded a minimum of two times because manual records are completed by the nurse in the operating room and then entered into the system at a centralized location. Depending on the OR system selected and the functions available, the entry of information into the computer eliminates redundant manual recording by the nurse into different log books and records. The computer will also generate the daily log, list each specimen per patient that is sent to the lab, maintain surgical-implant logs for all services, generate charges, and maintain inventory.

All nurses in the OR benefit when data can be sorted and used for many purposes. Clinical data can be used to research patient care outcomes and provide information and answers to clinical questions. Reference cards can be complete and up to date with minimal effort. Supplies and equipment can be properly requested, supplied, and charged. Personnel data can be used for education assessments, license and credentialing records, and productivity and performance appraisals.

Management Considerations

Health care professionals are in the business of managing the health care of their patients and clients. A great amount of information must be recorded and evaluated to accomplish this. Knowledge of operating room nursing, business and management skills, and computer technology are the key attributes every operating room manager of today and the next decade should possess. The OR manager faces increasing volume and complexity in procedures and associated patient care needs as well as requiring more sophisticated resources, from supplies, equipment, and instrumentation to personnel. In short, to be expert, the manager should be "someone who has been there," who understands the rapidly changing health care environment, can assess the potential impact for the OR, articulate the needs of the OR department, and determine what must be done to increase the level, safety, and effectiveness of health care each patient receives.

The OR manager of today deals with a new breed of patients and a new health care environment. Patients are increasingly better educated consumers of health care, and able to direct when and where their surgical care will take place. The patient is no longer a captive audience, but an activist that as a customer and consumer of health care needs to be cultivated, listened to, and sought after. Personnel working in operating room suites need patient feedback on their interactions and how the patient perceived them during the surgical experience. This type of information can readily be acquired and used to increase patient satisfaction through staff interaction.

The OR manager needs information to assist in the management decisions of running a major cost-and-revenue department, to monitor the quality of patient care, and to build and market new services and programs in a financially responsible way. Some information needs remain constant; but, as health care continues to change, information needs also change. Computer systems provide current, accurate, comprehensive, and variable information—information needed to make sound decisions, improve patient care, meet regulatory rules and standards, and identify staff learning needs.

System Acquisition

User Input

In preparing the groundwork for administrative approval, the OR manager must enlist key individuals to support acquisition. Most probably these include the director of nursing services and/or the vice president for nursing as well as directors or other influential persons in any or all of the following departments:

anesthesia
finance
quality assurance
infection control
data processing
materials management
medical records
admissions.

Each of these departments has a vested interest in the benefits of an OR computer system.

In addition, the chief of surgery, service chiefs, and other surgeons who are high-volume users can lend their power in support of a computer system acquisition. The OR manager may also find it helpful to identify surgeons who complain about the services, determine how the system could benefit them, and enlist their support if possible. Administration is always looking for ways to keep complainers happy, especially if the result could be increased operating room usage and revenues.

To gain administrative approval, the OR manager must prepare documentation that answers the question of how the system, once acquired, will support and contribute to achieving the goals and objectives of the operating room and the organization. The financial officer will require a cost justification document that clearly establishes the return on the investment.

Steps to Acquisition

Step 1. Determine the Needs of the Operating Room

The first step is to review the manual systems in use and to determine which could provide better and more timely information with automation. Systems appropriate for computerization include scheduling, materials management, patient billing, central processing, case cart pull lists, surgeons' preference cards, clinical data bases, surveys, and administrative and financial reporting (see Table 4-1 on p. 155).

Obtaining timely information about the costs of doing business is extremely important. The information is basic to arriving at pricing strategies, developing new services, changing or expanding hours of services, determining staffing patterns, and marketing the OR to surgeons.

Step 2. Conduct a Formal Needs Assessment

The second step is developing a needs assessment document from user input to establish departmental and interdepartmental needs. The OR manager plays a key role here, determining with the support people identified in step 1 how the OR interfaces with other hospital departments and existing hospital computer systems (Fig. 4-1). Surveys of the needs of the laboratory, blood bank, radiology, preadmissions, admitting, and marketing are also important. This information is critical to improving interfaces with other departments and thereby achieving maximum benefits of computerization.

Step 3. Establish a Computer Selection Team

The next step is to establish a team that will work with the OR manager to select a system. The team should include individuals knowledgeable in data processing and hospital-wide information systems, as well as

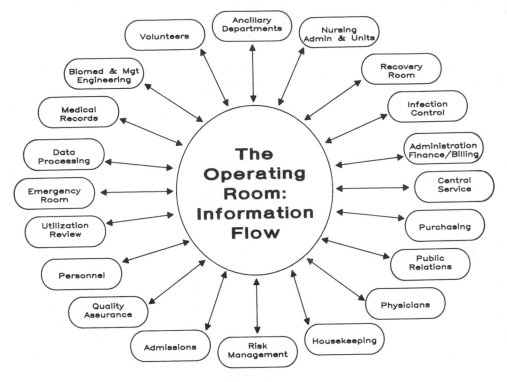

Figure 4-1
Operating room information flow.

OR staff who will be using the system, e.g., scheduler, materials manager, clinical instructor, circulating nurse, and evening charge nurse.

Step 4. Analyze Vendor Systems

An overview of the marketplace will permit the selection committee and the OR manager to assess how a system will fit a particular environment. It would be very time-consuming to review all systems in detail as there are over 25 vendors in the United States. To evaluate the systems efficiently and economically, the computer selection team should (1) list and prioritize the system requirements for the OR and the organization on the basis of the needs assessment completed in step 2, and (2) decide which vendors will be invited to demonstrate their product.

In evaluating vendor demonstrations, the selection team should consider how well the software meets the established criteria and identify any limitations and their potential effect on achieving the goals set for the system. The demonstrations should allow the team to narrow the field down to two or three vendors for further consideration.

The request for proposal (RFP) should now be prepared. The OR manager needs the help of the interdisciplinary selection team to develop the RFP, which will guide selection of the vendor. The hospital's consulting firm or an outside consultant knowledgeable about OR systems should assist in preparing the RFP, which details a method for the selection process and also specifies as precisely as possible what the system must do for the hospital. The vendors responding must indicate whether their system will meet the hospital's needs as stated in the RFP and in detail how it will do so.

In addition to stating system requirements, the RFP should request answers to questions on how and by whom the proposed system would be implemented and supported. Among these questions are the following:

Who inputs the hospital data into the computer to build the data bases?
What is the estimated time to build the data bases?
Is a system administrator necessary for efficient and effective implementation?
Should a permanent system administrator be assigned to the system?
What percentage of a full-time employee's time should be allocated to support the system; what is the job classification?
How many clients are installed with their full software package?
How many clients have fully implemented the system?

The questions about implementation are clearly important to potential users, but equal importance should be assigned to questions regarding the stability of the firm. The software industry is highly volatile, with many new young companies. The vendor that is no longer in business cannot serve the owner of its software. Measures of vendor stability and viability can be obtained by asking the following questions:

How long has the vendor been in business?
What is the viability of the company?
What is the financial status and backing of the company?
How many personnel are employed?
What are their qualifications and work within the company?
Do they interface with the client and if so how?

The RFP should also stipulate that each vendor provide a list of clients and a contact person for each client. The OR manager and the selection team should then communicate directly with clients that are actually using each system. Contact with these clients is essential to evaluate thoroughly vendor support services. Questions to ask such clients include the following:

How responsive is the vendor to problems, questions, and for support during and after implementation?

Does the implementation team (the people assigned from the company to work directly with the client in getting the system up and running) understand the workings of a surgical suite?

Will they try to tailor the OR to meet the software or tailor the software to meet OR needs?

How many people are on the implementation team, and who from the company manages them?

Organizational Impact of the OR

The operating room is the key to the overall hospital success in delivering excellent care to the surgical patient while containing costs. As the OR explores the opportunity for computerization, consideration should be given to the interfaces with other hospital departments. For each and every patient, concerted efforts by a number of departments must be the base for patient care in the operating room. Many persons throughout the hospital coordinate and function in a timely, efficient, responsive way to provide OR care, even for the shortest surgery.

One of these interdepartmental relationships exists between the operating room and the admissions area. In completing the needs assessment, it is helpful to consider how to integrate the OR with admissions. Multiple options exist. One possibility is to link the OR scheduling system with the hospital information computer to utilize prescribed criteria (including those for reimbursement by each individual patient's third-party coverage) and conduct searches for surgical beds. A second option is to have the admitting department enter the scheduling information and use the hospital information system to pass it to the operating room system. A third option is to place a terminal in the admitting department that is an extension of the operating room system. Whichever option is selected, integration has definite advantages. The admitting department is notified of the prospective bed reservation and the operating room has the patient prospectively scheduled for surgery. Integration with other departments offers additional advantages. The needs assessment step of the acquisition process should clearly identify patient and perioperative information needed by other hospital departments and incorporate these into the OR computer system requirements (Table 4-1).

Cost Justification of an Operating Room System

Analyzing the true costs of a care delivery system and how the implementation of an automated system can offset some of these costs is of particular interest to the financial administrator. The director of fi-

Table 4-1
Easily Computerized OR Functions

Patient Billing
Central Processing
Case Cart Pull Lists
Surgeons Preference Cards
Scheduling
    Showing first available time and/or following hospital policy
    Automatic resource conflict checking
Materials Management
    Complete inventory tracking
    Vendor profiles
    Property ledger
    Preventive maintenance log
    Service repair log
Clinical Data Base
    Pre-, intra-, and postoperative data
    Wound classifications
    Quality assessment
    Implant logs
    Specimen logs
    Outcomes
Surveys
    Postoperative follow-through
    Demographics
Administrative and Financial Reporting
    Case mix analysis
    Room utilization
    Overtime
    Physician utilization and procedure statistics
    Supply and equipment utilization and costs
    Procedure costs and charges by procedure codes
    Surgeon estimates versus actual procedure times
    Personnel case experience by resident, intern, and nurse
    Case cancellations, delays, and causes
    Average cost per case per surgeon (in comparison to other surgeons)
    Utilization and revenue by service

nance is charged with managing and allocating the financial resources of the hospital in the most prudent and advantageous way. The cost/benefit document should specify the real dollar benefits to the surgical suite and the hospital. Questions to be answered include:

Will acquiring the system require a price increase to the patient?
What is the return on investment?
Are additional short- or long-term employees needed to implement or maintain the system?
Is there potential for increasing revenue?

If so, how and by how much?
What is the life of the system?
What is the depreciation period?

Some of the costs of the system can be identified as potential cost savings, others as real savings. Potential cost savings include the estimated lost charges that will now be captured by using the system. Real cost savings address the costs of manually preparing reports, inventory overstock, and supply waste. Potential benefits and savings include increased utilization of the OR resulting from enhanced scheduling and reporting capabilities, based on the ability to rapidly access data and to run customized reports. Available software includes the following:

Comparative studies of costs
Resource utilization tracking
Trend identification by surgical specialty, groups of surgeons, or individual surgeon
Case mix volume by cost and charges

Along with the amount of data input, the actual OR system selected (including the data base and report generator) will determine how extensive, how finite, and how specific the reports will be.

Preparation of the cost/benefit documentation can be time consuming and frustrating. Cost justification can be difficult because many benefits are based on assumptions. Some vendors will assist the OR manager in this process. Because vendors do not usually quote all associated costs required for implementation, it is important to ask the vendor a number of questions:

How much manpower will be required, and at what job classification, to build the data bases? for example, preparation, input, and verification of doctor preference cards, procedure codes, and inventory.
If the vendor does data entry, what is the cost?
Will the amount of user training provided be adequate for training the system administrator and other trainers? If not, what additional costs will be incurred?
What is the estimated parallel run time and what costs will be incurred? (This is the time to verify that the system is working correctly and the users are making the transition from the manual system to the computer system. There will be some additional costs incurred in running the manual and computer systems simultaneously.)

It is extremely important to determine the hidden as well as publicized vendor costs in the evaluation. Other associated costs are the field trips the selection team makes to visit sites where the software systems have been installed and the use of consultants. Some vendors have consultants who will work with the client. The tasks the consultant will do and these associated costs should be clearly stated.

When preparing the documentation to support the purchase of a system, it is worthwhile to obtain a second opinion or help from a responsible source inside the hospital or an outsider familiar with computers and the operating room environment. In most hospitals, the cost/benefit documentation is the key to approval to purchase the system.

Contract Agreement

Once a vendor is selected, the next step is the contract or license agreement, which is drawn up by the vendor. The license agreement is a legally binding document between the vendor and the hospital. Negotiation and discussions about the license agreement will take place at the administrative level and involve the hospital attorney. Although the operating room manager will have little if any direct involvement in the contractual process, he/she should have a copy of the agreement to review and comment on before it is finalized. Areas on which the manager should focus are the implementation and training responsibilities of the vendor.

Benefits Realization

The interesting part begins after the system is installed in the OR— now the benefits must be realized. An ongoing evaluation asks certain critical questions:

Does the system do what the OR manager and selection team thought it would do?

Do initial audits of output show the statistical evaluations to be accurate?

What changes in procedures, practices, case carts, inventory, assigned block times, staffing patterns, etc. are indicated from the analysis of the reports generated by the system?

What are the financial implications of the changes?

What can be done now that could not be done before the system was installed?

The evaluation will serve two functions. First, it should validate the selection decision. If the right system was selected, benefits will be achieved. If the wrong system was selected, benefits will be limited. Second, the evaluation should determine what operational or organizational changes might optimize the benefits of the selected system, such as data handling. In addition, as users become more involved, software changes will be required to smooth use of the OR system. The monitoring of software capabilities will play a critical role in determining what these changes should be.

Summary

The important element in obtaining a system is to gain agreement among the key supporting individuals very early in the process. Agreement on assumptions is critical in determining what changes in the OR are desirable and achievable, as is agreement on how the OR manager and the selection team will analyze costs and estimate benefits. This requires marketing the project well and getting these individuals to agree to the acquisition/implementation strategy.

The ultimate usefulness of the system will depend on the number of applications available and implemented, the flexibility of the system in using and manipulating all data, and the structure of the data base in sorting and printing patient data in a seemingly infinite number of ways to meet the individual information requirements of each hospital. Further, the OR manager must use this system to its maximum capabilities and use the reports generated to promote and meet departmental goals and develop strategies to further increase the capabilities of the operating room department.

Implementation of a comprehensive system is a major undertaking and requires thoughtful planning and complete management support throughout the project. With the right system appropriately implemented and utilized, the benefits and rewards will be great.

Questions

1. Why has proliferation of computer systems in the operating room been slow?
2. How do you determine if a computer system is needed in the operating room?
3. What benefits can be gained from an OR computer system in the operating room?
4. What are some barriers in acquiring a system?
5. What steps are necessary to acquire a system?
6. What are reasonable expectations from a system?
7. What should you look for when evaluating a system?

References Cited

Ball MJ, Warnock-Matheron A, Hannah KJ, Douglas JV: The case for using computers in the operating room. *Western Journal of Medicine* 1986; 145:843–847.

Schrader ES: Big transition to OR automation still to come. *OR Manager* 1987; 3:1–7.

5—The Nursing Minimum Data Set: Effort to Standardize Collection of Essential Nursing Data

*Harriet H. Werley, Elizabeth C. Devine,
and CeCelia R. Zorn*

Abstract

The concept of the Nursing Minimum Data Set (NMDS), which is based on the concept of the Uniform Minimum Health Data Sets (UMHDS), is described in relation to its purposes and consensually derived elements and definitions. A brief report of pilot test findings is given, and implications for clinical practice, administration, research, and education are highlighted. The NMDS is viewed as a link in integrating computers into nursing care across all practice settings.

The Changing Clinical Scene

The Nursing Minimum Data Set (NMDS) is an initial effort to establish uniform standards for the collection of minimum, essential nursing data. It draws on the documentation of the nursing process that is exercised when nurses provide care to people in any setting. This establishment of uniform standards is crucial within the changing clinical scene as the dawn of the twenty-first century approaches.

Many factors are influencing all of nursing practice at an unprecedented pace. Nurses are practicing in more diverse settings than ever before. The move in health care from acute care settings to community settings is changing the employment practices of many nurses, especially those 2 or 3 years post graduation. With the movement to more autonomous practice comes a need for nurses to accept increased accountability. This accountability is not only for the use of resources, but also for specific interventions to achieve a desired client outcome.

There also are far-reaching effects resulting from the growth in the aging population and the increasing cost of health care. The increase in the elderly population in the United States is probably the most dramatic change in the twentieth century. Based on the 1980 census, 1 person in 9 is currently over 65 years of age compared to 1 person in 25 in 1900. Considering projected growth between 1976 and 2000, it is estimated that the 65- to 74-year-old age group will increase 23%, those aged 75 to 84 will increase 57%, and those 85 and over will increase by 91% (Rich and Baum, 1984). With the growing elderly population, an increase in chronic diseases and accompanying socioeconomic issues must also be addressed. Closely related to the increase in the elderly population are rapidly rising health care expenditures. In 1981, health care costs totaled $1,223 per person and comprised 9.8% of the gross national product. For Medicare alone, the costs were estimated at $57 billion in 1983, rising to $112 billion by 1988 (Barger, 1985).

As a minimum data set is established for nursing within the changing health care arena, its development must be geared to all of the nursing profession. A setting-specific data set would serve only that area of nursing practice, and it might result in a division of nurses based on health care settings. A minimum data set applicable to all of nursing would assist in the establishment and use of a common language, which is surely needed by the nursing profession and others in the health care field. In the spirit of increased acceptance of accountability by nurses, change in practice settings, increases in cost of health care, and the growth of the elderly population—coupled with an existing and projected shortage of professional nurses—the NMDS will be explored as a link in integrating computers into nursing care across all practice settings.

The concept of the NMDS as derived from the Uniform Minimum Health Data Sets (UMHDS) is described. Its purposes and elements, as they evolved from the NMDS national conference, are also discussed. After a brief overview of the pilot study findings, implications of the NMDS for clinical practice, administration, research, and education are identified.

NMDS Concept Derived from the Uniform Minimum Health Data Sets

A Uniform Minimum Health Data Set (UMHDS) has been defined by the Health Information Policy Council (HIPC) as "a minimum set of items of information with uniform definitions and categories, concerning a specific aspect or dimension of the health care system which meets the essential needs of multiple data users" (Health Information Policy Council, 1983, p. 3). The key here is "multiple data users," not only nurses. This concept was identified first in 1969 in an effort to develop national health data standards and guidelines (Murnaghan and White, 1970). Three patient-focused UMHDSs have been developed previously, in the areas of long-term care, hospital discharge, and ambulatory care (National Committee on Vital and Health Statistics

[NCVHS] 1980a,b, 1981). Of these, the Uniform Hospital Discharge Data Set (UHDDS), which was adopted first in 1972, is currently used widely in the United States (Health Information Policy Council, 1983, 1984, 1985).

The NMDS was built on the concept of the UMHDS and represents the first attempt to standardize the collection of essential nursing data. In this context, essential nursing data are viewed as those specific items of information that are used on a regular basis by the majority of nurses across all settings in the delivery of care.

Purposes of the NMDS

The purposes of the NMDS are to

- establish comparability of nursing data across clinical populations, settings, geographic areas, and time
- describe the nursing care of patients in a variety of settings
- demonstrate or project trends regarding care and allocation of nursing resources to patients according to their health problems or nursing diagnoses
- stimulate nursing research through links to the detailed data existing in nursing information systems and other health care information systems (HCIS).

Consensually Derived System

The NMDS was developed consensually through the efforts of a national group of experts, who participated in the 3-day invitational NMDS Conference held in Wisconsin in 1985 that was sponsored by the University of Wisconsin-Milwaukee (UWM) School of Nursing and funded largely by the Hospital Corporation of America (Werley and Lang, in press; Werley et al, 1986a,b). The participants at this conference included nurse experts in a variety of areas; health policy spokespersons; information systems, health data, and health records specialists; and persons knowledgeable about development of the UMHDS. These participants were charged with identifying the appropriate NMDS elements, or items, and developing the definitions for them.

Task Forces

The 65 conference participants were assigned to one of six task forces to work on identifying the elements of a particular category of the nursing process. The categories designated for these six task forces were as follows:

Nursing assessment
Nursing diagnoses

Nursing interventions
Nursing outcomes
Nursing intensity
Demographics.

The task forces also were asked to define their identified elements, and, where time permitted, to identify subelements and measures. A post-conference task force reviewed and refined the data set developed by the conference task forces.

The Data Set Elements

The NMDS includes three broad categories of elements:

Nursing care
Patient or client demographics
Service elements.

Elements that also are included in the previously mentioned UHDDS (Health Information Policy Council, 1985; National Committee on Vital and Health Statistics, 1980b) are indicated by an asterisk. Elements comparable to those already being collected need not be re-collected in hospitals, when they can be obtained through existing relational data base management systems. (Table 5-1).

Table 5-1
Elements of the Nursing Minimum Data Set

Nursing Care Elements

    1. Nursing diagnosis
    2. Nursing intervention
    3. Nursing outcome
    4. Intensity of nursing care

Patient or Client Demographic Elements

    5. Personal identification[a]
    6. Date of birth[a]
    7. Sex[a]
    8. Race and ethnicity[a]
    9. Residence[a]

Service Elements

    10. Unique facility or service agency number[a]
    11. Unique health record number of patient or client
    12. Unique number of principal registered nurse provider
    13. Episode admission or encounter date[a]
    14. Discharge or termination date[a]
    15. Disposition of patient or client[a]
    16. Expected payer for most of this bill (anticipated financial guarantor for services)[a]

[a] Elements comparable to those in the Uniform Hospital Discharge Data Set.

Nursing intervention was included in the NMDS during the pilot testing period so that the feasibility of adding it as an element could be assessed. Before this element can be recommended fully, there must be an acceptable, exhaustive, and mutually exclusive coding scheme for categorizing nursing interventions.

Pilot Test Findings

The pilot test of the NMDS, directed by Dr. Elizabeth C. Devine, included 116 subjects from four clinical sites: a hospital, nursing home, home health care agency, and two clinics affiliated with a teaching hospital. Overall intercoder agreement was a satisfactory 91%, with an item-specific range of 57 to 100%. The implication of these results is that the definitions and protocol for coding were generally acceptable, although a few elements need refinement. Most of the NMDS elements were available for more than 90% of cases. The exceptions were the unique number of principal registered nurse provider, which was never available; ethnicity, available 9% of the time; race, available for 71% of subjects; resolution status, available for 79% of the documented nursing diagnoses; and personal identification number of the client, which was available for 86% of subjects. A conclusion can be drawn from these results that existing records were an adequate source of most of the elements in the NMDS. For detail about the NMDS testing, see Devine and Werley (1988).

Perceived Benefits and Implications

The benefits for nurses and nursing are highlighted, because nurses need to work toward a system of ongoing collection of nursing's essential data. The benefits for nursing, if the NMDS were adopted nationwide with ongoing data collection, are as follows:

1. Access to comparable, minimum nursing care and resources data on local, regional, and national levels

2. Enhanced documentation of nursing care provided

3. Identification of trends related to client problems and nursing care provided

4. Impetus to improved costing of nursing services

5. Improved data for quality assurance evaluations

6. Impetus to development and refinement of nursing information systems

7. Comparative research on nursing care, including research on nursing diagnosis, nursing interventions, resolution status of client problems, and referral for further nursing services

8. Contributions toward advancing nursing as a research-based discipline.

The implications of the NMDS for clinical practice, nursing administration, research, and education follow.

For Clinical Practice and Nurse Clinicians

1. Stress complete, accurate documentation of nursing care according to the nursing process model.

2. Facilitate continuity of care of clients with transfer among health care settings through proper and accurate documentation of care provided.

For Nursing Administration and Nurse Administrators

1. Emphasize the need to measure nursing care and resources consumed.

2. Develop computerized nursing information systems (NIS).

3. Highlight the need to abstract core minimum nursing data across the four types of care delivery settings.

4. Recognize the trends about nursing practice and research needs that these core data can reflect.

For Nursing Research and Nurse Researchers

1. Promote descriptive research on nursing care of clients in various settings.

2. Stimulate efforts to compare nursing interventions for specific nursing diagnoses across settings—locally, regionally, and nationally.

3. Investigate the status of nursing diagnoses resolution and referrals for further nursing care.

4. Assess the patterns of outcomes for various nursing diagnoses.

5. Investigate the patterns of nursing care and costs in various types of care delivery settings.

6. Develop new nursing resources allocation methods.

7. Describe the differential staffing patterns of nursing personnel across types of care delivery settings.

For Nursing Education and Nurse Educators

1. Facilitate development of sensitivity in students to the necessity of careful documentation, reflecting use of the nursing process model.

2. Ensure the integration of information management in the undergraduate and graduate curricula for decision making in all areas of nursing.

3. Incorporate implications of the NMDS concept and elements as a link in integrating computers in nursing care in the undergraduate and graduate curricula.

4. Support continuing education for nurses on implementing the NMDS as an abstraction tool, thus requiring careful documentation of care provided and resources used.

Future Directions for the NMDS

These are essential aspects of this project to continue:

1. Develop guidelines and manuals for use in further studies of the NMDS.

2. Conduct a regional field study of the NMDS with a larger sample of health care settings of different types.

3. Conduct a national field study of the NMDS.

4. Plan for local, regional, and national sessions on nursing documentation per the nursing process and the NMDS definitions, to promote comparable data.

5. Encourage computerization nationally of NISs, to facilitate data audit trails from the NMDS to the more detailed raw data in NISs, HCISs, or health records, for research purposes.

6. Stimulate interest in and facilitate accomplishment of Resolution 24 on computerization of nursing services data, which was passed by the American Nurses' Association House of Delegates at the 1986 Convention.

Acknowledgment. Grateful acknowledgment is expressed to the Blanke Foundation for partial support in writing this chapter.

Questions

1. Describe the Nursing Minimum Data Set and its relationship to the Uniform Minimum Health Data Sets.

2. Identify the Nursing Minimum Data Set elements and their derivation.

3. What are some benefits of the Nursing Minimum Data Set to the profession of nursing?

4. State the implications of the Nursing Minimum Data Set for clinical practice, nursing administration, research, and education.

References Cited

Barger SE: Nursing centers: here today, gone tomorrow. In: McCloskey JC, Grace HK, eds. *Current Issues in Nursing*. 2d ed. Boston: Blackwell, 1985; 752–760.

Devine EC, Werley HH: Test of the nursing minimum data set: availability of data and reliability. *Research in Nursing and Health* 1988.

Health Information Policy Council: *Background Paper: Uniform Minimum Health Data Sets*. Washington, DC: U.S. Department of Health and Human Services, 1983.

Health Information Policy Council: *1984 Revision of the Uniform Hospital Discharge Data Set*. Washington, DC: U.S. Department of Health and Human Services, 1984.

Health Information Policy Council: 1984 revision of the uniform hospital discharge data set. *Federal Register* 1985; 50:31038–31040.

Murnaghan JH, White KL, eds: Hospital discharge data: report of the conference on hospital discharge abstract systems. *Medical Care* 1970; 8(4, Suppl).

National Committee on Vital and Health Statistics: *Long-term Healthcare: Minimum Data Set*. Hyattsville, MD: U.S. Department of Health and Human Services, National Center for Health Statistics (DHHS Publication No. PHS 80-1158), 1980a.

National Committee on Vital and Health Statistics. *Uniform Hospital Discharge Data: Minimum Data Set*. Hyattsville, MD: U.S. Department of Health, Education, and Welfare, National Center for Health Statistics (DHEW Publication No. PHS 80-1157), 1980b.

National Committee on Vital and Health Statistics: *Uniform Ambulatory Medical Care: Minimum Data Set*. Hyattsville, MD: U.S. Department of Health and Human Services, National Center for Health Statistics (DHHS Publication No. 81-1161), 1981.

Rich BM, Baum R: *The Aging: A Guide to Public Policy*. Pittsburgh: University of Pittsburgh Press, 1984.

Werley HH, Lang NM, eds: *Identification of the Nursing Minimum Data Set*. New York: Springer, 1988.

Werley HH, Lang NM, Westlake SK: Brief summary of the nursing minimum data set conference. *Nursing Management* 1986a; 17:42–45.

Werley HH, Lang NM, Westlake SK: The nursing minimum data set conference: executive summary. *Journal of Professional Nursing* 1986b; 2:117–224.

6—A Unified Nursing Language System

Kathleen A. McCormick

This chapter describes the concept of a unified language system in nursing as a part of a unified language system for the health care community. A unified language system is a standardized nosology and terminology for nursing with a defined structure and syntax. A unified nursing language system is needed as content in computer-based nursing information systems throughout the world. The focus of this chapter is to

- describe the concept

- describe previous work that may be appropriate for a unified nursing language system

- recommend further research and development required to move the nursing profession toward a unified language system.

The Concept

The Need for a Unified Language System

At this stage in computerization, efforts to implement computers in clinical settings—including the hospital, community, nursing home, and home—should be under way. A major impediment to more widespread use of computers in nursing has been the absence of a standard vocabulary for describing health care phenomena pertaining to patient care, nursing research, nursing education, and nursing administration. Vocabulary diversity within these areas has evolved from direct observations of signs and symptoms in clinical practice to basic science concepts in research and on to managerial, accounting, and business terminology in nursing administration. Nurses implementing documentation requirements on the computer are besieged by content-related problems (see *Essentials of Computers for Nurses*, the section on the implementation process of nursing information systems) (Saba and McCormick, 1986).

An Integral Part of a Minimum Data Set

A minimum data set is defined by the U.S. Department of Health and Human Services Health Information Policy Council as a minimum set of items or elements of information with uniform definitions and categories, concerning a specific aspect or dimension of the health care system, that meets the essential needs of multiple data users (Health Information Policy Council, 1983, p. 3). It is the answer to the question of how much information is needed to describe a component of the health care system. An integral part of the definition is the need for items with uniform definitions and categories. Some experts argue that the minimum data set will serve the profession to describe nursing practice in retrospect (Werley et al, 1986).

If the long-term goal of a minimum data set is computerization, then an essential integral part of that development is the need for a unified nursing language system. Guidelines have been presented for computerizing a minimum data set to make it useful for research (McCormick, 1988). One integral requirement is that the uniform language can be defined by the nursing profession. In addition, the concept of unified language system is the basis of content on nursing information systems and could be used for concurrent clinical decision making. The unified nursing language system would provide the framework, the taxonomy, and the indexing system that fits within a nursing information system and assumes the capability for minimum data extrapolation.

A Collaborative Language System

It is imperative that nursing perceives a unified language system as part of the health care language system developments. Previous research has described three-quarters of the nursing information system within a hospital information system as generated directly from doctors' orders (McCormick, 1983). The language of the doctors' orders usually follows medical diagnosis and the ICD-9-CM code, and is further taxonomized and indexed by the Medical Subject Heading (MeSH) vocabulary for publications related to the health care field.

A common language needs to be derived from a common conceptual framework. The MeSH vocabulary is one framework that seems to offer a great potential for a unified language system (National Library of Medicine, 1986). In an effort to develop a unified medical language system, the National Library of Medicine has proposed that the MeSH vocabulary system, which has been used to classify health care publications, be investigated as a language system. This system not only has special linguistic features in medical terminology that are used internationally, but it also has been effectively computerized. No substantive research in nursing has demonstrated that nursing terminology is compatible with the MeSH framework.

The MeSH System

MeSH is an indexing system used worldwide in the National Library of Medicine (NLM) MEDLARS for providing access to bibliographic citations of health care literature, including nursing journals. It is used by professionals in schools of nursing, hospitals, clinics, and the community. However, in order to be used as a standardized unified language system, MeSH would have to be expanded to better represent terminology used in clinical care and specialty areas of nursing. Nursing would also have to develop an indexing structure or framework within which nursing diagnosis could be classified.

Nursing Diagnosis Taxonomy

A recent attempt to taxonomize and classify the nursing diagnosis content established a structure that includes nine patterns of human responses. Developed by the North American Nursing Diagnosis Association (NANDA), and labeled Taxonomy I, it presents patterns following the Roy model:

1. exchanging
2. communicating
3. relating
4. valuing
5. choosing
6. moving
7. perceiving
8. knowing
9. feeling.

A recent critical analysis of Taxonomy I as recommended by NANDA determined that the taxonomy does not meet the necessary indexing capabilities of a taxonomy and is not capable of being integrated with the vocabulary used in other health care-related systems, including reimbursement systems (Porter, 1986).

The Integration of Computer Technology to Establish a Unified Language System

For a computer system to be integrated, the vocabulary used in the clinical setting must be linked to that used for clinical, research, academic, and administrative usages. It must also be linked to reimbursement systems. A major obstacle for the profession may be in valuing the integrated use of nursing information. However, the health care industry reimbursement mechanisms do seem to be driving much of the information systems that have developed around a nomenclature that accrues answers such as: Whom does the profession treat (census data), what were patients' common problems (diagnostic data), and how much do patients owe for services (cost data).

Computer technology provides methodologies for research into language that can be used in all areas of health care delivery. For example, retrieval systems can be used to search and analyze full texts of documents and files. This creates the opportunity to define the vocabularies used in clinical practice, to examine the role of syntax and context in determining the meaning of terms used, and to discover methods of language unification or linkage.

The use of computers in many hospitals and clinics throughout the world provides sufficient data bases to assemble large collections of computer-stored patient care records and nursing notes. Because much of the data in these computerized records exists in the form of machine-readable text, this creates the opportunity to consider the relationship of the clinical vocabularies to be correlated with other systems, e.g., the MeSH vocabulary.

The Essential Elements of a Unified Nursing Language System

A unified nursing language system needs to include five important elements (Table 6-1). For the system to be optimally effective, all five should be present, from the data bases replacing traditional thesauri to automated tools and programming capabilities.

The Criteria for Selection of Content in a Unified Nursing Language System

The criteria for selecting content in a unified nursing language system are listed in Table 6-2. They involve a high level of expertise in justifying and subsequently validating the inclusion with both users and advisors, as well as skill in arriving at precise definitions.

Table 6-1
The Essential Elements of a Unified Nursing Language System

1. Dictionaries and thesauri
2. Cross indexes
3. Automated tools for indexing and classification
4. Computer programs to process records and evaluate their conformance with standards
5. Programs to update and maintain files

Table 6-2
Criteria for Selecting Content in a Unified Nursing Language System

1. Frequency of usage of a term in nursing
2. A recognized need
3. Approval of an advisory panel
4. Ability to precisely and clearly define the term

Advantages of a Unified Nursing Language System

A major advantage of a unified language system would be the integration of patient data with scientific data, thereby increasing the ability of the nurse in practice to use literature and to rely on literature in decision making. A unified language system would also improve the efficiency of searching the literature. Another advantage of the unified language system is to facilitate the application of computer methods in nursing, and link different kinds of information sources. For example, a unified language system can facilitate the linking of practice data with cost data or of clinical with educational case simulation studies.

Previous Efforts toward a Unified Nursing Language System

Integrated Systems

Research has described the four headings within which nursing can be defined (McCormick, 1982):

- science

- remedial and therapeutic healing arts

- focus/direction

- professional conditions and controls.

Within these categories, the subheadings that represent nursing can be further evaluated (Table 6-3). These headings and subheadings can be correlated with the MeSH vocabulary system, nursing diagnoses, and the frequency of usage of terms in the many computerized nursing information systems throughout the United States, Canada, the United Kingdom, Sweden, Japan, and other countries with sophisticated nursing information systems. In this system, the commonalities of nursing with other health-related language systems would be the science and focus/direction headings and subheadings.

The expansion of systems like MeSH to accommodate nursing information would have to occur in the areas of remedial and therapeutic healing arts and professional condition and controls. Currently, the MeSH vocabulary includes subheadings related to nursing ethics,

Table 6-3
Headings and Subheadings of Nursing

I. Science
    1. Anatomy
    2. Physiology
    3. Pathology
    4. Biochemistry
    5. Information science
    6. Research methods
II. Remedial and therapeutic healing arts
    1. Rehabilitation
    2. Cure
    3. Maintenance
    4. Prevention
III. Focus and direction
    1. Cell
    2. Individual
    3. Society
IV. Professional condition/control
    1. Nursing laws
    2. Nursing ethics
    3. Nursing politics

nursing laws, and the nursing profession. However, presently it does not include the remedial and therapeutic healing arts components of either medical or nursing care. The science and remedial and therapeutic healing arts components of care comprise clinical judgment, which has been neglected in any current indexing systems. This system of headings and subheadings has not been correlated with nursing diagnosis, has not been evaluated in clinical practice, and has not been correlated with the MeSH vocabulary system.

Nursing Intensity Index

Another system that has been described and correlated with reimbursement systems is the Nursing Intensity Index (Reitz, 1985). The headings and subheadings of this system are listed in Table 6-4. This system does not have extensive subheadings categorization, has not been correlated with nursing diagnosis, and would need expansion. However, it is an example of heading and subheading indexes that could be correlated with the MeSH vocabulary system and fit within a unified health language system. The categories of this index system are a combination of the science and remedial and therapeutic healing arts, which were previously described.

Although this system has been used to evaluate reimbursement strategies, it has not been tested in community health settings, the home, or in nursing homes. This intensity index does not include the

Table 6-4
Reitz Nursing Intensity Index[a]

I. Functional health parameters: biophysical health
1. Nutrition
2. Elimination
3. Sensory function
4. Protection
5. Neurologic function
6. Circulatory function
7. Respiratory function
II. Functional health parameters: behavioral health
1. Emotional response
2. Social system
3. Cognitive response
4. Health management pattern

[a] From Reitz J: *Nursing Management* 1985; 16:21–30.

Table 6-5
Gordon's Functional Health Pattern Areas[a]

1. Health perception/health management
2. Nutritional/metabolic
3. Elimination
4. Activity/exercise
5. Sleep/rest
6. Cognitive/perceptual
7. Self-perception/self-concept
8. Role relationship
9. Sexuality/reproductive
10. Coping/stress/tolerance
11. Value/belief

[a] From Gordon M: *Nursing Diagnosis: Process and Application.* New York: McGraw-Hill, 1982.

element of nursing's professional practice, i.e., the ethics and laws that govern nursing practice.

Functional Health Patterns

The system that has been perhaps most carefully correlated with nursing diagnoses is the system that identifies 11 functional health pattern areas (Gordon, 1982) (Table 6-5). While these patterns have not been thoroughly defined and evaluated, it would appear that they could be studied and with some modifications correlated with the MeSH vocabulary. From the description of the previous two systems, it appears that the functional health patterns described by Gordon are compatible with the Science and Remedial and Therapeutic Healing Arts components of McCormick's categories. The similarity of concept within the Gordon and Reitz categories implies that the Gordon Functional Health Patterns could also be evaluated for reimbursement potential. Again, the Gordon categories exclude the concept of Focus and Direction, as well as Professional Conditions and Controls. These categories need to be considered in the unified nursing language system, because all health care policies must reflect the professional standards, ethics, and laws of practice.

Research and Development Needs

Coordination and Collaboration

Achieving a unified nursing language system will require a substantial coordinated national effort of many organizations representing nursing. The coordination task will need a highly committed professional organization and specialty organizations representing nurses in hospital-based practice, community health, nursing home care, and home care. Essentially every environment where nurses work must be represented on national panels and commissions so that standard terminologies and nomenclatures can be developed, with related development of electronic dictionaries and thesauri linked through computer-based indexing technologies. The companies that have been involved in indexing nursing journals and collaborated with the National Library of Medicine also need to be included in the development of a unified nursing language system. The major health care organizations and foundations that support research and development need to be involved in addressing the research and development issues of such a system.

Research will need support from federal and private foundations related to language attributes, terminology, representation, and refinement of computational tools for testing and implementing the products developed. Informatics societies with international memberships need to participate in program design, implementation, and dissemination of information. The informatics community needs to establish standards and develop specialized software tools for knowledge and data exchange over large national communication networks.

Establish Data Base Networks

A mechanism to develop a unified language includes the establishment of a large national data base network. Already in existence for the medical community is an electronic system called ARPANET. If a unified language system could be developed on such a system, then expansion of a system might grow from nurses in academic and research environments to the hospital and communication-based machines. Finally, nodes could be established within localities so that local needs could be specifically met.

Research and Development Advantages

Such development and dissemination will require education of health care professionals and specifically the nursing profession. The advantages of a unified system need to be evaluated and demonstrated in problem solving, in quality care provision, and in cost savings in health care delivery. Currently, the lack of unified language in nursing information systems and the sheer volume of data collected on patients in the health care setting make the data available elusive and often irretrievable. The potential for research is lost because the validity and reliability of the data are lost. The end product has been previously described as a "data cemetery" (McCormick, 1981). The potential exists to describe the science of nursing, the efficacy of nursing actions, and the organization and delivery of care.

Need for Evaluation

The correlation of information obtained from large nursing information systems needs to be searched for syntax and terminology in the MeSH vocabulary system. For example, if the clinical data base is in machine-readable form, then the use of terms and vocabulary used in clinical practice can be linked to MeSH terms. If the MeSH terms are not adequate for the nursing profession, then either the MeSH terms have to expand to represent nursing phenomena, or nursing phenomena need to be more precisely defined, or another taxonomy that reflects nursing needs to be developed.

Summary

A concept of a uniform nursing language system, as well as the implications of this concept for future research and development needs of the profession, has been described. Without a unified language system that is integrated into other health care standard initiatives, the nursing profession will not be able to use the standard language developed in collaborative health care initiatives. Nor will the unified language be capable of being integrated with other developments in clinical practice, reimbursement formulae, or case simulation models without a collaborative health care initiative.

The nursing profession has done much in identifying nursing diagnosis as a conceptual framework, the need for a nursing minimum data set, and now needs to go beyond that framework in developing an index and definitions of terms. The National Library of Medicine's

MeSH vocabulary system is a proposed index format because it has had extensive terminology evaluation and has been computerized. Basic criteria and guidelines are presented to guide the development of a unified nursing language system.

Questions

1. Define a unified language system.

2. Describe one reason why a unified language system is needed in nursing.

3. Name an international taxonomy from the National Library of Medicine that could be evaluated for a unified language system.

4. What is an important usage of a unified language system?

5. List the five important elements of a unified nursing language system.

6. Describe the criteria for selecting content for a unified nursing language system.

7. Discuss one previous effort of nursing taxonomy that could be evaluated for a unified nursing language system.

8. What is the advantage of perceiving a unified language system of nursing within a larger concept of a unified language system for the health care community?

9. What further research and developments are needed to move the nursing profession toward a unified language system?

10. What is the major advantage of having a unified language system for computerization?

References Cited

Gordon M: *Nursing Diagnosis: Process and Application.* New York: McGraw-Hill, 1982.

Health Information Policy Council: *Background Paper: Uniform Minimum Health Data Sets.* Washington, DC: Department of Health and Human Services, 1983; 3.

McCormick K: Nursing research using computerized data bases. In: Heffernan HG, ed. *Proceedings of the Fifth Annual Symposium on Computer Applications in Medical Care.* New York: IEEE Computer Society, 1981; 738–743.

McCormick K: Preparing nurses for the technologic future. *Nursing and Health Care* 1982; 4:379–382.

McCormick K: Computerizing theoretical frameworks. In: *Proceedings of the First National Computer Conference in Nursing*, Vol. 83. Bethesda: National Institutes of Health, 1983; 51–57.

McCormick K: Conceptual considerations, decision criteria, and guidelines appropriate to the development of a nursing minimum data set: from a research perspective. In: Werley H, Lang N, eds. *Identification of the Nursing Minimum Data Set*. New York: Springer, 1988.

National Library of Medicine: *Report of Panels 1–5*. Bethesda: National Institutes of Health, 1986 (unpublished).

Porter E: Critical analysis of NANDA nursing diagnosis taxonomy, I. *Image Journal of Nursing Scholarship* 1986; 18:136–139.

Reitz J: Toward a comprehensive nursing intensity index: part I, development. *Nursing Management* 1985; 16:21–30.

Saba V, McCormick K: *Essentials of Computers for Nurses*. Philadelphia: Lippincott, 1986.

Werley H, Lang N, Westlake S: Brief summary of the nursing minimum data set conference. *Nursing Management* 1986; 17:42–45.

Section 2—Where Caring and Technology Meet

Unit 2—Administrative Systems

Unit Introduction

This section on Administrative Systems focuses on the **A** of our **CARE** concept. In the first chapter, Peterson and Gerdin Jelger explain the information needs to be met in a functional hospital information system. Next M. Peterson and Hannah focus on specific nursing information management systems needs. Ball then looks at the general responsibilities of nursing in selecting a computerized hospital information system. Mills reinforces the nursing role in the selection process and gives an overview of a nursing request for proposal (included in detail in Appendix A). In the next chapter, Jenkins explains the role nursing must take in implementing an information system. Lafferty and Sheffield emphasize the design aspects of health care information systems with a helpful questionnaire on how to do a site visit as part of the selection process. The unit concludes with a literature review by Kjerulff, who looks at the impact of computerization on various aspects of nursing.

1—Hospital Information Systems

Hans Peterson and Ulla Gerdin Jelger

Information Needs in Health Care

Trends in Patient Care and Information Access

All treatment of patients is founded on access to information about the patient and the patient's problems. Thus, the most important resource in all health care work is this access. The physician and the nurse have always collected information about the patient by questioning, by observing, and by conducting different kinds of clinical investigation. The information collected in this way is the foundation for the diagnostic, therapeutic, and nursing process.

Formerly, the physician and the nurse collected all information. They also performed all necessary clinical investigation and examination themselves. The documentation was very brief, and the handling of the information was simple. Because all information derived from contact with the patient, there was no problem with the documentation or with the communication.

In modern health care, the situation is completely different and much more complex. The amount of information collected is more extensive and the documentation is much more voluminous. Although the amount of information collected by physical examination of the patient has not grown substantially, the number of members of the treatment team has grown markedly, and all have responsibility for collecting information and documentation. Different diagnostic tests and procedures have drastically increased the amount of information gathered about each patient, which is compounded by the fact that the patient is transported to numerous laboratories and facilities within the hospital for testing, and the resulting data must be transferred to a staff member in another location before it can be used in the patient care decision-making process. Thus, the problem arising for the health care field is how best to handle the increasing amount of information.

This increasing volume of data can be demonstrated in another way.

Measured in the amount of paper put on a shelf, the patient information collected during 1 year within one health care organization such as Stockholm County, responsible for 1.5 million inhabitants, is 2.4 shelf-kilometers, or nearly 1.5 shelf-miles. Shelf-kilometers can be used to estimate the space needed for hospital archives. A governmental committee in Sweden determined that every year Swedish hospitals produce 14 shelf-kilometers, or almost 9 miles, of new patient records.

Health Care Organization

The organization of health care has changed over the years, and the demand for information and documentation has changed accordingly. Today, there are new medical specialties and more categories of staff. No longer can the physician's documentation remain separate from the nurse's. Modern health care requires that work be done in treatment teams. New procedures and increasing specialization have reconfigured and reassigned the tasks performed by that treatment team. Today the nurse is often responsible for what was once done only by physicians. All the members of the team must have equal access to the patient's record, in whole and in part, and that record must accompany the patient throughout the hospital and the health care delivery system. Recently, it has become common practice to request a copy of previous records when the patient is treated in a hospital. This further increases the size of the patient record in an almost uncontrolled way.

Communication Systems

Other problems arise. A patient's record may be needed at several places at the same time in the hospital. Often there are difficulties in finding the record when it is needed. Elsewhere in this book, the issue of minimum data sets as well as the issue of unified medical language, extremely important issues that the informatics community will be addressing in the years to come, are discussed (see Werley et al [Chapter 5, Unit 1, Section 2] and McCormick [Chapter 6, Unit 1, Section 2]). One of the goals for developing hospital information systems is to guarantee access to the patient record when and where it is needed, using a recognized, unified language common to the health care community.

An essential aspect of communication within the hospital is the transmission of information from the laboratories to the wards and outpatient departments, as well as among the different members of the treatment team. This can be both slow and subject to error. Studies of manual paper information systems show that up to 15% of the results reported from the pathology laboratory do not agree with the laboratory's measurements. This could include anything from a transcription error of one single digit or a single decimal place to the entry of a result on the wrong line or even in the wrong patient's medical record. Time used for this manual information transfer at the ward unit varies between 1 and 1.5 hours per day.

Development of Hospital Information Systems (HIS)

The term hospital information systems (HIS) is commonly used to refer to different types of computer systems used in the health care field. HIS build upon the ability of computers to handle large amounts of information, to manipulate and store the information, and to make it available as needed, and the primary goal of current HIS is to supply patient care areas with this information. Another goal is to supply administrators and planners with needed information. Clearly, an efficient HIS is not developed and introduced in a short time. Rather, it involves a lengthy process by which the different parts, one by one, grow from observed needs and requirements.

Early HIS

Early hospital information systems used a central computer with terminals in a star network. Those computers were large, expensive, and difficult to program. Systems were rarely customized or modified to fit the environment, regardless of where they were used. Flexibility was impossible to build in because of technical and economic constraints. Moreover, these inflexible systems were designed to collect financial data for operational activities only, not for planning and statistical analysis.

Modular Development

In the late 1970s, the large inflexible HIS gave way to a new concept, which addressed the needs of individual institutions by allowing for the development of modules in specific areas. Hospitals could adapt available modules or develop modules tailor-made for specific units and thus attempted to develop modules to support operational functions. Information needed by administration for staff and financial planning functions was also available in the operational systems. The advantage of this concept and the resulting strategies was that information generated in the day-to-day work was significantly more accurate and could be collected and condensed to serve other levels and meet common needs.

Today, HIS are built in a modular fashion. The usual HIS is made up of a large number of modules assembled to fit specific requirements. These modules very somewhat from country to country in accordance with each country's health care delivery organization. Countries that offer nationalized health care may utilize a special type of HIS; such a health care information system may provide basic HIS functions that can be used by a group of hospitals or by all health care activities in a specific geographic area. Modules in these special systems provide for preventive medicine and early detection of diseases, and operate with the health care information system's file that contains all residents of the area.

Features of Modern HIS

Hospital information systems are developed to respond to the problems arising from the organization of modern health care, notably those in the areas of information and communication. Features of modern HIS that address these problems include:

- Structure and content of the documents to be processed by the system
- Flexible adaptation to the needs of different categories of staff
- Transfer of information between internal and external units, laboratories, and ward units.

A modern HIS must satisfy the need for information and follow-up in the areas of

- Operations
- Finances
- Treatment.

Modules

A modern HIS includes several modules or components. Although technical solutions may differ, those modules currently include the following:

- Patient record
- Admissions/discharge/transfer
- Order entry/results reporting
- Drug profile
- Care planning
- Personnel/staff planning
- Financial.

Patient Record

Patient record-handling systems consist of rules and functions for input of text, results and diagnoses, and manipulation, retrieval, output, and storage of information. These systems assume great significance as the largest module in any HIS. The patient record, i.e., patient-centered information, constitutes about 80% of the information handled in a hospital, requiring between 20 and 30% of a hospital's running costs. These percentages make it easy to understand why the rationale for developing patient record-handling modules was so strong.

Patient record-handling modules were among the first to be targeted for development, yet they have taken the longest time to develop. Every unit argues that it is unique and needs its own module for handling patient records. Although for economic reasons it is impossible to develop a separate module for every unit, functionality dictates not all units can use the same one. The solution of this seemingly insoluble problem lies in the development of main functions, those functions in a patient record-handling system that are alike and must be alike within one institution or within one organization with several hospitals. The critical elements are

- Access control functions
- Input and presentation functions
- Document-handling functions
- Information-handling functions
- Electronic mail functions
- Help functions
- Communications functions
- Functions for follow-up of the activities.

If these functions can be developed so that they accommodate all the individual units, 80% of the total development costs for the system are covered. If the system is developed using fourth-generation languages, the remaining 20% of development can be done at the unit using the system. About half of this 20% can be developed by staff working at the unit; the other half must be done by computer specialists.

Admissions/Discharge/Transfer (ADT)

The patient admissions component stores basic facts about patients. This information is used during the treatment period to locate the patient in the health care delivery system for the necessary financial transactions and required statistics. The admissions system is different for outpatient and inpatient care. Modules appropriate to each type of care should be provided.

Outpatient Care Modules

Scheduling of appointments with physicians and nurses
Registration of the visit
Financial functions
Statistics
Data transfer to the hospital financial system.

Inpatient Care Modules

Waiting list
Preadmission data
Admission and discharge
Diagnosis
Hospital statistics
Data transfer to the hospital financial system.

Order Entry/Results Reporting

It is important to keep track of examinations and diagnostic procedures performed on a specific patient and hospital resources used by the patient during treatment. Systems to order drugs, food, and laboratory or surgical supplies are, therefore, part of an HIS.

In actuality, there are two subsets to the order system. First is the order entry system, which includes all orders for a patient and links that system to the hospital financial routines. Second is the referral reply system, the order for a procedure or an examination, usually connected with an appointment scheduling module. This system also checks that all referrals are handled and the results signed and included in the patient record.

Drug Profile

Drug information systems are relevant to both inpatient and outpatient care. These systems may include modules for retrieving information about drugs as well as for indicating what drugs a patient is using at a given moment. They may also provide formulations for specific prescriptions, allow data manipulation, and link to the hospital financial system.

Care Planning

Systems for giving every patient an individual care plan and following it up also contain functions that assist in selecting the appropriate care plan, evaluating follow-up, and manipulating data for further analysis and study.

Personnel/Staff Planning

Another component includes systems for personnel and staff scheduling. These systems handle individual unit requirements in assigning staff; they also provide follow-up reports, assist in daily planning for staff allocation, and link to the hospital financial routines.

Financial

As each individual local unit becomes more and more responsible for its own budget, it needs routines for planning financial transactions and for evaluating their effectiveness. Linkages with the main financial system eliminate the need to duplicate data input and to refer to separate systems.

Implementation of HIS

A number of conditions must be fulfilled if an HIS is to function satisfactorily. Experience has shown these aspects should be addressed if not resolved before developing a new system:

Access Control System. If the question of who is allowed to access what part of the patient information is not adequately resolved, a computer support system for health care activities should not be developed.

Patient Identification System. By using different types of numbering systems in which the numbers are connected to the patient's date of birth, name, race, religion, place of birth, etc., a very secure patient identification system can be developed, and the number of the patient or patient record can be retrieved with the help of the data base. Certain countries have national numbering systems that also can be used, depending on their legislation.

Patient Admission, Discharge, and Transfer System. These routines should be accepted by all units within the organization or institution.

Data Communications Standards. Because different system modules are developed using different computers, often from different manufacturers, standards for data communications become increasingly important. For health care to achieve integration of information, standards are essential.

Other processes and decisions are critical to the success of any HIS. Because computerization requires information be handled differently than in a manual system, responsibilities for information handling must be delineated and distributed. All involved must realize the nature of their new individual responsibility, and the new responsibility must be accepted. It may be difficult to do this before the system is developed, but it is almost impossible when the system is ready to be implemented. Time and effort required for education and training of staff are always underestimated. Without solid programs for staff, even excellent systems will fail when implemented.

Last, but perhaps most important, is planning for the implementation process, with an eye to organizational involvement. Those directly responsible for the implementation must know who is doing what tasks. Review of the process as it occurs is as essential to an effective implementation as the subsequent evaluation in allowing for the inevitable modifications and adjustments. If this phase of the work is neglected or mismanaged, the new HIS not only will not produce the desired benefits, but also will increase costs.

Future HIS

The prototype of the future HIS is already in existence. It consists of a system for each unit, department, or laboratory connected to common systems, such as word processing, appointment scheduling, and storage, all connected in a local area network. The local area network also has access to a host of central functions, including administration, finance and budget, and stock control as well as to external data base systems. Local area networks allow communication between individual units as well as with central systems. External access also can extend to smaller units outside the hospital. Every unit's system is constructed from a number of modules. Departments often can use identical modules, but sometimes a unit needs a specially customized module.

Other technical developments are addressing long-standing problems and needs. Although large amounts of information are too expensive to store on magnetic disks, new laser optic disks provide inexpensive storage. Laser technology also has the potential to store the patient's record on a machine-readable "smart card" that resembles plastic credit cards. Communications technology is solving compatibility problems, linking multiple equipment and systems.

Governments are recognizing the potential of computing, as the development of policies, laws, and regulations in many countries demonstrates. In Sweden, for example, as of January 1, 1986, the patient records act requires that all categories of staff participating in the treatment of the patient are responsible for documenting the activities in one and the same patient record. The act also requires that all members of the treatment team and the patient have access to the patient record. Storage of the record on computers is allowed in place of storage on paper or microfilm.

To date, the success of hospital information systems has been limited. Although many are in place, no one system has had general acceptance. Their future is promising, however. The technology is available to develop functional local systems; costs have decreased to a realistic level; new tools speed up development work and allow users to do the maintenance themselves. Computing and health care are inseparable. Hospital information systems are well established, yet their potential is not fully revealed.

Questions

1. Give five ways in which a computerized hospital information system differs from a manual hospital information system.

2. How has hospital management changed over the past years to warrant a difference in information management?

3. List the hospital information system features you feel are the most important to improve your present current institution.

4. What are some major issues involved in handling the patient record most effectively in the hospital? Where do the major problems lie?

5. Give a brief description of how the implementation issues must be addressed when satisfactorily installing a hospital information system. Cite specific examples if possible.

6. Can you add one new concept to the hospital information system of the future? Try to be futuristic and creative in your response!

2—Nursing Management Information Systems

Mary Peterson and Kathryn J. Hannah

Introduction

In health care organizations, as in other fields, the first computer-based management information systems implemented were typically limited to financial applications. Quantitative financial data are easily automated, and the benefits are readily observable and measurable. However, the role of management information systems in today's nursing departments continues to expand as nursing managers recognize the value of information as an essential resource. The increasing complexity of patient care problems, combined with the pressures for efficiency and effectiveness in patient care, have prompted nursing managers to require quick access to useful, reliable information.

With these kinds of demands, manual data processing has become increasingly ineffective in supporting management decision making. The advantages of automation extend far beyond the ability of a computer to crunch numbers. While it is true that more data can be processed at a greater speed, automated management information systems provide for enhanced accuracy, increased detail, and flexibility in reporting, as well as standardization of the information reported.

In this chapter we examine how computers can assist nursing managers in decision making. We propose a definition of management information systems (MIS), and discuss the potential role of MIS in nursing administration. Following a review of MIS applications currently available to the nursing manager, we present some considerations to ensure the information obtained from the applications is useful and relevant.

Management Information Systems: A Definition

The concept of management information systems is not unique to nursing. While it has been developed largely in the business and industrial sectors by management scientists, the notion of MIS is relevant to any discipline. This is perhaps best evidenced in the description, which begins by defining each of the words in the term management information system:

Management: The process of directing and controlling resources, and their application toward the achievement of specific objectives.

Information: The result of transforming data into elements of knowledge that are directly useful and applicable.

System: An array of components designed to accomplish a particular objective according to a plan.

MIS: An array of components designed to transform a collective set of data into knowledge that is directly useful and applicable in the process of directing and controlling resources and their application to the achievement of specific management objectives (Hanson, 1982).

To put this more simply, a management information system is a system that provides information to assist the manager in the decision-making process. The level of involvement in the decision-making process varies. In many instances, the role of MIS is limited to the processing, storage, and retrieval of information. Other systems allow the user to estimate the outcomes of alternative decisions through modeling. Finally, one group of applications assists the nursing manager in communicating a decision once it has been reached. Applications that fall in the latter category are referred to as office automation systems.

While the definition presented here could apply to both manual and automated systems, the following review will be limited to automated management information systems.

MIS Applications

Increasingly, the nurse administrator's role is being facilitated by the use of management information systems to assist in the management of nursing resources. In the past, the nursing manager's involvement with MIS was limited to receiving various budget reports produced by the accounting department's financial system. Until recently, very little information appeared in the literature regarding MIS applications for nursing managers with the exception of articles relating to the area of nurse scheduling. With advances in computer software, nursing management applications have been expanded to the extent that they are now beginning to support decision making and strategic planning. Computers currently play a critical role in fiscal resource management, workload measurement, personnel management, staff scheduling, quality assurance, and office automation.

Fiscal Resource Management

Computers are well suited to store and manipulate the range of data required for budgetary purposes. In most hospitals, staffing the nursing division represents a major portion of the hospital's operating costs, accounting for 40% or more of the entire hospital budget. Management information systems play a key role in providing accurate, relevant information for use in administrative decision making related to the largest component of the hospital budget. Through the use of hierarchical reporting, information can be extracted and summarized for use at all organizational levels from the individual nursing unit level through the department and board levels to external agencies. Because budgets typically involve many figures, the principle of exception reporting is routinely applied in management reports. That is, the computer will flag information that falls outside (above or below) a specified range. This feature avoids overwhelming the manager with the volume of the reports and focuses attention on potential problems.

The major advantages provided by fiscal resource applications relate to the speed with which the computer is able to organize, summarize, and retrieve stored data. The information generated can be used to monitor past performance, as in the case of variance analyses, or to predict future performance. Accumulated data can be analyzed for the development of trends that can then be extrapolated to project future expenditures. Necessary reallocations and budgetary adjustments can then be made on the basis of these projections.

Workload Measurement and Staffing Requirements

Because nursing salaries do represent a significant portion of the institution or agency budget, much attention has been directed toward systems that aid in the efficient utilization of nursing resources. The challenge for nursing managers is to ensure that nurses are available in just the right mix to meet patients' needs and yet be cost effective.

Traditionally, patient census has been used as an indicator to estimate workload and forecast an appropriate level of nurse staffing. The weaknesses of this measure have become more evident with the increasing complexity of patient care problems. Patient demands for care are highly variable. Consider, for example, the differences in care required by patients presenting to an emergency department. Their concerns range from the aches and pains of a common cold to multiple trauma with multisystems failure. To add to this uncertainty, patient care demands represent only one of many factors that must be considered in defining nurse staffing needs. Other factors are not only difficult to measure; in some instances they cannot even be identified. Those commonly referred to in the literature include

personnel factors
administrative support
environmental factors
physician practices
philosophy of care
organizational mode for delivery of care.

In an attempt to respond to these multivariant circumstances, various workload measurement and staffing methodologies have been developed and aimed at the effective allocation of nursing resources. Workload measurement and the determination of staffing requirements make excellent use of the ability of the computer to rapidly store, manipulate, and retrieve large volumes of data. The information generated assists nursing managers in planning, monitoring, and evaluating use of nursing resources on a daily basis and in the longer time frame. This information is also used in conjunction with personnel management information to generate staff schedules.

Personnel Management

While workload measurement systems attempt to weigh the requirements for patient care, personnel management systems perform a similar function for the staffing side of the formula. We often hear the expression "a nurse is not a nurse is not a nurse." Using a personnel management system data can be accumulated regarding each staff member's employment and educational history. This may include diplomas and degrees obtained, professional registration, inservices and continuing education programs attended, certification status for medically delegated functions, special skills possessed, and career goals and interests.

If maintained, these personal data bases can supply information to fulfill a variety of functions. Managers will have current access to records for performance appraisal purposes; an employee with a special mix of skills can be located. Records are readily accessible if needed for accreditation purposes or to monitor contract compliance. The information may also be retrieved on a daily basis for use in conjunction with workload measurement and contract requirements to plan staffing assignments.

Staff Scheduling

Over the years, nursing managers have invested an incredible amount of time in producing and maintaining rotations. Instead of getting easier with experience, manual scheduling has become increasingly difficult as more variables must be addressed by the nursing manager in planning assignments. Contract requirements are more stringent. Patient care needs dictate a more particular mix of nursing skills. Even the nursing staff themselves are more difficult to plan around as they reserve more time for continuing education as well as personal professional development. These variables have helped to put staff scheduling applications high on the MIS priority list for nursing managers.

As a result, numerous diverse systems have been developed for automated nurse scheduling. The complexity of these systems varies considerably. Cyclical systems simply repeat a given schedule for a given position or nurse. "Intelligent" systems have the capacity to adjust staff schedules in an interactive fashion on a shift-to-shift basis. Because staffing requirements are driven by workload, these systems must be linked with those for workload measurement. The staff scheduler then can create a schedule that incorporates nursing requirements (determined through workload measurement), the various levels of staff expertise (based on data from the personnel system), contractual specifications, and personnel policies.

The benefits of an effective automated scheduling system are also numerous. Nursing managers are able to plan schedules in advance with considerable time savings. Staff are informed well ahead of time, and the computer is generally more able to meet their individual needs for time off. Staffing records, if maintained, provide useful information for monitoring absenteeism, scheduled time off, and turnover. Finally, with the pressure for maximum efficiency, information can be retrieved on a shift-to-shift basis to assist with variable staffing.

Quality Assurance

Over the last two decades quality assurance, the process of establishing and maintaining the quality of care provided, has become a key issue in the delivery of nursing care. Increasingly sophisticated quality assurance programs have been implemented in organizations in response to increased consumer awareness regarding health care, more stringent accreditation guidelines, rising costs in the health care industry, and the pressure for peer review to support the growing professionalism of nursing.

The first step required in a quality assurance program is the establishment of minimum acceptable standards for patient care. These standards must be reviewed periodically to ensure they are consistent with current nursing practice standards. Indicators must then be defined relative to each standard. Observing for the presence or absence of the various indicators in the process of patient care delivery will then determine if the standards have been met—or, better yet, surpassed!

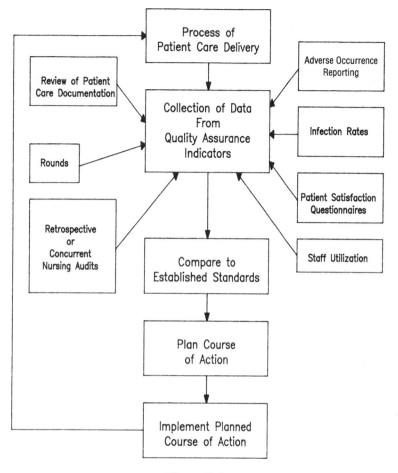

Figure 2-1
Components of a quality assurance program.

Figure 2-1 illustrates the various steps of a quality assurance program. The model includes some of the common sources of data used to evaluate quality of care. When one considers the wealth of data that is involved, the role for computers becomes readily apparent.

While several automated tools to measure quality of care are currently available, users frequently experience difficulty substantiating the validity of the tool within their own organization. Although the standards for care prescribed by the vendor are generally consistent with those established by the organization, there are frequently concerns regarding the appropriateness of the indicators used to evaluate those standards. Cognizant of these concerns, many nursing administrators have carried on with their existing audit practices while taking advantage of the computer to process and summarize the data collected. However, the real opportunities for automated quality assurance applications exist with integrated hospital information systems. Relying on computerized nursing care plans and patient care documentation, organizations with integrated systems have the capability to retrieve online concurrent data for nursing audit purposes, which saves considerable time.

Office Automation

The proliferation of office technologies that began more than 10 years ago in business and industry has finally started to make its way into health care institutions and agencies. While electric typewriters and dictation machines have made work easier in the past, the computer is changing the work environments and habits of all office workers, administrative and clerical. Office automation is the application of computer and communications technology to office activities. It is by no means restricted to administrative offices. The technology is being employed throughout some organizations, in inservice and continuing education, in research offices, even in systems departments. It has the potential to affect almost any aspect of office work, including text processing, filing, telephone communications, personal planning, messaging, and meetings. The major office automation systems currently utilized in some nursing offices are word processing and electronic office communication systems.

Word Processing and Electronic Filing

The bottle of "white-out" may soon become an office aid of the past. Word processing involves the automated manipulation of text to produce office communications in a printed medium. The mode of entry remains the same (the keyboard) and the final output will look similar (the hard copy), but some innovative technology has revolutionized the steps in between. Data entered on the keyboard is recorded on electronic media and simultaneously displayed on a video screen. Errors can be corrected by simply typing over the error, and any number of characters or words can be inserted, moved around, or deleted. Margins, line endings, and indentations are automatically adjusted. Some systems have dictionaries to automatically correct spelling errors. Storing activities include filing the completed document on a diskette in an organized manner so it can be easily retrieved if necessary (Fig. 2-2).

Word processing offers many advantages. It reduces the time and expense invested in correcting or retyping text material and shortens

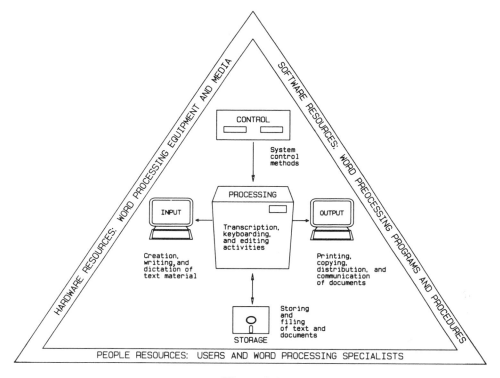

Figure 2-2
Word processing resources.

turnaround time for completion of the final hard copy. Storage and retrieval of documents can be handled quickly and efficiently.

Electronic Office Communication Systems

When one considers the profusion of systems already available to transmit communications, one wonders if there is really need for yet another. However, the critical factor is that although some electronic systems generally work, others often do not. How long is required for the articles deposited in the outbasket to make it to the right inbasket? Some of us have relinquished precious documents to the pneumatic tube system only to find out later it was jammed. We all have played seemingly endless games of telephone tag at one time or another (this is the process of calling someone, finding them unavailable, leaving a message, and then being unavailable when the call is returned). Electronic office communication systems enable the user to send text of any type electronically. The receiving location can view the information on a video screen or print it. Electronic mail services are now available to transfer the same kinds of electronic messages to sites around the world. More recent technology allows communication through voice mail. Instead of using a keyboard for data entry, voice messages are digitized so they can be transmitted and stored by the recipient voice mail system.

Things may seem a little overwhelming. New technology does take some getting used to, but it can make worklife a whole lot easier, sometimes even a little bit fun! The recommendations discussed in the remainder of this chapter should assist potential users of nursing management information systems in determining that the information obtained from the various applications is indeed helpful in meeting their needs.

Software Selection: The "Make-or-Buy" Decision

There are two basic alternatives once the decision has been made to invest in a management information system, regardless of the application. The first option is to develop the application in house. Although this process usually does not require large software expenditures from the capital budget, it may require considerable expenditure from the operating budget for the time of the individuals involved in design and development. For organizations without a computer services department, this likely involves outside contracting for systems design services. Regardless of the source of systems design and computer programming staff, liaison with the user group of nurse managers is essential. This is best achieved by having one designated nursing manager who clearly understands the desired outcomes of the system working in close association wit the systems staff. Although in-house development involves considerable start-up time, the end product is generally unique to the needs of the particular nursing organization, its philosophy and practices. Further, the decision regarding the level of integration of the application with existing information systems remains within the organization.

The second option is to purchase a software package from a commercial vendor. These fall into two categories. General-purpose software (such as Lotus 1-2-3 or Jazz) provides a framework that the user can then modify or further develop to meet specific needs. Special-purpose software, on the other hand, is designed for a particular application or group of applications. In most cases, purchased software packages are designed for stand-alone microcomputer-based systems. A few currently available have the capability to integrate with a hospital-wide information system or with other microcomputer systems. Purchased systems are usually package deals, providing a variety of supports during the implementation phase. The support offered generally refers to user training and, in some instances, software program modifications to customize the applications to the unique requirements of the organization. Some vendors for an additional cost extend these services into the future. However, caution should be exercised in these agreements. Prospective buyers may be lured into a contract by promises for technology and innovation currently under development that in fact never materialize. The system should be evaluated based on its existing potential, not on what it may or may not be capable of doing in the future.

While it is confusing to talk about modifying a system before it is even purchased, this aspect does present a significant concern. One of the major drawbacks of commercially available systems is their lack of flexibility. Because changes are often difficult if not impossible to make, the system may either fall short of meeting the needs within the organization or necessitate changes to existing practices to conform to the needs of the system! Often this is not readily apparent at the time of trial or purchase, but things change: Patient care becomes more complex, technology unfolds, and nursing practice must evolve with these changes. Inflexible systems quickly become obsolete. Before considering a commitment to purchase, nursing administrators would be well advised to take a thorough look at the future. If a purchased system is still an option, advertisements in nursing management journals provide general information on a number of commercial management information systems for a variety of applications.

Flexibility is only one essential characteristic of a useful management information system. To assist in the selection process, nursing administrators and those people involved in the decision should define the criteria that will be considered in evaluating the available alternatives. While these criteria will vary for different organizations evaluating different kinds of applications, important factors to assess include

- Validity: To what extent do the tools incorporated measure what they are supposed to measure?

- Reliability: How consistently do the tools incorporated measure the attribute they are supposed to be measuring?

- Ease of use: How simple and cost-effective is the system to use?

- Comparability: To what extent can the information produced be compared over time, both internally and externally with other organizations?

- Conformity: How well does the system conform to existing nursing practices?

- Performance targeted: To what degree is the information produced evaluated against predetermined standards?

- Action orientation: To what degree does the information obtained promote an active decision-making process as opposed to merely listing strings of data?

- Sensitivity: How useful is the information in providing a discriminating and meaningful comparison for nursing managers?

- Timeliness: How timely is the information? Is it made available before decisions are required?

A number of criteria must be considered in the selection process, and judging from the foregoing list, few are readily measurable. To help make an objective decision, many organizations use a rating scale. Each of the systems under consideration is rated on its effectiveness for each of the defined criteria. Because these are not necessarily equally significant, it is also useful to weight each of the criteria based on their relative importance. Table 2-1 illustrates this kind of decision-making process applied using the criteria described. Incorporating the input from the key decision makers into a model such as this helps simplify a relatively complex process.

Table 2-1
System Selection Model

Criteria	Relative weight of criteria	In-house system rating (1–10)	In-house system rating × Relative weight	Purchased system A rating (1–10)	System A rating × Relative weight	System B rating (1–10)	System B rating × Relative weight	System C rating (1–10)	System C rating × Relative weight
Validity	5	6	30	8	40	9	45	8	40
Reliability	5	8	40	9	45	8	40	8	40
Comparability	4	5	20	7	28	8	32	9	36
Action/ orientation	3	8	24	5	15	7	21	8	24
Timeliness	3	9	27	6	18	6	18	7	21
Conformity	4	9	36	5	20	6	24	9	36
Ease of use	4	7	28	7	28	5	20	6	24
Sensitivity	3	8	24	6	18	7	21	8	24
Performance target	3	4	12	7	21	6	18	8	24
Total points (of possible 340)			241		233		239		269

Implementation

A successful plan for the implementation of a management information system must begin well before the selection process described. Unfortunately, nursing administrators with little systems experience often limit planning activities to picking a system and following the vendor's instructions to get things going. In most instances, these attempts result in systems that are ineffective in meeting the needs of the nursing managers. Selection and implementation of management information systems require comprehensive planning that includes feasibility assessment, analysis, design, development, implementation, and maintenance.

Feasibility Assessment

There must be a preliminary understanding of the information needs of the potential users and the feasibility of the proposed system. Initially, objectives must be stated in measurable terms that specify what functions or tasks are to be accomplished by the system. The feasibility assessment is an attempt to then determine whether or not it is possible to achieve the objectives. Are there sufficient interest, commitment, and skill among the people involved? Does the organization have the financial resources to undertake the project? Are the anticipated benefits derived from the system worth the investment? Are the objectives technically feasible, that is, does the technology exist to perform the job?

If the project is approved at this level, the level of investment will now begin to increase sharply. The commitment is made and cancellation becomes difficult.

Information Analysis

To define the product, information required for the application must be determined. This demands a thorough understanding of the roles of the various users of the system and the decisions they make. Who generates the data and where? Who receives the data? Who will use the information generated by the application? For what purpose? In what format? Consideration should be given to the current situation as well as to future goals and needs.

Systems Design

A design for the system is produced that meets the requirements of the application established in the information analysis stage. The design includes specifications for hardware, software, people, data resources, and information requirements. It is at this point that a decision is made with regards to designing the system in house, purchasing general-purpose software and modifying it to a specific purpose, or purchasing commercially produced special-purpose software.

The approved or selected design must be evaluated to ensure the system achieves the stated objectives and endorses the needs of management. A checklist (e.g., Table 2-1) developed to assist in system selection can also prove an invaluable component of the review process. In addition to conforming to system specifications, the systems staff must be confident that if implemented the system will perform as specified. At this point there is no system, only a design, so it is not too late to make many of the changes desired.

Software Development

In this stage, the designs are translated into a working application on a computer. For purchased systems, the vendor incorporates the necessary modifications requested by the user organization. If the system is being developed in house, this is usually the most costly and time-consuming stage. Complex applications are best divided into steps with unique time estimates. The progress of development can then be monitored to maintain adherence to the schedule. Once the software is in a completed form, it should be validated using test data to ensure the program does indeed work.

Implementation

While the development stage draws heavily on systems resources, implementation has a major impact on the nursing department. The key issue in the actual automation of the application is user satisfaction. Involving nursing staff and managers throughout the selection and implementation process is a significant factor in achieving success. The tactic is to determine where support exists and build on it. A thorough orientation program to train users to correctly retrieve and enter information is essential to prevent errors (i.e., to maintain data integrity) as well as to foster commitment. Some applications (such as workload measurement and quality-monitoring tools) will require judgment and rating decisions by qualified data gatherers among whom interrater reliability must be established. Implementation requires consistent feedback to determine where problems exist and to get the system working smoothly.

Maintenance

Most of the bugs in an application should be resolved by the end of implementation, but constant attention is required to maintain data integrity. Orientation programs are ongoing as new users access the system. Initial interrater reliability must be reconfirmed at regular intervals. Equipment and software require maintenance to stay in good working order. Inevitably, as time goes on, users will suggest refinements of the application to improve efficiency and support current practices.

A critical aspect of the maintenance stage is evaluation. After implementation, an evaluation should be conducted to determine the extent to which the application meets the objectives defined at the outset. Users will want to ask a number of questions: Did we get what we wanted? On time? Within budget? Can we learn anything else from the project?

While these steps do not come with a written guarantee, thorough planning and tight control help secure project success. It is best described as a building process, with each stage dependent on the foundation laid in prior stages.

Information versus Data: A Word of Caution

In the introduction to this chapter, it was proposed that the advantages of automated management information systems lie in their ability to process more data at a greater speed. This statement suggests that more is equated with better in the realm of management information. To qualify this, a distinction must be made between data and information. A description describing data as a string of characters or uninterrupted patterns assists in this differentiation (Murdick, 1980). Information is distinguished from data in that it acts as a signal which predisposes a person to take action (recall the criteria for action orientation from Table 2-1). The role of the computer, therefore, is to process data so that it takes on a useful and relevant form. The actual benefits achieved through automation are ultimately dependent on the action taken by the manager as a result of the information generated.

Implications for the Future

While nursing administrators are realizing the benefits of automated management information systems, the rapid pace of technologic change continues to present new opportunities and issues. As more computer applications are developed for use by nursing managers, many users will be confronted by the problems associated with incompatible systems. Integration of the previously described management applications with each other as well as with the hospital information system is currently a key focus for hardware and software development.

Existing systems are also suboptimal in supporting decision making.

As nursing managers become more familiar with statistical methods and operations management, standard reports and strings of numbers will be replaced by integrated data bases and analytical models that will allow an interactive decision-making process. The emphasis on quantitative data will evolve to focus on the realm of qualitative information, which plays a far more significant role in the decisions of nursing managers. The volume of output currently produced will be streamlined and displayed visually in condensed form through the use of graphics systems.

Questions

1. In your own words, explain what a management information system is.

2. List and define the six major areas in which computer supported management information systems are being used. Identify the advantages of each for the nurse manager.

3. Based on the material in this chapter, would you prefer to buy management information system software or generate your own for your organization? Why?

4. What is the difference between data and information?

References Cited

Hanson R: Applying management information systems to staffing. *Journal of Nursing Administration* 1982; 12:5–9.
Murdick R: *MIS Concepts and Design.* Englewood Cliffs, NJ: Prentice-Hall, 1980.

Bibliography

Batchelor G: Computerized nursing systems: a look at the market-place. *Computers in Healthcare* 1985; 6:55–58.
Carpenter C: Computer use in nursing management. *Journal of Nursing Administration* 1985; 15:18–23.
Courtemanche J: Gearing up on an automated nurse scheduling system in a decentralized setting. *Computers in Nursing* 1986; 4:59–63.
Finkler S: Microcomputers in nursing administration: a software overview. *Journal of Nursing Administration* 1985; 15:18–23.
Johantgen ME, Parrinello K: Microcomputers: turning the database into unit management information. *Nursing Management* 1987; 18:30–38.
Kiley M, Halloran EJ, Weston JL, et al: Computerized nursing information systems. *Nursing Management* 1983; 14:26–29.

Meyer D, Sunquist J: Selecting a management system. *Computers in Healthcare* 1986; 7:22–24.

O'Brien JA: *Computers in Business Management*. 4th ed. Illinois: Richard D. Irwin, 1985; 464.

Schifiliti C, Bonasero C, Thompson M: Lotus 1-2-3: a quality assurance application for nursing practice, administration, and staff development. *Computers in Nursing* 1986; 4:205–211.

Somers J: Information systems: the process of development. *Journal of Nursing Administration* 1979; 9:53–58.

3—Responsibility of Nurses in Selection of a Computer System

Marion J. Ball

Introduction

Two forces are converging on nursing today, and both carry tremendous implications for the profession. The first is the demand for accountability, both of quality and of cost. The reimbursement revolution and the malpractice crisis together create a need for increased data collection for ongoing and retrospective monitoring of standards of care and of cost. The second is the force of technology in the fields of biomedicine and information. These technologies are changing the way nursing is practiced, posing new challenges and offering new opportunities.

This presentation focuses on the responsibilities of the nursing profession in the selection of computer systems, from small specialized systems such as surgical software to large hospital information systems (HIS). It is imperative that nursing be actively involved at every stage in the process, from the beginning through the evaluation. Whatever the size of system, the selection should be determined by a formal decision-making process, involving top-level management as well as the users themselves.

The Request for Proposal (RFP)

Hospital Information Systems (HIS)

The process is most elaborate in the selection of the HIS, partly because of the expense involved in such an acquisition. This process also achieves prominence because of the many phases involved. First, detailed information and statistics describing the institution must be gathered. Then, information forms and flows must be defined and subsequently refined in anticipation of installation of the new system. Clearly, this involves a wide range of personnel from varied departments and provides the base for definition of specifications in an HIS that go to the vendors in a request for proposal (RFP).

Nursing is critically involved in the generation of such information, from census, staffing, and other administrative data to patient-specific data such as care plans and acuity indices. Thus, nursing must participate in the process accompanying computer system acquisition, because this offers the opportunity to examine existing information flow and usage and to take remedial action. Often an existing system is cumbersome and inefficient. Evaluation can identify areas needing minor improvement, modification, or major revision; adjustments can be made before acquisition of a new computer system. For example, the information analysis done by nursing may reveal that no standard format for patient care plans is followed by all patient units within the institution. Remedial action can be taken during the acquisition process. Thus, the computerized information system subsequently installed can incorporate all enhancements. In short, the better the initial information-handling system and the better its documentation, the better the final product of a computerized information system.

The final RFP is prepared using vendor-provided information in conjunction with the description and documentation of information use and flow developed by the institution and assembled either internally or with the assistance of outside consultants. Every area must review the final document before it is issued; no department in a hospital can work in isolation. For example, admitting must work with medical records and then in turn with nursing, and they in turn with the various ancillary areas. Thus, nursing is responsible for addressing a number of areas during the generation of specifications for the RFP.

The order entry, result reporting, and communications system should allow physician and/or nursing order entry from all areas of the hospital. This requires the installation of remote terminals in all nursing units, patient care areas, and ancillary departments to provide the users in these areas with data entry and inquiry capabilities. Outstanding or queued orders should be approved and verified against a written order before their release to the system for processing.

A generalized communication should provide a standard interface that any future subsystem can use to obtain all required patient demographic and medical information captured by some other subsystem. Additionally, the communications system should allow each subsystem to transmit captured data, both medical and financial, to a central patient-oriented data base for the purpose of storage or transmittal to a financial system. The capability of a future problem-oriented medical record must be displayed.

The second major area the nursing section of the RFP should address is result entry, also called result reporting. The system should provide the ability for on-line result entry by selecting the patient and then entering the results for that patient.

Other requirements include scheduling systems for nursing staff and for patient appointments. The capability to provide each patient with a complete schedule for ancillary service and treatment areas such as x-ray (radiography) and physical therapy eliminates conflicts in appointments and maximizes the efficiency of those units. These systems must be able to schedule at least 7 days in advance and allow rescheduling by authorized personnel only.

Specialized Microcomputer Systems

Software systems are now available to support applications that are smaller in scale than full-scale hospital information systems. These systems build on the increased capabilities of microcomputers to store, process, and communicate data. The operating room is seeing particularly intensive development of such software. Many vendors offer surgical software packages that address a number of functions, all of which impact the operating room nursing staff.

These specialized systems provide nursing with data-gathering capabilities which in turn support monitoring and analytic activities. System features generally include operating room scheduling, surgeon preference case cards, and operating log recording. Other features less uniformly provided are equipment control, implant information, and such medical items as patient care plans, recovery room, and clinical data. The most frequently provided cost-related item is a case cost/patient billing feature; vendor and market analysis are infrequently offered. A patient assessment subsystem is now offered by a limited number of vendors.

Clearly the operating room is just one area in which the microcomputer will assume a more integral role in providing and monitoring health care. As such applications are more commonly used and accommodated by links to major HIS, nursing will be involved in an increasing number of acquisitions. Although the process of selecting these smaller and more specialized applications packages will most likely involve fewer departments within the institution than the process of bringing in an HIS, nursing should play a key role.

The Selection Process

When the vendors' responses to the RFP have been received, the institution makes a preliminary review and selects bids that merit further evaluation. Site visits to view proposed computer systems in operation are in order. Nursing should insist on being included in these site visits, and should prepare a structured interview schedule in conjunction with other users. Site visits are essential to making a selection, as they enable the users to see the system, to clarify understanding of the system, and to verify the vendor's claims.

Additional Step in the Evaluation Process

One final step should be added to the traditional evaluation process. At the time of the best and final offer,the vendor must be required to demonstrate each function addressed in the request for proposal to the satisfaction of the selection committee. A scoring system of 1 to 3 can be employed, awarding 3 points if the function is fully demonstrated, 2 points if the function is demonstrated with some difficulty, 1 point if the intent to develop the function is clear and beta test data are available, and 0 point if the function is totally lacking. This approach to evaluating the product ensures that "what you see is what you get," and establishes the confidence level required for success. This method was employed by the University of Maryland Medical System in their selection of an HIS. Howard Massingill, the Director for Information Systems, provided the author with the details of his methodology and permission to reference his work.

Nursing Issues in Selection

In approaching selection process, nursing will confront certain vital issues, among them the following:

- justification and/or modification of the current operation of the nursing department

- specific management or technical problems

- financial and organizational implications of alternative systems under consideration

- planning for long-range needs in the department.

Consultant Role

Given the complexity of these issues, and the impact that they may have both on the selection and on the nursing department itself, those nurses in decision-making positions may elect to seek assistance beyond that available in their department or provided by computing vendors. Nursing may choose to involve a knowledgeable individual from elsewhere witin the institution or to retain an independent professional consultant. Quite possibly, nursing may choose to tap all sources of expertise, using an internal consultant to serve as liaison with those from outside.

In turning to health care computer consultants for assistance, nursing should not expect definitive decisions but rather a set of viable alternatives. The final selection of a computer system rests with those in nursing, who possess the knowledge of nursing practices and issues required to make an intelligent and informed decision.

Contract Negotiations

The final stage is the negotiation of a contract that defines the HIS or the smaller specialized system. In addition to stipulating ownership of the software source code and other issues such as warranties and liabilities, this document must clearly and comprehensively describe the responsibility of vendor and buyer for software, maintenance, and support functions, as well as technical and legal standards for measuring the success or failure of the implementation. Legal counsel of an information technology-literate attorney is an absolute must from the very beginning of negotiations.

Linking Nursing and Health Care Computing

Today computing offers much-needed capabilities in the field of health care. Advances in information technology provide the ability not only to collect and store data, but also to monitor, analyze, manipulate, and communicate the resulting information. To have a successful information system, whatever its scope, good communication must exist between and among the various professionals, technicians, and administrators within a health care organization.

Working Relationships

In short, the nurses and the computer systems department must establish an effective working relationship. Nursing management must ask how the health professional can best utilize the computer analyst. To do so, nurses must grasp the basic principles and methods of information processing that affect the design and production of computer-compatible records. In corollary fashion, the computer professional must learn the terminology and practice of modern nursing. Together these two groups of professionals can then address the demanding task of managing computerization, optimizing its benefits and minimizing its risks.

The task is not an easy one, but when it is successfully accomplished nursing can meet the pressing issues of cost containment and quality assurance. Enhanced information handling will provide more precise records of cost as well as new mechanisms for monitoring patient care on both an individual and an aggregate basis. As responsible professionals, nurses have great need for sophisticated information processing. The technology now offers the power; nursing must work to realize its potential.

Nursing Informatics

Nationally and internationally, nursing informatics is a new and growing field. A general knowledge of computers and data processing is now required of nurses in almost every setting. Those in management positions are being called on to maintain their nursing orientation while communicating and participating with data processing professionals in developing solutions for computing problems related to nursing. And the change masters in nursing are making major commitments to computing and data processing, by acquiring training in both nursing and computer science and becoming involved in developing and initiating new computer systems.

These changes in the profession deserve and demand the attention of nurses. Today the leading schools of nursing are moving to institute programs in nursing informatics. The next few years will see major advancements in the development of curricula and appropriate learning materials.

Medical informatics, dental informatics, nursing informatics— these new and growing fields will bring the full benefits of information technology to health care. They will provide the map to the future for the health professions.

Questions

1. What are two major forces affecting nursing today?
2. What particular aspects of a hospital information system request for proposal require nursing input?
3. Identify the steps in the selection process.
4. What should nursing expect from consultants?
5. What must nurses and computer professionals each learn about the alternate profession?

Bibliography

Ball MJ, Boyle TM: Hospital information systems: past, present and future. *Hospital Financial Management Journal* 1980; 10:12–24.

Ball MJ, Hammon GL: Hospital information systems: a ten year follow up. In: Lindberg DAB, Collen MF, eds. *AAMSI Congress 1984—Proceedings of the Third Spring Joint National Congress*. Bethesda: American Association for Medical Systems and Informatics, 1984; 37–42.

Ball MJ, Hannah KH: Nursing and computers: past, present, future. *Journal of Clinical Computing* 1984; 12:179–184.

Ball MJ, Hannah K: *Using Computers in Nursing*. Reston: Reston Publishing, 1984.

Ball MJ, Hannah K: Computerization—the experts say it's working. *Canadian Nurse* 1985; 81:21–23.

Ball MJ, Shannon RH: Vertical and horizontal curricula: how they can work together in the integration of medical computer science and the classic medical sciences. *Medical Informatics* (London) 1984; 9:281–288.

Ball MJ, Snelbecker GE, Schechter SL: Nurses' perceptions concerning computer uses before and after a computer literacy lecture. *Computers in Nursing* 1985; 3:23–32.

Ball MJ, Warnock-Matheron A, Hannah KJ, et al: The case for using computers in the operating room. *Western Journal of Medicine* 1986; 145:843–847.

Petroski S, O'Desky RI, Ball MJ: Innovative technologies for healthcare enhancement. *Computers in Healthcare* 1985; 6:20–28.

4—Nursing Input to the Selection of Hospital Information Systems

Mary Etta Mills

Introduction

Health care facilities are increasingly exploring and incorporating computer-based information systems as a method of managing complex patient care and financial data. Because this type of information management is indeed structured to integrate all sources of data, it is the rare department head that is disinterested in the process of deciding what, how, and by whom information will be collected, dispatched, and utilized. For this reason, the best received evaluation and selection process will include a systems steering committee that is fully representative of all major health care facility departments.

Nursing is frequently likened to the hub of a wheel, with which all patient care activities, like spokes, have a connection. Nursing often is the network by which patient care is not only delivered but coordinated. In this role, a critical linkage is provided that extends from the provision of care itself to the communication of that care. While departments such as pharmacy, radiology, dietary, and clinical laboratories have a primary concern with order communication and reporting, nursing uniquely interacts with these departments to integrate the multiple facets of information produced.

The initial evaluation and selection of an information management system is critical to identifying a system that will best meet the needs of the institution it is to serve. Criteria on which an overall evaluation is based will generally include system function and features, functional architecture, references, quality of documentation, system design, risk, vendor support, vendor background, hardware and system software, and cost. Nursing is key to this evaluation process. Data systems personnel and financial analysts can assess the technical, mechanical, and cost feasibility of various systems, but nursing has the broad clinical and administrative perspective by which to critique the system's programs and information flow. An example of nursing input to

Table 4-1
Order Communications/Nursing System Requirements[a]

Enter Orders
Manage Orders
Update Standard Orders Directory
Produce Billing Transactions
Update Procedure Directory
Enter Results
Manage Results
Update Procedure Directory
Update Abstract Code Directories
Print/Display Order/Result Directories
Inventory Control
Patient Scheduling
Care Planning
Infection Control
Determine Patient Care Requirements
Compute Nurse Staffing Requirements
Display/Print Nurse Staffing Requirements
Maintain Patient Care Directories
Maintain Nurse Staffing Conversion Directory
Performance Reporting

[a] See Appendix A for detailed nursing content to a request for proposal.

a request for proposal (RFP) is summarized in Table 4-1 and included in detail in Appendix A.

The knowledge that nursing brings to the administrative selection process includes detail relevant to the interaction of departments participating in patient care management, the degree of systems enhancement that will or will not be necessary, the ease or difficulty of implementation based on system complexity, the expense of educational preparation of staff, and the potential for fully integrating system components. Most importantly, nursing can ascertain the system's potential to improve patient care. In this role, nursing provides a critical balance in facilitating the selection of a technically capable system that also yields maximum utility in a patient care environment.

The decision to implement an information management system represents a major financial commitment on the part of any institution. The potential of an information system to meet the unique needs of any specific health care facility is an essential ingredient for its long-term success in that environment. Nursing can be an invaluable component both formally and informally in structuring the evaluation process, making recommendations for mandatory and desirable components, assessing a system's potential relative to the needs of practicing professionals, and making a selection with both the present and the future in mind.

Computer-based information systems will revolutionize communications in health care and markedly impact nursing practice. The context of communications must be structured to clearly define and facilitate the documentation of the nursing process, to streamline the clarity, availability, and integration of essential information, and to conserve nursing time so that it can be spent with the patient. The only way nursing can ensure the system selected will facilitate these goals is to participate actively in the administrative selection process.

A priority role for nursing will serve the best interests of the health care facility and the nursing profession. Where that role has been a reality, information system selection has proven to be farsighted and positive. Implementation likewise has proceeded in a productive way. Working closely with other technical and professional members of the health care system, nursing is critical to the selection, design, and implementation of an optimum clinical information system.

5—Nurses' Responsibilities in Implementation of Information Systems

Suzanne Jenkins

Selecting Hospital Information Systems

The influence of nursing on the decision-making process of the selection of hospital information systems (HIS) is increasing. Systems planning and implementation are based on not only the capabilities of information technology but also forces in the environment that impact health care.

Computer decisions in the 1970s were primarily financially oriented. Hospitals saw the need for automating their patient billing process and other key systems such as general ledger and accounts payable. Advanced technology led to increased sophistication of hardware and software capabilities, and concurrently the information needs of the hospital increased. More extensive reporting requirements, as well as the need for management reporting on productivity, became the norm.

The decisions in the early 1980s focused primarily on ancillary systems. Many of them were not integrated with the rest of the system and were categorized as stand-alone systems. As a result, redundant patient information had to be entered in each system. The laboratory, pharmacy, and radiology generally had their own systems, including an order entry function typically done by their own departmental staff. If terminals were placed on the nursing unit, clerks or nursing staff could enter the orders.

The trend for the mid-1980s through the 1990s is taking patient care back to the bedside. Although terminals at each bedside can be an expensive venture for the hospital, many vendors are claiming both reduced nursing costs and increased quality of patient care. Terminals provide on-line flow charting, vital signs, and nursing care plans. The vendors claim that nurses can spend more time delivering care and less time charting.

Nursing has now defined additional needs and requirements for information systems. For many institutions, the ultimate goal is to have a "paperless" system. The entire medical record can be stored and accessed on line from a terminal device. This concept allows consolidated accurate information to be available at the user's fingertips. Patient charts need not be tracked down. Lab slips need not be filled out. Patient medication records can be easily accessed on-line. On-line order entry means no more order/charge slips—all information can be captured automatically.

Also influencing the computer systems of the 1980s and 1990s is the need for quality assurance and utilization review modules. Expedient, timely information about the patient is critical. Diagnostic related groupings (DRGs) are having a major impact in the financial area and the patient's length of stay. This ultimately impacts the type and quality of care provided.

Meeting the Challenges

The implementation of any hospital information system (HIS)—from selection through installation—is never 100% problem free. Problems to solve and challenges to face are what make every implementation unique and exciting. Problems can occur at any stage of the implementation cycle, beginning with the selection of a system and moving through the next phases, i.e., installation, training, parallel testing, "going live," and even into the postimplementation evaluation. The key to resolution is the identification of existing resistance factors. Once they are identified, plans can be made to eliminate them through teamwork, transitional strategies, and educational offerings. The acquisition of a complete HIS is an expensive venture for a hospital to undertake, and requires a large commitment from administration to support and guide the installation.

Common barriers to overcome range from general mistrust of computer systems to misgivings regarding a specific system. Potential users may fear that implementation of a system will result in an increased workload without tangible benefits. These fears and inhibitions are some of the most difficult barriers to overcome. Together they elongate the normal learning curve, increasing the time it takes to become familiar with the new system.

Often, the politics surrounding a major acquisition such as a computer system can slow or stall it. The very idea of change is sometimes threatening and can stall the implementation process. Interestingly, though, the people most resistant to a new system often become its best promoters once they are knowledgeable about and comfortable with it.

Changing from a manual mode to an automated system can generate insecurity and distrust, and even changing from one automated system to another automated system often elicits resistance. A common complaint is "the old computer system didn't do it that way," regardless of comparative merit. It is sometimes easier to train people who have never used a system than to retrain people who are constantly making comparisons to previous systems.

An automated system should not only assist in expediting accurate patient information throughout the hospital, but should somewhat reduce paper generation. Most of the necessary information can be viewed on a terminal, and only legal documents of the medical record must be printed. Yet for some people, seeing is believing. They derive a sense of security from the paper generated by the system. When they are no longer required to fill out manual requisitions and charge slips, they need the reassurance of the hard copy (paper) form before they believe that their orders have reached the designated department.

During the implementation process, therefore, it is advisable to allow generous amounts of paper printing to promote security that reliable information is being transmitted throughout the system. A postimplementation evaluation should expose unused printed reports. This indicates that either the information is not displayed in a usable format, or more commonly, the information can be adequately accessed on line and may no longer need to be printed.

Throughout the process, teamwork and cooperation among decision makers are essential to a smooth implementation. Otherwise, in-house politics can have the largest negative impact on system implementation. Power plays among people and/or departments can bring implementation to a virtual standstill. If one person on a committee of decision makers is following a different agenda from everyone else, all will experience frustration. Education and communication can prevent many of the negative perceptions. There is a great sense of satisfaction and accomplishment at the completion of a successful implementation.

Defining the Requirements

The request for proposal (RFP) is one of the preliminary steps a hospital takes when selecting a computerized information system. The hospital produces a checklist of needs for each department, or alternatively employs a consultant to assist in succinctly defining and communicating those needs to many vendors. In either case, nursing defines the requirements to support the philosophy and practice of their department. It is vital that nurses are involved in the definition process of requirements necessary to meet the needs of the nursing department as information input comes from ancillaries and other hospital departments (Table 5-1).

Table 5-1
Sample Specifications for Requests for Proposals (RFPs) by Area

Registration
1. Automatically utilize outpatient and emergency room data for inpatient registration
2. Utilize an on-line card embosser
3. Automatically utilize patient information from a previous visit recorded in the system
4. Allow in the admission/discharge/transfer (ADT) system for the following fields: patient name, patient street address, city, state, zip, home phone, birthdate, sex, marital status, ethnic origin, social security number, religion, financial class, occupation, employer, employer address, guarantor information, etc.
5. Have a bed-hold feature for a specific time period for patients on leave of absence
6. Provide the ability to add and delete beds and medical service units

Medical records
Master patient index
1. Contain the following data elements: patient name, medical record number, date of birth, address, phone number, previous names, admit and discharge dates, physicians
2. Identify the location of any record at any given time
3. Track the incomplete record and amount of time the record has been incomplete
4. Integrate the DRG grouper with admission/discharge/transfer module
5. Provide built in edits for Medicare code, sex-specific information, etc.
6. Maintain multiple diagnosis and procedure data, per patient, for each outpatient encounter (emergency, outpatient surgery, outpatient department visits)
7. Provide concurrent and discharge abstracting capabilities for inpatient and outpatient cases

Order entry
1. Provide on-line ordering and results reporting
2. Provide on-line real time patient-centered scheduling
3. Access patient information on the system using patient name, patient location, and/or patient number
4. Access status of tests/procedures offered
5. Change/cancel patient orders with audit trail
6. Display possible conflicts between any current orders and those previously entered, including drug incompatibilities and other hospital-defined criteria
7. Charge orders at time of placement
8. Prompt to verify all elements are included in the order, such as route of administration, dose time, frequency, and any special instructions
9. Prompt to flag all STAT orders or special instructions
10. Record the time an order is received and completed, as well as who completes the order
11. List all orders not yet completed, available at each nursing unit
12. Produce standard reports, including

Occupancy summaries	Pending discharges
Admissions by physician	Vacant bed census
Transfer lists	Scheduled preadmissions

Table 5-1 (*continued*)

Nursing management
1. Provide a library of nursing care plans to which care items can be added, deleted, or otherwise made more specific
2. Provide a predefined format for individualized care plans developed at the unit level
3. Allow users to enter free text into the nursing care plan
4. Give worksheets for day-to-day and shift-to-shift planning of individual patient care
5. Schedule nursing staff at the unit level and centrally
6. Accommodate multiple versions of patient classification systems, for example, obstetrics, critical care, medical/surgical
7. Report in terms of specific nursing care hours per day and per shift
8. Maintain records for each employee, including credentials, competence verification, continuing education units, illness and absence profile, CPR certification status, and expiration dates
9. Store, update, and print nursing policies and procedures

Utilization review
1. Identify on a daily basis those patients who have met hospital-defined criteria for concurrent admission review
2. Allow on-line completion of utilization review worksheet including discharge date, length of stay, number of reviews, physician referrals, denials, diagnosis, and disposition of patient
3. Allow editing of utilization review data for accuracy and completeness
4. Generate a monthly log of patient discharges and the number of patient-days denied as specified by outside review agencies
5. Maintain utilization review statistics reflecting monthly activity, for example, total numbers of discharges denied, discharges with denials by insurance carrier, admissions and discharges, emergency and elective admissions
6. Maintain a log of denials by third-party intermediaries

Quality assurance
1. Set up defined criteria to which a patient treatment can be compared
2. Generate a list of exceptions when patient data fall outside the established range
3. Override previously defined criteria for the purpose of performing projects or reviews
4. Log incident reports including patient information, type of incident, place, etc.

Nursing's involvement in defining requirements reflects its critical role as key integrator in the provision of patient care. When patients are admitted to a hospital, they are deluged with questions, many of which are asked and documented more than once. It is the nurse who must integrate and collate all the information in a logical format and develop a comprehensive plan of care for the individual patient. Information the nurse collates is captured by registration, medical records, physicians, laboratory, pharmacy, radiology, physical therapy, dietary, and many other departments. The same information is fundamental to the utilization review and quality assurance functions.

Integrating Systems

An integrated system should capture information once, sort it, and generate output in a readable, cohesive format. The point of information capture is most logically determined by nurses; they know what type of information should be captured at registration and what information should be captured by nursing. They can determine the critical points of integration that will improve the quality of information and eliminate duplication.

For example, many registration systems ask height and weight during the admission process. Regrettably, admissions personnel are not the most accurate source of this information. And inaccurate information, once entered into the system, may be accessed throughout the entire hospital. It is the nurse who can best provide accurate information—information critical for the pharmacy to calculate drug dosages appropriate for the patient.

All of the departments that make up a hospital are important and vital to the care of the patient, but they are generally focused on just one area (their own) and may tend to be myopic in their view of the patient. The nurse, on the other hand, is the focal point as care-giver for the patient, compiling all pertinent patient information and disseminating appropriate data to a department or person. It is imperative

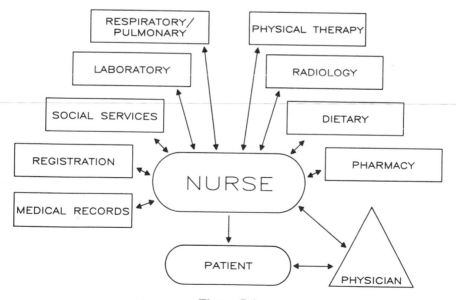

Figure 5-1
The nurse acts as the "hub" for patient information processing.

that the nurse as the integrator of an HIS work with the ancillaries in determining their requirements for computer systems and make sure those requirements are met.

Ancillaries interact with the patient on an individual basis, but the nurse coordinates the activities to best benefit the patient. Social service consultations are generally initiated by nursing based on the patient's need for financial assistance, postdischarge placement, or general counseling. Dietary consultations are also usually initiated by nursing. Nurses inform the laboratory of any pertinent medications prescribed for the patient that might affect normal results; for example, coumadin affects PTTs. Registration and medical records information are often corrected and/or updated by nursing personnel. Nursing also interacts with departments that indirectly affect the patient's care, such as central supply, housekeeping, and transportation. Physicians write orders that direct the care provided to the patient, but nurses play an interpretive role for the physician and assure that the care is coordinated and integrated.

The nurse needs access to ALL this information to provide quality care, so who is the most logical person to function as the integrator of the system? Of course, the nurse.

Implementing the Selected System

The implementation of a hospital computer system begins almost immediately after a vendor has been selected. Nurses can play an extremely valuable part in that implementation, because nurses have more direct, hands-on interaction with and knowledge of the different departments than perhaps any other member of the implementation team. Thus the nurse can be a direct source of information to facilitate the implementation of a system—whether a stand-alone, single application, or multiple applications—in ways that might not be intuitively obvious to implementation planners. Nurses also provide helpful input into the restatement of procedures, roles, and workflow within hospital departments during a system implementation. By contributing in these two ways, nurses can move a step closer to their primary objective: making optimal use of resources to provide quality care to their patients.

These contributions by nursing begin in the selection process, when requirements are first established. They continue throughout the standard cycle of implementation, once a selection is made.

Phase 1: Installation. During this phase, the software is loaded onto the computer and a complete system demonstration should be given by the vendor. The need to understand the system fully at this point cannot be stressed too heavily. For the implementation to be successful, definition of software modifications to meet the hospital's needs should be undertaken at the same time, and through the same process, as the definition/redefinition of policies/procedures to meet the systems requirements. Both serve as a basis for discussion with the vendor to determine the time frames for completion of implementation and to delineate vendor/client responsibilities.

Phase 2: Training. Once installation is complete or at least well under way, training begins. There are many approaches to training all the users of the system. Because nursing is generally the largest group of employees in a hospital to be trained and because accommodating multiple shifts is necessary, planning is of the utmost importance. Typically the vendor is responsible for training the trainer(s). Often a designee from each unit or department is responsible for making sure the training is complete and thorough. All future problems and issues, as well as requests for changes to the system, will be funneled through that designee. Training is most effective if taught in multiple short segments 1 to 2 hours long. Depending on the complexity of the application as well as previous user experience, the sessions can be shortened or lengthened.

Phase 3: Parallel Testing. This involves a simulated dry run of what actually happens during the daily routine of a department. It is important to test the validity and reliability of the software, as well as to make sure new policies and procedures support the designed intent of the system. Information is sometimes duplicated during parallel testing. Patient orders may be entered into the system and may also be sent to the ancillary for verification purposes. Parallel testing may last from a few days to a few weeks to thoroughly test cumulative summaries.

Phase 4: "Going Live." This is a term commonly used at the time the system goes into actual production. The parallel testing is complete and data are being communicated on line, real time. This step typically requires handholding support from the vendor. The users should be well trained and fairly comfortable with the system. This is the phase in which all the effort and hard work pay off.

Phase 5: Postimplementation Evaluation. There may be a temptation to shortchange the evaluation phase. This clearly is shortsighted. If all is going well, this final phase will help to fine-tune the system just implemented. If problems exist, evaluation will help to avoid problems in implementing additional applications in the future. In either case, evaluation can provide valuable insights to the hospital and its many departments, especially nursing. Questions to be raised in evaluation include the following:

- What reports are being printed and why? Is there a functional use for them?

- What problem areas are procedural? Who are the problem users and why? Is it because they don't understand the system? Do they need additional training? Do their problems result from not being involved in the implementation process?

- Is the system doing what the specifications say it is supposed to do? Is the workflow smoother? Is communication improved? Is there any increased efficiency in staff?

Nursing Involvement

In assisting throughout the entire process of implementation integrated hospital information systems, nurses can apply the familiar nursing model of assessment, planning, implementation, and evaluation. Each is discussed here in detail.

Process Model

Assessment. The scope of the project, the players, the time frame, and the needs of the hospital are all analyzed and documented. Documenting the current workflow in any department will assist in determining the impact the computer system will have during and after the implementation. For example, it will show that because the system automatically notifies the nursing unit when a patient is admitted, a phone call from the admissions department can be eliminated. Similarly, orders entered into the system will eliminate the need for order requisitions to be manually completed and the need for the transport function to deliver the requisition to the respective ancillary. The requisitions will automatically print in the ancillary. These and many other time-consuming tasks are flowcharted during the analysis of the department workflow and identified as areas that will be eliminated with an automated system.

Planning. When the assessment phase is completed, roles and responsibilities are defined. The liaison nurse works closely with the vendor to identify checklists and checkpoints and to establish detailed training plans. The vendor will often suggest two or three options that best suit the hospital's resource situation. Another important step is establishing correct courses of action to follow when system problem arise. Nurses can help to determine who should be called when a problem has been identified, as well as the chain of command. The vendor may be involved if the problem is software- or hardware-related. A solid plan is imperative to facilitate a smooth transition during any implementation.

Implementation. This is the third point at which nurses can contribute. Implementating the plan(s) coincides with the actual implementation of the system. The system implementation consists of many logical and sequential steps; but with the proper plan in place, a successful implementation will ensue.

Evaluation. Postimplementation analysis ensures that all the defined requirements have been met. Comparing the specifications of a system provided by the vendor to the actual system functionality will identify any delinquent areas. For example, if the specifications indicate that the system will generate a certain report, and the system clearly does not produce the report, the nurse must decide how important the report is to the overall functioning of the department. The identified areas must be assessed as to the nature of the deficiency and prioritized. Plans must then be created and implemented to resolve any deficiencies.

Roles Played

Nurses play a variety of roles during a system implementation, roles that can be accomplished without a programming or technical background; it is far more important that the nurse have a solid understanding of hospital policies and procedures and the ability to change those procedures to improve workflow of the departments. Probably the two most important roles are communicator and coordinator. Other critical roles include mediator, decision maker, and politician/marketeer. Let's look at each of these roles.

Communicator. The role of the nurse as communicator starts before the implementation begins and does not end until the postimplementation phase is completed to the satisfaction of all participants. Many different tasks occur simultaneously during the implementation phase. If one link is lost in the shuffle, it can cause great distress and distrust of the system as well as delay to the implementation. The nurse can smooth the process and reduce confusion by identifying tasks and communicating with other involved hospital staff members. Many people need to be kept informed of the status of the project, but at varying levels.

Coordinator. Nurses spend much of their time prioritizing needs and coordinating the care of the patient. This experience lends itself to making them the focal coordinators of an HIS implementation. Responsibilities of coordination include training, meetings with ancillaries, setting target dates, and defining a plan. It is important to keep issues focused and to observe priorities. The nurse/coordinator may delegate as needed to ensure timely implementation.

Mediator. Many decisions must be made during the implementation process of a computer system. When multiple departments are involved, many issues cross departmental boundaries. An individual should be designated to mediate and facilitate compromise. Because nurses interact with and understand so many of the hospital departments, they are the ideal choice for this role. A side benefit of this arrangement is that it gives nurses a chance to see what happens on the other side of a STAT lab result or the process involved in dispensing therapeutic medications or transcribing radiology reports. Conversely, the arrangement allows the ancillary departments to better understand nursing responsibilities. The first few times all department representatives meet to discuss system needs may be like hungry lions sharing a meal. A mediator can be essential. An effective mediator can help create a spirit of cooperation and a vision of how the rest of the hospital operates, greatly facilitating the implementation process. Ultimately, one person should be responsible for seeing that decisions are made and are made appropriately.

Decision Maker. The role of decision maker during the implementation of a system is highly important. The input of many people must be considered, because the outcome affects the entire institution. A nurse with authority to make decisions is essential to keep the project moving forward. Knowing hospital policies and procedures aids the nurse during the decision-making process. Questions to be answered in decision making center on access to information:

- Who are the authorized users?
- Who should print reports? Where? When?
- Will nursing enter orders of ward clerks?
- What is the sign-off process?
- Will orders be held in the system until a RN reviews them?
- Or will orders be automatically released to the ancillary with verification taking place later?

These questions are just a few examples that require decisions. Ultimately, one person should be responsible to make sure that decisions are made, and should be held accountable for them.

Politician/Marketeer. The nurse's role as marketeer of the system should be a fun one. It is the responsibility of nursing to propagate positive information, solicit support, and promote the system. There are no hard-and-fast rules to follow to make this role successful. A feeling of ownership of the system clearly helps in establishing a positive attitude toward the system. Getting people involved is imperative, but also difficult when considering the activity and workload that occur in a hospital. Videotapes, buttons, and coffee socials are all methods of encouraging staff participation and support of the system. Skepticism may be prevalent initially, but curiosity usually overcomes the skeptics and there is opportunity to get everyone involved.

Keys to a Successful Implementation

All the roles the nurse play during a system implementation have an impact on how well the system is received and utilized by the entire hospital staff. For the implementation to be truly successful, six key factors must be in place.

1. Make sure nursing is involved in the decision-making process of the HIS selection. If hospital administration makes an independent decision without consulting nursing, system implementation can be greatly inhibited. The system will change how nurses create orders, generate staffing needs, and communicate with ancillaries.

2. Solicit upper-management support. Strong support from upper management positively impacts the implementation process. Nurses feel more confident and are more open to change if they know management is supporting their decisions. A positive attitude at the top will generate a positive attitude throughout the institution.

3. Make sure that the time schedule is appropriate for success. Ask questions to determine whether adequate time has been allotted:

    What is the commitment of the hospital?
    Is staffing adequate for training and coverage?
    Does the hospital want to implement the system on one or multiple pilot units?
    Does the hospital want to implement the system in one ancillary at a time or in multiple ancillaries?

    The action plan should be closely coordinated with the vendor. It is important to define the responsibilities of the hospital staff and the vendor up front.

4. Realize that mindset and attitudes can make or break a system. If the leaders of each unit are upbeat and enthusiastic, their positive attitudes will create a general feeling of security and support. No implementation is problem free. Every implementation presents different challenges, but all problems can be overcome by working as a team.

5. Designate a liaison person from the hospital. Nursing representatives are often the best candidates for this key role. The selected nurse should preferably be one who understands the hospital's

policies and procedures and who has the authority to make decisions. Subcommittees and working committees are great, but tend to drag out the decision-making process and can delay the installation of a system. Nurses can accurately define the requirements of a system to meet the needs of the nursing department. Nurses also add valuable experience of interaction with ancillaries, administration, and physicians.

6. Highlight communication as an essential ingredient in the implementation process. Keeping the right people informed is a monumental task, but one that should be addressed. Weekly or monthly newsletters and/or meetings can be instrumental in a successful implementation. Misinterpretation of issues is decreased and negative rumors are squelched. The project will also be more focused on critical issues that need immediate attention and resolution.

New Opportunities for Nurses

The increasing involvement of nurses in the implementation of hospital information systems may be partially responsible for the current shortage of hospital nurses. Today, nurses are moving away from the bedside and into the boardroom. In some major metropolitan areas, per diem nurses are earning up to $24 per hour. Certainly there are at least as many nurses graduating from school today as there were 10 years ago, and there are more professional working women than ever before. Where are these nurses going and why?

Many nurses are choosing to use their hard-earned degrees and experience to move into the business side of the health care industry. They are putting away their white caps and shoes, donning business suits, and entering the health care market through a different door. This seems to be a natural path for many nurses, as they are familiar with the process, politics, and terminology that occur in a hospital. This can be accomplished in many different ways and through many different roles.

Some are taking the experience they have gained from being part of an implementation team of an HIS, updating their resumes, and joining the corporate world. Others are part of the increasing enrollment in master's programs for computer sciences. It doesn't require technical brilliance to earn a degree in "Management Information Systems." This is just what it implies—managing information—and it's making nurses marketable in the computer health care industry.

The computer industry is fast paced and forever changing—not an unfamiliar situation for nurses. Unlike nursing, it offers many opportunities for growth and promotion in a short period of time. Nurses associated with the computer industry can impact bedside nursing by facilitating the information process relating to patient care.

Nurses never give themselves credit for the multifaceted roles they play every day. They have marketable skills of which they are not even aware. They are analysts, consultants, politicians, and problem solvers. They are also logical thinkers and skilled communicators with experience in priorization and organization. These roles nurses fulfill in traditional patient care areas can effectively be transferred to the computer health care industry.

Analyst. Nurses are trained to observe, to make decisions, and to act on decisions. Nurses have trained eyes for clinical and psychosocial situations. They have been taught to analyze the situation thoroughly before making those critical decisions. They are adept in dealing with change—they do so every day. They have learned to be nonjudgmental and to ask critical questions to get to the heart of the matter. In short, nurses are analytical. Their skills translate well to the role an analyst plays in the implementation process. An analyst must logically look at how the system works and how the hospital will be impacted. Together, the hospital representative and the analyst make decisions as to the least intrusive method to accomplish any modifications that are required.

Programmer. Nurses who enjoy the technical side of nursing—where things are concrete, and planned actions produce anticipated results—may be interested in learning to program. Many of the analytical skills developed through bedside nursing can be transferred, but some structured training is usually required to become a programmer. This is a highly sought-after combination in the health care computer marketplace today. It is much easier to teach a nurse how to program than it is to teach a programmer about the inner workings of a hospital. Nurses quickly lose their stereotype in this industry, but learn to keep an aspirin bottle handy for colleagues who come to them for a "professional" opinion on everyday maladies.

Consultant. The doors are beginning to open for nursing in the consulting field. Almost every hospital purchasing an information system today is using a consultant to aid in the selection process. Consulting is a multimillion dollar business. The nurse is the best resource for determining a hospital's needs and deciding what vendor meets those needs. Consulting contracts range from remote question and answer support to extensive analysis of the current workflow and requirements of a hospital. Extended contracts may include long-range planning and marketing tactics for the hospital to employ in attracting patients to their facility. Nurses provide expert assistance in determing system requirements for a hospital. The nurse's ability to take a large amount of data and organize it into a "big picture" is a positive asset in the consulting field. A certain level of detail is required, but the key is to take all the pieces and assimilate them into a big picture concept.

Developer. Experience gained from being part of an installation team (either the hospital side or the vendor side) provides credentials to develop new systems. The development of a system requires a healthy balance of technical expertise and practical user experience. The technical design by programmers is important to ensure efficiency of computer resources without degrading response time. Nurses can provide the workflow design and requirements of a system, as well as contribute to the human factor influence of how the screens should be designed. Neither side can work independently in a vacuum. Teamwork is essential to provide success of a newly developed system.

Sales/Sales Support. Nurses provide a tremendous amount of credibility and knowledge of hospitals in the sales cycle of an HIS. Health care professionals feel more comfortable talking to peers who understand the issues facing hospitals today. Medical jargon can be overwhelming to a nonhospital person. Nurses provide the link of interpretation and commmunication between the nonhospital person (sales representative) and the hospital professional. Other sales skills that nurses possess include the ability to handle many different personalities and to use different approaches with people as the situation dictates. Product demonstrations require knowledge of that product as well as teaching skills that nurses have practiced and perfected over the years.

Marketeer. Nurses can apply their creative side to marketing special products or total hospital information systems. The strengths of interpreting medical terminology and knowing what hospitals want to hear will assist any business in appealing to the marketplace. Having an inside track to the future of hospitals makes nurses a valuable commodity. Suggestions to help develop some background with computers include

- attending health care computer trade shows
- subscribing to journals (these will identify trade show dates and locations)
- getting involved in a hospital system implementation as an insider
- attending classes at the local community college or university
- joining a local network group (in larger cities, nursing groups exist that are predominantly computer-oriented).

Summary

Nurses today have the opportunity to affect health care in many ways. They may choose to remain at the bedside, using handheld terminals to deliver better care. They may elect to enter into the decision-making arena, working to integrate information systems. Or they may move over into the corporate world and represent the interests of health care there. But wherever nurses go, the computer will not be far away. Nurses will become more and more involved with information management and the technologies that support it.

Questions

1. Identify three roles the nurse can play during a system implementation.

2. Identify four key factors to ensure a successful implementation.

3. Assimilate the nursing process (assess, plan, implement, and evaluate) with the implementation of a computer system.

4. Name four new career avenues for the professional nurse.

6—The Nursing Function in Designing Health Care Information Systems

Karen D. Lafferty and S. Denni Sheffield

Introduction

In recent articles and seminars on the subject of nursing automation, there is a recurring theme: "We in nursing should no longer ask if we should automate, but when." The intent of this popular phrase is to inspire nursing activism in the age of automation.

It is interesting to note that a profession oriented toward deliberate interventions to achieve measurable results would pose such an undefined strategy. Does this strategy infer automation for automation's sake, regardless of potential benefit? Further, does this strategy infer that we simply automate a manual nursing process complete with redundancies, lack of nursing definition, and as many different interpretations of nursing practice as there are practitioners? Perhaps a more pragmatic rhetoric would be: "We in nursing need to decide not only when to automate, but what should be automated."

Perhaps not all components of nursing practice can or should be automated. Not only are there issues of ready access to terminals and the method of data entry (which are being addressed by a few companies with handheld terminals or bedside terminals and light pen or touch data entry), but there are many other significant concerns. These include:

- What is "practical" and "beneficial" information to be entered into a computer?

- Can the information be entered into the system as quickly as written on a well-designed flowsheet charting tool, and if not, who is caring for the patient while the nurse is entering data?

- How efficiently and effectively can the data be maintained by the nurse in the dynamic arena of patient care?

- Who benefits from the information entered?

- What kind of tools does the computer afford the nurse in providing patient care?

"Prospective reimbursement demands for cost accounting at the individual patient, diagnosis, and nursing task level have substantially defined what a nursing information system is and should be, before nursing research has had time to develop a conceptual model" (Lenkman, 1985, p. 577).

In today's health care environment, attention must be focused on the development of information systems that effectively balance the needs of the nursing care provider with the needs of nursing administration. Who are those responsible for making these many decisions? Who is responsible for designing nursing computer systems that are currently available in the marketplace? Essentially, software vendors are taking on the role of direction setters for automated nursing information systems. But how are vendors making the design decisions for the development of current and future nursing software?

Design of the System

Most hospital systems purchased today are turnkey systems, meaning the design of the system is basically preestablished. The hospital determines the content of files, tables, and to a lesser extent, the screens. For illustrative purposes, let us explore in a practical way what is meant by setting a direction for the design of nursing information systems.

The information system vendor will determine that the design of the patient plan of care, for example, will incorporate a particular nursing model. The design will further allow a variety of functions, such as the initiation, modification, and evaluation of a care plan. The flow of the screens is predetermined by the software delivered by the vendor. The screen design is somewhat more user defined, depending on the vendor selected, but many times the vendor's software mandates meeting certain requirements; i.e., a screen of two columns, 20 items per column, 35 characters per item. The user then determines the actual items and where they are to be placed on the screen, which minimizes the vendor's role in dictating the practice of nursing.

The vendor's software is typically already defined with extremely important help screens and from where they may be accessed, user instructions for using the screens, and in many cases, what information is available to the nurse for inquiry during the care planning process, what ancillary information can be integrated into the care planning process without redundant entry, and what the actual care plan presentation looks like on the screen and in printed form.

A multitude of other design decisions have been made before the system is delivered to the health care facility. A few more general examples include the duration of time in which the care plan will be available on line after the patient has been discharged, the specific patient population supported by care planning software (e.g., perhaps only inpatients), and whether or not discharge care planning uses the same inpatient care plan design or a design more specific to its unique requirements.

Within this brief overview, it is clear that software vendors are making major design decisions regarding available software in the marketplace today. It is not within the scope of this article to evaluate this process. Rather, it is the objective of this article to present a profile of those responsible for providing leadership in the design of the nursing applications developed by leading hospital information system companies.

Several articles are available advising nursing administrators on the selection of information systems. Some appear elsewhere in this book. Others are cited in the selected bibliography, representing various opinions on important systems selection criteria. The credentials of the vendor's staff, especially the design and support staff, should be a major consideration. The vendor's design philosophy should also be considered.

In a more global sense, nursing as an organized professional group needs to recognize the importance of the role of nurses within the vendor ranks, not only to support that role but to assist in its direction. "There is a certain reluctance within nursing circles to see nurses in vendor roles as working toward mutual professional goals. If nurse vendors of information systems are not seen as peers supporting identical professional goals and objectives as nursing administrators, much valuable time and information can be lost" (Lenkman, 1985, p. 564).

The Nursing Dimension in System Design

Designers, installers, product line managers, and users and promoters of hospital information systems are often curious about and sometimes stymied by the design of a product for hospital users. It is not always possible to feel confident that an expert in the clinical specialty for which the system was developed played an integral role in developing, designing, and testing of that computer application.

To profile those responsible for influencing nursing development within the framework of hospital information systems (HIS) vendors, 13 leading HIS vendors were contacted. Ten agreed to participate in the interview process. The interview was conducted with the designated person most involved in the design of the vendor's nursing information system. Thirty questions were posed to each interviewee for response. A majority of these questions are represented directly in the three matrices and narrative that follow.

Background of Vendor Representatives

In the following matrix, the credentials of those influencing nursing information system design are presented. Additionally, the interviews revealed that 7 of 10 interviewees approached their current employer versus other methods for securing their positions. The overall theme when asked what specific systems training was acquired, in order to secure these influential positions within the organization, was that additional coursework was specifically sought on an individual basis and/or experience had been acquired on the job, sponsored by the current or previous vendor. The specific results of this interview segment are given in Table 6-1.

Vendor Background

Table 6-2 presents a profile of the various HIS companies interviewed. This profile reveals basic components of design philosophy practiced by the respective vendors. In addition, information is provided about the development direction of these leading vendors.

Nursing Involvement in Product Design

Table 6-3 reflects nursing involvement in three key areas of system design. The percentage of the total research and development budget dedicated to nursing information systems provides insights into the perceived importance of the nursing information system to the overall success of the HIS by the respective company's upper management.

These data may also provide an indication as to the quality of nursing information systems to be expected over the next several years. It was revealed in this segment of the interviews that although several vendors are currently focusing on completing current installations of financially oriented products, other companies are concentrating on completing the development cycle of the nursing management product, as well as linking financial and clinical data into an integrated data base.

Summary

It is clear from the profile of leading vendors of hospital information systems and from the bibliographic resources that nurses are actively involved in today's design decisions for nursing information systems. The backgrounds of these decision makers vary greatly, bringing a diversity of clinical and educational experiences to the task.

The data collection results provide some generalizations that describe nurses in the vendor role:

Table 6-1
Profiles of the Nursing System Designers

Vendors	1	2	3	4	5
Title	(Product) Nursing advisor	Marketing clinical product specialist	Product manager	Marketing consultant	Product manager
Credentials	RN	RN	RN	RN	RN
Degree	BSN, MSN	BSN[a]	0[b]	BSN[c]	BSN, MBA
Publications	Yes	No	No	No	No
Years of health care experience/positions	12 (staff nurse; home health coordinator; assistant director of nursing)	18 (staff nurse; consultant; education coordinator; unit manager)	11 (staff nurse; computer project team leader)	4 (staff nurse; inservice educator)	11 (staff nurse; nurse; operating room director)
Years of health care systems experience	5 (3 years with current company)	6 (4 years with current company)	9 (7 years with current company)	1 (1 year with current company)	3 (2 years with current company)
Was previous position systems related?	Yes	Yes	Yes	No	No

[a] MBA coursework completed.
[b] Coursework: BSN.
[c] Coursework: MBA.
[d] Coursework: MBA.
[e] Coursework: Ph.D.

Table 6-1 (*continued*)

Vendors	6	7	8	9	10
Title	Director of development	Corporate marketing manager	Clinical health care specialist	Director of clinical system design	Director of professional services
Credentials	RN	0	RN	RN	RN
Degree	BSN, MSN	BS	BS[d]	BSN, MSN[e]	BSN, MN
Publications	No	Yes	No	Yes	Yes
Years of health care experience/positions	25 (staff nurse)	3 (admitting clerk; supervisor)	6.5 (staff nurse)	13 (instructor; researcher; systems liaison)	18 (staff nurse; administrator; researcher; instructor; consultant)
Years of health care systems experience	7 (5 years with current company)	8 (5 years with current company)	3 (3 years with current company)	9 (3 years with current company)	3 (3 years with current company)
Was previous position systems related?	Yes	Yes	No	Yes	No

Table 6-2
Profiles of the Hospital Information System Vendors

Vendors	1	2	3	4	5
Size of company	1,800	650	600	300	40,000
Number of RNs	N/A[a]	14	20	13	3
Number of MSNs	N/A	2	2	0	1
Number of DNSc	N/A	0	2	0	0
Other health care staff	Laboratory, radiology, pharmacy, medical records, patient accounting	Laboratory, radiology, pharmacy, respiratory therapy	Laboratory, radiology, pharmacy, physical therapy	Laboratory, radiology, pharmacy, medical records, physical therapy	Laboratory, pharmacy, medical records
Market size (beds)	700–2,000 +	150–650	100	45–500	200–1,000
Client base (accounts)	11	275	85	210	30–40
Applications available[b]	1, 3, 4, 5, 6, 7, 9, 10, 11, 13, 14, 15	1, 2, 6, 7, 8, 9, 11, 12, 13, 14	1, 3, 4, 6, 7, 9, 11, 13, 14, 15	1, 5, 7, 9, 11, 13, 15, 17	1, 4, 5, 6, 7, 9, 11, 12, 13, 14, 15, 17
Applications in development	12, 16	10, 16, 17	16, 17	N/A	16
Applications scheduled for development	2, 8, 16	4, 16	8, 16	N/A	N/A

[a] N/A, data not available.

[b] Applications symbols defined:

1 Admission/Discharge/Transfer	9 Order Communication
2 Bedside Support	10 PC Interface
3 Decision Support	11 Pharmacy
4 Dietary	12 Quality Assurance
5 Laboratory	13 Radiology
6 Medical Records	14 Utilization Review
7 Nursing Management (Care Plan, Acuity,	15 Financial Management
Staffing and Scheduling, Kardex)	16 Enhancement of Existing Applications
8 Operating Room Management	17 Other.

Table 6-2 (*continued*)

Vendors	6	7	8	9	10
Size of company	26	160	3,000–4,000	160	100
Number of RNs	1	7	3–5	10	20
Number of MSNs	0	0	2	3	3
Number of DNSc	0	0	0	0	0
Other health care staff	Medical records	Laboratory, pharmacy	Medical records, patient accounting	Laboratory, radiology, pharmacy, dietary, physical therapy	Laboratory, pharmacy, physician, occupational therapy, respiratory therapy, administrator
Market size (beds)	75–300	No limits	>200	>300	>200
Client base (accounts)	17	32	4	65	12
Applications available	1, 6, 9, 11, 14, 15, 17	1, 4, 5, 6, 7, 8, 9, 10, 11, 12, 13, 14, 15	1, 6, 7, 9, 15, 17	1, 4, 6, 7, 9, 11, 12, 13, 14, 15	1, 2, 3, 5, 6, 7, 9, 10, 11, 12, 13, 14
Applications in development	16	16	16	2, 16	16, 17
Applications scheduled for development	7, 16	3, 16	17	16	17

Table 6-3
Nursing Involvement in Product Design

Vendors	1	2	3	4	5	6	7	8	9	10
Are nurses involved in writing specifications?	Yes	Yes	Yes	Yes	Yes	Yes	Yes	Yes	Yes	Yes
Are nurses involved in designing screens?	Yes	Yes	Yes	Yes	Yes	Yes	Yes	Yes	Yes	Yes
Are nurses involved in writing documentation?	Yes, review and edit documentation; written by technical writers	Yes	Yes	No; written by technical writers	Yes	Yes	Yes	No	No	Yes
Percent of research and development budget dedicated to development of nursing products	20–25%	50%	10%	N/A[a]	N/A	66%	15%	N/A	N/A	100% through 1986

[a]N/A, data not available.

- Nurse decision makers in the vendor role are highly motivated to initiate advanced and specialized coursework related to computerization. A high degree of motivation is also evidenced by the many who are published authors and by the approach utilized by the nurse decision makers in securing their role with the vendor.

- The average number of years invested by these decision makers in their respective organizations is approximately 4.5. This reflects a high degree of commitment to the task on the part of the nurse decision makers, as well as on that of the vendor in supporting these roles.

- The nurse decision makers have an average of 12 years of health care experience. This provides a strong representation of clinically based goals for the design of nursing information systems.

This is especially important when considering that "the screen design must involve organizing data specific to the intended end users. The data must be presented in a meaningful way. This means that HIS screens should consider the way medical professionals think" (MacArthur and Sampson, 1985, p. 474).

Mychelle Mowry of Health Data Sciences Corporation (HDS) agrees. She states that design decisions at HDS are a collaborative effort among the large percentage of clinical staff employed by the company. Ms. Mowry emphasizes that the nurses at HDS have an average of 18 years of clinical, educational, or administrative experience in nursing and that HDS prioritizes a commanding knowledge of the nursing process among required traits of nurses employed.

The evidence indicates that highly motivated, articulate, and qualified nurses are having an impact on the design and direction of nursing information systems.

References Cited

Lenkman S: Management information systems and the role of the nurse vendor. *Nursing Clinics of North America* 1985; 20:557–565.
MacArthur AM, Sampson MR: Screen design of a hospital information system. *Nursing Clinics of North America* 1985; 20:471–486.

Bibliography

Anreoli K, Musser L: Computers in nursing care: the state of the art. *Nursing Outlook* 1985; 33:16–21.
Bursley HM, Tindal CL: Using nursing expertise for non-nursing computer systems. *Nursing Clinics of North America* 1985; 20:595–603.

Ginsburg DA, Browning SJ: Selecting automated patient care systems. *Journal of Nursing Administration* 1985; 15:16–21.

Hales GD: Shopping for hardware. *American Journal of Nursing* 1984; 84:1292, 1294.

Hoffman FM: Evaluating and selecting a computer software package. *Journal of Nursing Aministration* 1985; 15:33–35.

Lafferty KD: Patient care systems versus financial systems: the cost justification battle. *Nursing Management* 1987; 18:51–55.

Mowry MM, Korpman RA: Evaluating automated information systems. *Nursing Economics* 1987; 5:7–12.

Romano CA: Development, implementation, and utilization of a computerized information system. *Nursing Administration Quarterly* 1986; 10:1–9.

Schmitz HH, Ura S: New technology considerations in system selection. *Software in Healthcare* 1985; 3:14–15.

Zielstorff RD: Cost effectiveness of computerization in nursing practice and administration. *Journal of Nursing Administration* 1985; 15:22–26.

7—The Integration of Hospital Information Systems into Nursing Practice: A Literature Review

Kristen H. Kjerulff

Introduction

When a hospital information system (HIS) is implemented, the nursing department is frequently the last department, or one of the last, to begin using the system. A recent survey indicates that with only 20% of currently implemented HIS is there nursing interaction. Of that 20%, one-fourth have computer systems with specific applications for nursing such as patient classification systems, nursing notes, or nursing care plans (Grams, 1983). Thus, only about 5% of American hospitals have computer systems with specific nursing applications.

Research Studies

Although a nursing department is often slow to begin using an HIS, the nursing literature is replete with articles extolling the benefits nursing departments have derived from utilizing the information and capabilities an HIS can provide (Blaufuss, 1986; Cook, 1982; Edmunds, 1982, 1985; Hambley, 1985; Muirhead, 1982; Pluyter-Wenting et al, 1986; Skydell and Stone, 1986).

There are enough fully functioning HIS sites with extensive nursing use to document and validate the notion that computers can be a useful part of a hospital nursing practice. The National Institutes of Health (NIH) in the Washington, D.C., area and El Camino Hospital in California are two well-known and highly publicized sites.

The Impact of Computerization on Clinical Nursing

Numerous studies have examined changes in the percentage of time nurses allocate to various activities as a function of the implementation of some type of information system (Barrett, 1975; Farlee and Goldstein, 1972; Schmitz et al, 1976; Simborg et al, 1972; Tolbert and Pertuz, 1977). All of these studies report significant decreases in time spent on clerical activities. Only one of these studies found a significant increase in direct patient care activities (Simborg et al, 1972). In general, nurses seem to utilize their increased free time by spreading it out across all other nursing activities so that there is no category of activity that changes significantly. Although it is interesting to note that information systems decrease nursing time spent in clerical activities, it is not particularly surprising. It is much more pertinent to ask how an information system affects patient care.

One study reports that a ward information management system resulted in a significant decrease in errors in carrying out physicians' orders (Simborg et al, 1972). A second study compared a computerized versus a noncomputerized cardiac ICU (Tolbert and Pertuz, 1977). The two ICUs were carefully matched for staffing and patient characteristics. This study indicated that nurses spent less time in direct patient care activities, and more idle time, on the computerized unit. However, patients on the computerized unit had shorter lengths of stay. There was also "evidence of earlier recognition of cardiac arrhythmias and finer hemostatic monitoring (resulting in better blood management)" on the computerized ICU (Tolbert and Pertuz, p. 84).

Clearly a well-designed and implemented HIS should improve the quality and quantity of patient information available to medical professionals. The nursing literature reports increased legibility of patient records (Beckman et al, 1981; Brennan, 1983; Greene et al, 1982), more complete records (Brennan, 1983; Greene et al, 1982; Cook, 1974), and more organized patient records (Martin, 1982).

If computerization appears to be beneficial to patients, nursing staffs, and hospitals, why are there computerized nursing systems in only 5% of American hospitals? There are many factors that can account for this low rate, particularly the lack of appropriate software (Study Group, 1983) and a hesitancy on the part of hospitals to invest the amount of money needed for clinical systems. It has also been suggested that nurses have not been, in the past, overwhelmingly enthusiastic about the use of computers as part of nursing's clinical practice (Rosenberg et al, 1967; Hannah, 1976; Grobe, 1984).

The Attitudes of Nurses and Nursing Students toward Computers

Early research on attitudes found nurses and nursing students markedly negative toward computers (Reznikoff et al, 1967; Friel et al, 1969; Rosenberg et al, 1967). In more recent studies, nurses and nursing students were less positive toward computers than were medical students or faculty (Startsman and Robinson, 1972; Thies, 1975). A replication of the Startsman study reported that nursing students were more positive toward computers than any other group, although nurses were the least positive (Melhorn et al, 1979).

Several studies have examined attitudes toward computers among occupational groups using an HIS. Findings have been contradictory. Barrett (1975) reported that nurses were the group most positive toward computers, while Edwards and Shartiag (1973) found that nurses were the least positive toward the HIS in comparison to other occupational groups.

Studies examining attitude change over time in relation to the implementation of a particular HIS report present conflicting results. Results range from a reported increase in favorability over time (Barrett, 1975) to a decrease in favorability over time (Counte et al, 1984; Thies, 1975; Farlee and Goldstein, 1972).

Individual Differences in Attitude

Although there has been at least a moderate amount of research examining the impact of computerization on clinical nursing practice, there has been very little research focusing on individual differences in the use of an HIS among nurses. However, several studies report marked individual differences in HIS use among physicians (Anderson et al, 1981, 1985, 1986; Dlugacz et al, 1981, 1982).

Research on physician attitudes indicates the influence of social networks on patterns of adoption of medical innovations (Coleman et al, 1966; Counte and Kimberly, 1974). A study of physicians' positions in the referral and consultation network indicated that they were a major predictor of medical information system use (Anderson and Jay, 1984).

Possibly nurses have less freedom than physicians in choosing not to use an HIS or to use it in idiosyncratic ways, but anecdotal evidence suggests that some nurses refuse to use an HIS for extensive periods after implementation (Farlee and Goldstein, 1972). Research on adaptation to MIS among clerical employees indicates considerable variability in use of the system, incorporation of the system into clerical work, and perceived problems with the system (Kjerulff et al, 1982, 1983). Some employees persisted in using the manual system long after the MIS had been fully implemented. Anecdotal evidence indicated that the attitudes of the department directors seemed to have a major impact on adaptation patterns exhibited by employees in various hospital departments. If clerical employees exhibit considerable variability in use of an HIS, it is logical to assume that nurses will also exhibit variability in use and adaptation to HIS, particularly since nurses have considerable professional autonomy as to how they perform their jobs.

A study measuring adaptation to an HIS among nurses reported that there were considerable variations in compliance with medication orders and strong differences as a function of nursing units (Farlee and Goldstein ,1972). Two studies also examined the impact of the type of nursing unit on changes in time allocated to various nursing activities as a function of implementation of an HIS (Farlee and Goldstein, 1972; Barrett, 1975); both reported differences between units. A study at El Camino Hospital found significant differences between units in terms of the impacts of several very sophisticated HIS nursing subsystems, including a nursing care plan subsystem and a patient care audit subsystem (Gall, 1980).

Current Research

Kjerulff and colleagues are currently studying the impact of an HIS on nine nursing units at the University of Maryland Hospital. The primary goal of this research, funded by the National Center for Health Services Research, is to examine the process of incorporating an HIS into nursing practice. Because HIS are generally implemented in stages, with implementation occurring over the course of several years, this study will follow the same nurses through the entire implementation process. Nursing attitudes toward the system, use of the system, problems and perceived benefits, and utility of each aspect of the HIS will be measured after each component is implemented. In addition this study will measure changes in the way that the nurses process patient information, changes in the organizational structure of the nursing units, and changes in the way that nurses use the HIS as they become more comfortable with it.

Because nursing units differ greatly in the type of nursing required and the demands made on the nursing staff, a variety of unit level characteristics such as patient acuity levels, nursing hours per patient day, and complexity of patient needs are also being measured. In this way it will be possible to relate differences in nursing unit characteristics to differences in use of the system across units. Preliminary evidence suggests that the nursing units differ markedly in the extent to which they regularly do care planning, discharge planning, and ordering of medications, tests, and procedures for their patients. Clearly these types of differences should affect the use that the different units make of the HIS and the perceived utility of its various functions.

Hospital information systems with nursing-specific functions, such as care planning and nurse documentation, clearly have the potential to decrease the amount of time nurses spend in clerical activities and make life easier for nurses in many respects. The extent to which nurses are able to realize these benefits will depend on the extent to which they utilize fully this new technology and incorporate it into nursing practice.

Questions

1. Select and read one of the major research topics referenced in this paper and be prepared to lead a discussion for your class.

2. Put together a brief questionnaire addressing the questions in which you yourself are interested regarding the use of computers in nursing practice, education, research, or administration (no more than five questions). Have your classmates answer them and do a mini-analysis on data gathered.

3. Formulate a well-thought-out research topic you think should be addressed pertaining to the use of computers in nursing. This might be a dissertation topic.

References

Anderson JG, Jay SJ: The diffusion of computer applications in medicine: the relative impact of network location on innovation adoption. In: Cohen GS, ed. *Proceedings of the Eighth Annual Symposium on Computer Applications in Medical Care.* Washington, DC: IEEE Computer Society, 1984; 549–552.

Anderson JG, Gray-Toft P, Lloyd FP, et al: Factors affecting physician utilization of a computerized hospital information system: a social network analysis. In: Heffernan HG, ed. *Proceedings of the Fifth Annual Symposium on Computer Applications in Medical Care.* New York: IEEE Computer Society, 1981; 791–796.

Anderson JG, Jay SJ, Schweer HM, et al: Perceptions of the impact of computers on medical practice and physician use of a hospital information system. In: Ackerman MJ, ed. *Proceedings of the Ninth Annual Symposium on Computer Applications in Medical Care.* Washington, DC: IEEE Computer Society, 1985; 565–569.

Anderson JG, Jay S, Schweer H, et al: The role of communication networks in physicians' adoption and utilization of computer technology. In: Salamon R, Blum B, Jorgensen M, eds. *MEDINFO 86—Proceedings of the Fifth Conference on Medical Informatics.* Vol. 5. Amsterdam: North Holland, 1986; 1052–1056.

Barrett JP: *Evaluation of the Implementation of a Medical Information System in a General Community Hospital: Final Report* (NTIS #PB-248 340). Columbus: Battelle-Columbus Laboratories, 1975.

Beckman E, Cammack BF, Harris B: Observation on computers in an intensive care unit. *Heart and Lung Journal* 1981; 10:1055–1057.

Blaufuss J: Promoting the nursing process through computerization. In: Salamon R, Blum B, Jorgensen M, eds. *MEDINFO 86—Proceedings of the Fifth Conference on Medical Informatics.* Vol. 5. Amsterdam: North Holland, 1986; 585–586.

Brennan LE: Computerized, professionalized, utilized. In: Dayhoff RE, ed. *Proceedings of the Seventh Annual Symposium on Computer Applications in Medical Care.* Silver Spring: IEEE Computer Society, 1983; 556–560.

Coleman JS, Katz E, Menzel H: *Medical Innovation: A Diffusion Study.* Indianapolis: Bobbs-Merrill, 1966.

Cook M: Introduction of a user-oriented THIS [Total Hospital Information System] into a community hospital setting—nursing. In: Anderson J, Forsythe JM, eds. *MEDINFO 74—Proceedings of the First World Conference on Medical Informatics.* Amsterdam: North Holland, 1974; 303–304.

Cook M: Using computers to enhance professional practice. *Nursing Times* 1982; 78:1542–1544.

Counte MA, Kimberly JR: Organizational innovation in a professionally dominated system: responses of physicians to a new program in medical education. *Journal of Health and Social Behavior* 1974; 14:188–198.

Counte MA, Kjerulff KH, Salloway JC, et al: Implementing computerization in hospitals: a case study of the behavioral and attitudinal impacts of a medical information system. *Journal of Organizational Behavior Management* 1984; 6:109–122.

Dlugacz YD, Siegel D, Fischer S: Physician/computer interaction. In: Heffernan HG, ed. *Proceedings of the Fifth Annual Symposium on Computer Applications in Medical Care.* New York: IEEE Computer Society, 1981; 797–801.

Dlugacz YD, Siegel C, Fischer S: Receptivity toward uses of a new computer application in medicine. In: Blum BI, ed. *Proceedings of the Sixth Annual Symposium on Computer Applications in Medical Care.* New York: IEEE Computer Society, 1982; 384–391.

Edmunds L: Computer assisted nursing care. *American Journal of Nursing* 1982; 82:1076–1079.

Edmunds L: Hospital information systems for nursing problems and possibilities. In: Ackerman MJ, ed. *Proceedings of the Ninth Annual Symposium on Computer Applications in Medical Care.* Washington, DC: IEEE Computer Society, 1985; 785–789.

Edwards SA, Shartiag J: *Demonstration and Evaluation Results: Final Report* (HSM.110.70.368). Vol. 1. Chicago: Health Services Research Center of the Hospital Research and Educational Trust and Northwestern University, 1973.

Farlee C, Goldstein B: *Hospital Organization and Computer Technology: the Challenge of Change: Final Report* (NTIS #PB 80.188 287). New Brunswick: Rutgers University Press, 1972.

Friel PB, Reznikoff M, Rosenberg M: Attitudes toward computers among nursing personnel in a general hospital. *Connecticut Medicine* 1969; 33:307–308.

Gall JE: *A Patient Care Quality Assurance System: Final Report* (#HS02027). Hyattsville: National Center for Health Services Research, 1980.

Grams R: *National Survey of Hospital Data Processing.* Gainesville: University of Florida, 1983.

Greene R, Karr H, Likely N, et al: Computer and patients: the user system. *Canadian Nurse* 1982; 78:34–36.

Grobe SJ: Conquering computer cowardice. *Journal of Nursing Education* 1984; 23:232–239.

Hambley S: Using the microcomputer for nursing care plans. In: Ackerman MJ, ed. *Proceedings of the Ninth Annual Symposium on Computer Applications in Medical Care.* Washington, DC: IEEE Computer Society, 1985; 763–767.

Hannah K: The computer and nursing practice. *Nursing Outlook* 1976; 24:555–558.

Kjerulff KH, Counte MA, Salloway JC, et al: Predicting employee adaptation to the implementation of a medical information system. In: Blum BI, ed. *Proceedings of the Sixth Annual Symposium on Computer Applications in Medical Care.* New York: IEEE Computer Society, 1982; 392–397.

Kjerulff KH, Counte MA, Salloway JC, et al: Measuring adaptation to medical technology. *Hospital and Health Services Administration* 1983; 28:30–40.

Martin K: A client classification system adaptable for computerization. *Nursing Outlook* 1982; 30:515–517.

Melhorn JM, Legler WK, Clark GM: Current attitudes of medical personnel toward computers. *Computers and Biomedical Research* 1979; 12:327–334.

Muirhead R: Happening now: the decline and fall of paperwork. *RN* 1982; 45:35–40.

Pluyter-Wenting E, Bakker A, Nieman H: Computers in nursing practice: why? In: Salamon R, Blum B, Jorgensen M, eds. *MEDINFO 86—Proceedings of the Fifth Conference on Medical Informatics.* Vol. 5. Amsterdam: North Holland, 1986; 597–601.

Reznikoff M, Holland C, Stroebel C: Attitudes toward computers among employees of a psychiatric hospital. *Mental Hygiene* 1967; 51:419–425.

Rosenberg M, Reznikoff M, Stroebel CF, et al: Attitudes of nursing students toward computers. *Nursing Outlook* 1967; 15:44–46.

Schmitz HH, Ellerbrake RP, Williams TM: Study evaluated effects of new communication system. *Hospitals* 1976; 50:129–134.

Simborg DW, MacDonald LK, Leibman JS, et al: Ward information management system—an evaluation. *Computers and Biomedical Research* 1972; 5:484–497.

Skydell B, Stone E: Using hospital case mix data bases to manage nursing services. In: Salamon R, Blum B, Jorgensen M, eds. *MEDINFO 86—Proceedings of the Fifth Conference on Medical Informatics.* Vol. 5. Amsterdam: North Holland, 1986; 587–591.

Startsman TS, Robinson RE: The attitudes of medical and paramedical personnel toward computers. *Computers and Biomedical Research* 1972; 5:213–227.

Study Group: Special report: computerized nursing information systems: an urgent need. *Research in Nursing and Health* 1983; 6:101–105.

Thies JB: Hospital personnel and computer-based system: a study of attitudes and perceptions. *Hospital Administration* 1975; 20:17–26.

Tolbert SH, Pertuz AH: Study shows how computerization affects nursing activities in ICU. *Hospitals* 1977; 51:79–84.

Section 2—Where Caring and Technology Meet

Unit 3—Research Frontiers

Unit Introduction

In this section we explore the **R** of the **CARE** acronym—Research Frontiers. Jacox and Meyer-Petrucci address the matter of support for research in nursing informatics. Hannah provides an overview and categorization for the various types of decision support systems. In the final two chapters, Brennan explores the concept of decision modeling and Ozbolt describes the use of knowledge-based decision support for clinical nursing practice.

1—Support for Research in Computer Applications in Nursing

Ada K. Jacox and Kerry E. Meyer-Petrucci

Introduction

In many respects, the coming of age of nursing research and of computer technology in health care occurred simultaneously over the past 25 years. While there was development in both fields before the middle 1960s, growth since that time has been considerably accelerated. The strengthening of nursing research and its beginning integration into the broader scientific community should be useful to nurses interested in seeking support for research in computer applications. This section addresses some of the recent changes in nursing research and their relationship to research in computer applications in nursing and health care.

Strengthening of Nursing Research

The idea that nurses do research is not so strange as it was 20 or 30 years ago. As doctoral programs in nursing have increased from a handful to more than 40, the pool of doctorally prepared nurses has grown remarkably. Additionally, many nurses prepared at the master's level also are engaged in nursing or interdisciplinary research. Accompanying the growth in the number of nurses involved in research has been an increased political sophistication in nurses generally, including nurse researchers.

The American Nurses' Association Council of Nurse Researchers has provided leadership in promoting nursing research at the federal level. Since the mid-1970s, major efforts have been made to increase the budget for nursing research and the education of nurse researchers and also to move nursing research into the mainstream of the federal scientific enterprise. Until 1986, major nursing research activities at the federal level were located in the Division of Nursing, in the Health Resources Services Administration. The federal budget for nursing research was held constant at $5 million for research and $1 million for research training from the mid-1970s to the early 1980s.

In June 1983, representatives from the American Nurses' Association, the American Association for Colleges of Nursing, and the National League for Nursing met in Washington, D.C. and agreed to lobby for legislation to establish a National Institute of Nursing within the National Institutes of Health (NIH). The bill quickly received bipartisan support and was passed in both houses, but was pocket-vetoed by President Reagan in October 1984. The legislation was reintroduced when Congress reconvened, with a Center for Nursing Research substituted for an Institute for Nursing Research. The legislation again passed both houses of Congress and again was vetoed by President Reagan in November 1985. This time, the veto was overwhelmingly overridden in both houses (380 to 32 in the House, and 89 to 7 in the Senate), creating a National Center for Nursing Research within the National Institutes of Health. This represented a major achievement for nursing and is contributing to the interpretation of nursing research to the rest of the scientific community. The nursing research budget, while still representing less than 1% of the total federal health budget, has gradually increased to approximately $19 million in fiscal year 1987.

As the research budget increased, the number of proposals submitted doubled, tripled, and then quadrupled. Clearly, the activities leading up to and culminating in a nursing presence in the National Institutes of Health represented an important achievement for nursing in its scientific coming of age.

Nurses have not only demonstrated their ability to strengthen nursing research at the federal level, but have also expanded their own private support. The American Nurses' Foundation, an affiliate of the American Nurses' Association, increased its support for grants to nurses from a few each year before 1976 to 32 in 1985. Sigma Theta Tau, the national nursing honorary society, also is in the process of expanding its nursing research programs.

Research in Nursing Informatics

There has been an exponential growth of the nursing informatics literature, discussing where we are with computers, what we are doing, and what we should be doing. Research in nursing informatics is less well developed, however. The achievements described should contribute to the development of research in nursing informatics (NI), a need that has been acknowledged in nursing. In 1984, the American Nurses' Association approved the establishment of a Council on Computer Applications in Nursing, which had been sponsored by the Cabinet on Nursing Research. This action was prompted by a special interest group that had formed while participating in the programs of the Annual Symposium of Computer Applications in Medical Care.

To date, the majority of NI research has been on computer-assisted instruction (CAI). A review of the research literature on CAI found that 45% of the studies showed achievement gains in favor of CAI, 40% of the studies showed no difference in achievement, and 15% showed mixed results (Edwards et al, 1975). The majority of studies on CAI have been done in university settings with undergraduate nursing students and in hospitals where CAI is used for continuing education. CAI has been demonstrated effective in student achievement and in saving of instructional time in studies of professional nursing students (Ronald, 1979). In addition to studies on CAI, there has been at least one study examining nurses' perceptions concerning computer uses before and after a computer literacy lecture (Ball et al, 1985).

Although numerous reports have described the implementation of computers in the clinical setting, little systematic research has been done on nursing. Unfortunately, the research that has been implemented has rarely been done by nurses. Many studies are the product of systems analysis performed by vendors and computer consultants and remain unpublished. The focus of such studies has been the implementation process of the computer system, the automation of care plans, and the reaction of nursing personnel to the computer technology.

Examples of research that have been published include a study done by Stein on the development and use of automated nursing reports (Stein, 1969). As described in Chapter 7 of Unit 2, Section 2, Kjerulff has examined the reactions of hospital employees, most notably of nurses, to computerization.

Probably the best-known computer-related research in nursing information systems is the testing and refinement of the nursing minimum data set developed at the University of Wisconsin-Milwaukee School of Nursing (also described in this book; see Chapter 5, Unit 1, Section 2) (Werley et al, 1986). This research is concerned with standardizing the collection of essential nursing data, viewed as those specific items of information that are used on a regular basis by the majority of nurses across all settings in the delivery of care. It is a collaborative study by nurse researchers, many of whom have computer expertise. The data base will facilitate investigation of

- nursing diagnosis and treatment of human responses to health problems

- outcomes and quality of nursing care

- use, management, and cost of nursing resources.

The study represents an important effort to determine what nursing variables should be included in health care computer systems.

Another kind of nursing research is that done to determine the kinds of decisions that nurses make (Ozbolt et al, 1985). Although the study of nurse decision making is not new, increased interest has been stimulated by the development of symbolic programming languages. Symbolic programming languages are highly sophisticated computer systems that have the potential to act as nurse experts (Charniak and McDermott, 1986). The COMMES system at Creighton University, for example, is an artificial intelligence nursing knowledge base that can serve as an expert clinical decision-support system in such areas as standards of care and care plans for patients with medical and nursing diagnoses (Ryan, 1985). Other examples of studies on nurse decision making include research on intuition (Benner and Tanner, 1987), examination of nursing inferences within a framework of information processing theory (Westfall et al, 1986), and development of an instrument to measure the ability to make clinical nursing judgments (Dinger and Stigder, 1976).

There have also been a few studies evaluating the effectiveness of computerized decision-support systems (Lagina, 1971; Goodwin and Edwards, 1975; Wessling, 1972; Ropper et al, 1981). These studies were conducted when attempts were being made to program complex decision-making systems on lower level languages. The new age of symbolic programming should stimulate increased research on computerized nursing assessment. Some of these studies are published (Roncoli et al, 1986). In addition, Brennan is now actively conducting research on decision-support systems for nursing with a focus on modeling (Brennan, 1985, 1986, in press).

Considering the progress made in nursing research and in nursing informatics, we should be optimistic about the future growth of computer-related nursing research. Models for nursing research in NI are being developed (Schwirian, 1986; Ozbolt et al, 1985), and the effectiveness of various kinds of computer literacy programs is being explored (Ball et al, 1985). Computer systems such as NURSENET and the National Nursing Data Base are available to assist researchers in sharing current information (Morey, 1985; Happ, 1986). Nurses are learning computer technology, both hardware and software, and sharing their expertise in national computer conferences such as the Symposium on Computer Applications in Medical Care (SCAMC), in special interest groups, and with personal resource-sharing networks (Armstrong, 1985). And, along with other areas in nursing, the research base is being strengthened.

Funding for Research in Nursing Informatics

As in any area of nursing research, finding the appropriate funding agency can pose a challenge. Fortunately, there are several federal and private agencies particularly appropriate for the funding of research in nursing informatics, such as the National Center for Nursing Research (NCNR) at the National Institutes of Health. One branch of the NCNR is Nursing Systems and Special Programs, which deals with "investigations of promising approaches to nursing management and nursing care delivery, for example ... use of automation to improve the effectiveness of nursing care" (Merritt, 1986).

Another federal agency supportive of research in nursing informatics is the National Center for Health Services Research and Health Care Technology Assessment (NCHSR). NCHSR "seeks to create new knowledge and better understanding of the processes by which health services are made available, and how they may be provided more efficiently, more effectively, and at lower cost" (National Center for Health Services Research and Health Care Technology, 1986). This agency has supported research in nursing informatics in the past and presently is supporting the study by Kjerulff.

In the private sector, both the American Nurses' Foundation and Sigma Theta Tau offer funding opportunities, primarily for pilot research. The proposals generally are limited to $2,700, but the scope of research supported by both organizations is broad. Finally, a number of nurses and other health professionals have had grants, primarily of hardware and software, from computer companies to carry out specific research and demonstration projects.

These are only some of the major sources of potential funding for research in nursing informatics. Nurses interested in this area should work with their personnel in university offices of sponsored programs to identify other possible funding sources.

Once an appropriate funding agency has been identified, it is important that the researcher take care to match the proposal to the mission and priority statements published by the agency. Reviewers of the proposals must be able to see how the proposed research relates to their stated funding priorities. This requires that the researcher state very clearly the problem to be addressed, including research hypotheses and questions. Methods for carrying out the research should be developed in sufficient detail so that reviewers know the researcher has the necessary understanding of research methods to carry out the proposed study. In developing the proposals and later implementing the research, investigators should make every attempt to locate consultants, either in informatics or in research design and data analysis, who can lend strength to the proposed research. Successful funding for research in nursing informatics is built on the same formula as successful funding in other areas of nursing research—a significant problem for study, a clear description of the methods to be used, and a strong research team.

New Opportunities

This discussion has emphasized research in nursing informatics. However, in this area as in others, health research is becoming increasingly interdisciplinary. Nurses should seek out opportunities for interdisciplinary research in informatics by meeting and interacting with researchers in informatics in other disciplines, and by being alert to requests for proposals that seek interdisciplinary research teams.

Nurses are being acknowledged as competent to do research, and nursing research is gradually becoming integrated into the mainstream of science. This progress is becoming increasingly evident within the field of nursing informatics.

Questions

1. List the historical dates leading to the establishment of the National Center for Nursing Research within the National Institutes of Health.

2. List the kinds of research being conducted in nursing informatics.

3. What agencies are identified as sources of funding for nursing informatics research?

4. Identify the elements of "grantsmanship" and discuss their implications for successful funding of nursing informatics.

References Cited

Armstrong ML: Techniques of networking in the computer world. *Nursing Clinics of North America* 1985; 20:517–528.
Ball MJ, Snelbecker GE, Schechter SL: Nurses' perceptions concerning computer uses before and after a computer literacy lecture. *Computers in Nursing* 1985; 3:23–32.
Benner P, Tanner C: How expert nurses use intuition. *American Journal of Nursing* 1987; 87:23–31.
Brennan PF: Decision support for nursing practice: the challenge and the promise. In: Hannah KJ, Guillemin EJ, Conklin DN, eds. *Nursing Uses of Computers and Information Science.* Amsterdam: North Holland, 1985.
Brennan PF: The effects of a computerized decision aid on the decision making of nurse managers. Doctoral dissertation. Madison: University of Wisconsin, 1986.

Brennan PF: Computerized decision support: beyond expert systems. *Health Matrix* 1987; 5:31–34.

Charniak E, McDermott D: *Artificial Intelligence*. Reading, MA: Addison-Wesley, 1986.

Dinger JR, Stigder SI: Evaluation of a written simulation format for clinical nursing judgment. *Nursing Research* 1976; 25:280–285.

Edwards J, Norton S, Taylor S, et al: How effective is CAI? A review of research. *Educational Leadership* 1975; 33:147–154.

Goodwin J, Edwards B: Developing a computer program to assist the nursing process, phase one: from systems analysis to an expandable program. *Nursing Research* 1975; 24:299–305.

Happ B: Computers: integrating information world into nursing. *Nursing Management* 1986; 17:17–20.

Lagina SA: A computer program to diagnose anxiety level. *Nursing Research* 1971; 20:484–492.

Merritt DM: The national center for nursing research. *Image* 1986; 18:84–85.

Morey J: Guest viewpoint, Reach out and touch someone ... *Computers in Nursing* 1985; 3:101–139.

National Center for Health Services Research and Health Care Technology: National Center for Health Services Research and Health Care Technology Assessment: functions and program. Rockville, MD: NCHSR, USDHEW, 1986.

Ozbolt JG, Schultz S, Swain MA, et al: A proposed expert system for nursing practice. *Journal of Medical Systems* 1985; 9:57–68.

Ronald JS: Computers in undergraduate nursing education: a report of an experimental introductory course. *Journal of Nursing Education* 1979; 18:4–9.

Roncoli M, Brooten D, Delivoria-Papadopoulos M: A computerized system for measuring the effect of nursing care activities on the clinical indices of energy expenditures. *Computer Methods and Programs in Biomedicine* 1986; 22:53–60.

Ropper A, Griwold K, McKenna D, et al: Computer-guided neurologic assessment in the neurologic intensive care plan. *Heart and Lung* 1981; 10:54–60.

Ryan SA: An expert system for nursing practice. *Journal of Medical Systems* 1985; 9:29–42.

Schwirian PM: The NI pyramid—a model for research in nursing informatics. *Computers in Nursing* 1986; 4:134–136.

Stein RF: An exploratory study in the development and use of automated nursing reports. *Nursing Research* 1969; 18:14–21.

Werley HH, Devine EC, Weslag SK, et al: Testing and refinement of the nursing minimum data set. In: Salamon R, Blum B, Jorgensen M, eds. *MEDINFO 86—Proceedings of the Fifth Conference on Medical Informatics*. Vol. 5. Amsterdam: North Holland, 1986; 816–817.

Wessling E: Automating the nursing history and care plan. *Journal of Nursing Administration* 1972; 2:34–38.

Westfall UE, Tanner CA, Putizer D, et al: Activating clinical inferences: a component of diagnostic reasoning in nursing. *Research in Nursing and Health* 1986; 9:269–278.

2—Classification of Decision-Support Systems

Kathryn J. Hannah

Introduction

Nursing publications on the use of decision-support systems in clinical practice are just beginning to appear. Unfortunately, this small body of literature already suffers from confusion and lack of clarity because of the various definitions and conceptualizations of decision-support systems. It is characterized by authors who use the same term to refer to different concepts or who use different terms for the same concept. However, there is consensus among authors that decision-support systems should be used to extend the nurse's decision-making capacity rather than to replace it. The care planning systems now in use are not decision-support systems. Standardized care plans, whether manual or computer-based, only provide care for standardized patients! Standardized care plans do not enhance nursing decision making; on the contrary, their cookbook approach discourages active decision making by nurses.

A decision-support system for nursing practice is intended to support nurses by providing them with information to facilitate rational decision making about patients' care. In other words, decision-support systems help nurses to maintain and maximize their decision-making responsibilities and to focus on the highest priority aspects of patient care. Decision-support systems can be described as tools that provide nurses with "strategies to analyze, evaluate, develop and select effective solutions to complex problems in complex environments" (Brennan, 1985, p. 319).

Types of Decision-Support Systems

Formatting Tools

The purpose of these rudimentary decision aids is providing a format for organizing, integrating, and manipulating data for predecisional analysis. Their function is data aggregation, compilation, and representation. Formatting tools present data in a fashion facilitating quick access to information and more rapid understanding of data. In general, the approaches utilized are data bases and spreadsheets.

Decision-Modeling Systems

According to Brennan (see Chapter 3, Unit 3, Section 2), the purpose of decision modeling systems is to elicit the decision problem. These systems assist nurses as they aggregate defining characteristics or cardinal indicators to produce statements of nursing diagnoses, identify new options for creative nursing interventions (i.e., problem solving), and select an appropriate course of action. Decision-modeling systems function as either stand-alone decision-support tools or as the basis for an advisory decision-support system.

Brennan characterizes decision-modeling systems as having domain-independent decision templates (i.e., they are content free and have no data associated with them) with a focus on analysis rather than advice. Brennan further emphasizes that the purpose of such systems is to augment rather than replace the judgment of the nurse.

Specifically, decision-modeling systems reflect and structure the nurse's knowledge base by a process-oriented approach with emphasis on detailed understanding of the problem, rather than on the recommendation of a solution. Brennan identifies two approaches to decision-modeling systems: decision-analysis modeling systems and multiple criteria modeling systems.

Decision-Analysis Modeling Systems

Brennan argues that this category of decision-modeling systems is designed to help nurses structure problems, explicitly consider risk and uncertainty, and make selections consistent with objectives. Decision-analysis modeling systems provide structure to a decision problem in which the choice of a present course of action depends on the outcome of some future event. Components of such systems include actions, events, outcome states, and probabilities. Normative decision theory dictates that the best action is the one with the highest expected value (probability of success). These systems provide a visual display on the computer screen of the acts/events sequence encountered in a problem and compute the desirability of each action on the basis of data entered by the nurse.

Multiple Criteria Modeling Systems

Brennan indicates that this type of decision-modeling system is used when decisions must simultaneously satisfy numerous values and objectives (i.e., meet several criteria). Multiple criteria modeling systems reduce complex decisions to their elemental parts, establish the relative importance of each component, and help the nurse select the alternative that performs best on all criteria.

Advisory Systems/Expert Systems/Knowledge-Based Systems

The terms advisory system, expert system, and knowledge-based system are synonymous. For the sake of simplicity, the term expert system will be used here; however, use of this term in this chapter encompasses advisory systems and knowledge-based systems as well. As Brennan explains, the purpose of expert systems is to recommend solutions to nursing problems, solutions that reflect the judgment of nurse experts regarding the most expedient response to nursing situations. The most succinct definition is that expert systems generate decisions an expert would make (Butler, 1985). The purpose of expert systems is to capture or encapsulate in a computer system the knowledge of a human expert. Their function is to mimic the clinical reasoning and judgment of one specific human expert in the aggregation and interpretation of data in a precisely defined area of practice.

Expert systems are characterized by use of artificial intelligence principles; specifically, these are

- symbolic representation of specialist knowledge to make decisions within a specified domain
- the capacity to interrogate the user sensibly
- explanation of reasoning (rationale) underlying a decision on request by the user
- incorporation into the knowledge base of systematic feedback about the effects of decisions.

General approaches used as the basis for expert systems are

- knowledge-engineering elicitation of a knowledge base and decision rules from an expert
- actuarial data based on numerous observations of patient encounters
- objective probability based on the subjective judgment of multiple experts
- use of heuristics to determine what a reasonable professional nurse would decide in a particular situation.

The components of an expert system include a knowledge base, inference engine, patient data base, and user interface. The knowledge base may incorporate empirically validated research, clinical experience-based heuristics, authority, tradition, and textbooks. An inference engine is the interpretation of knowledge using such techniques as logical deduction (decision rules), semantic networks, or logical relationships (Bayesian, probabilistic, or "fuzzy" logic). The patient data base is the data gathered from the patient who is the subject of the decisions. The user interface provides the capacity for natural language communication with the system so the user can ask questions and enter and receive information.

COMMES

COMMES was originally designed to support nursing education. Redesigned, COMMES is marketed as an expert system for use in nursing practice. Nurses can enter patient-related questions and receive information from the stored knowledge base (founded on the undergraduate nursing curriculum at Creighton University) in the form of bibliographic references from specified reference books. The inference engine for this system is based on a semantic network with the ability to incorporate new information. The COMMES systems can provide references on a wide variety of topics at the introductory (undergraduate) level.

Ozbolt identified the major limitations of COMMES: its present inability to be connected to a hospital information system for purposes of access to patient data, the need for lengthy dialogue to elicit responses that could be easily accessed directly from the standard reference books included in the accompanying library, and an illness-specific and procedurally oriented knowledge base. Additional limitations include the orientation to undergraduate level as "expert" and the inadequate interactive capacity to discriminate nursing concepts beyond a macroscopic level. (In a recent personal experience, the author's query regarding postoperative complications of a cholecystectomy produced prolonged scrolling of references across the screen instead of a system request for further discriminating criteria from the user.)

CYBERNURSE

CYBERNURSE is a prototype system developed at the University of Michigan. Ozbolt explains that it is based on "conceptual models and theories that provided a logical structure for the elements and relationships in nursing's knowledge base, ... production rules to prompt the nurse for client data, analyze the data, and propose nursing diagnosis ... [and] aids to formulating objectives and interventions."

Artificial Intelligence

Artificial intelligence can be defined as "making a computer behave in ways that mimic intelligent human behavior" (Feigenbaum and McCorduck, 1983). Artificial intelligence systems can provide users with open-ended decision support. Those systems, like intelligent human behavior, possess characteristics supportive of self-modification and a cumulative knowledge base. They mimic the human abilities to learn from experience, justify reasoning, and effectively handle inconsistencies in the knowledge base. How then is artificial intelligence different from the expert systems?

Artificial intelligence provides prescriptive and directive output in the absence of human professional expertise and judgment. Situations demanding nursing expertise in which a professional nurse expert would be unavailable might arise in an arctic outpost, in a space laboratory, or on a nuclear submarine submerged for prolonged periods of time. Artificial intelligence would have a huge knowledge base encompassing a comprehensive body of nursing knowledge and derived from a synthesis of the accumulated knowledge of numerous nurse experts. It is capable of substituting for a human expert, ultimately functioning as an autonomous agent.

The components of artificial intelligence systems would be the same as those found in expert systems: a data base of problem information, a knowledge source of accumulated knowledge, an inference engine for process control, and a user interface. The differences would be in the size and sophistication of the knowledge base and inference engine and in the type of output available through the user interface.

Interface between Hospital Information Systems and Decision-Support Systems

A decision-support system must generate a patient care plan, not merely a nursing care plan. One analysis of nursing activities identified three global categories for nursing tasks (Campbell, 1978). The first includes managerial tasks and clerical activities, such as order entry, results reporting, requisition generation, and telephone booking of appointments, as done by current hospital information systems. The second category is physician-delegated tasks. Current systems are capable of capturing these from the physicians' order entry set and incorporating them into the patient care plan. It is the third category, autonomous nursing functions, on which a nursing decision-support system would focus. All three categories, managerial/clerical, physician-delegated, and autonomous nursing functions, are required for a fully operational system. This third category of autonomous nursing interventions is critically lacking in the hospital information systems now marketed.

A patient care planning system or a decision-support system allows nurses to enter assessments at the bedside and use the computer for analyzing assessments and recommending nursing diagnoses. The nurse then accepts or rejects the recommendations and chooses the nursing interventions appropriate for the patient. This provides a tailor-made care plan and a personalized care plan. It must integrate with care plans generated by other health care professionals.

Such a system requires the technology for source date capture and considerable work by nurses on the development of the nursing knowledge base. Until recently it was not possible to even consider such a system. The technology did not exist, and nursing as a profession did not have sufficiently well-developed nomenclature. As that nomenclature develops, building a decision-support system will point out areas of the nursing nomenclature that require further definition or refinement. Clinical judgment that considers contextual factors as well as the recommendations of decision-support systems must be exercised. In addition, because the current status of computer technology and understanding human cognition restricts the performance of such systems, nurses must be discriminating users and ensure that the systems are providing appropriate recommendations (Blum, 1986) before acting on their output.

Conclusion

Nurses are identifying and developing new ways of using computers and information science as tools in the performance of their duties. At the same time, computers and information science are facilitating a more sophisticated and expanded level of nursing practice. Thus, there is an interactive and synergistic effect between nursing informatics and nursing practice. The goal of nursing informatics is to guide the design, use, management, and evaluation of computer systems that will meet the needs of nurses for use in health care agencies and institutions. The boundaries of nursing informatics are contiguous with those of nursing. Like the boundaries of nursing, the boundaries of nursing informatics are dynamic.

Questions

1. Identify the types of decision-support systems.

2. For each system identified, describe the purpose, characteristics, and function.

3. Discuss the integration of decision-support systems for nursing with existing hospital information systems.

4. Describe the prerequisites for development of decision-support systems.

References Cited

Blum BI: *Clinical Information Systems.* New York: Springer-Verlag, 1986.

Brennan PF: Decision support for nursing practice: the challenge and the promise. In: Hannah KJ, Guillemin EJ, Conklin DN, eds. *Nursing Uses of Computers and Information Science.* Amsterdam: North Holland, 1985; 315–319.

Butler EA: A direction for nursing expert systems. In: Hannah KJ, Guillemin EJ, Conklin DN, eds. *Nursing Uses of Computers and Information Science.* Amsterdam: North Holland, 1985; 309–313.

Campbell C: *Nursing Diagnosis and Intervention in Nursing Practice.* New York: Wiley, 1978.

Feigenbaum EA, McCorduck P: *The Fifth Generation.* Reading: Addison-Wesley, 1983.

Sonnenberg FA, Pauker SG: Decision Maker 6.0. In: Salamon R, Blum B, Jorgensen M, eds. *MEDINFO 86—Proceedings of the Fifth Conference on Medical Informatics.* Vol. 5. Amsterdam: North Holland, 1986; 1152.

3—Modeling for Decision Support

Patricia Flatley Brennan

Modeling for Decision Support

Computerized decision-support systems link computer technology with decision-making algorithms to augment, extend, or replace the judgment of the nurse. Decision modeling is one approach to computerized decision support with implications for clinical nursing. Nurses use decision-modeling systems when further analysis, rather than more data, is needed to solve a decision problem. Implemented primarily on microcomputers, these systems use decision-analytic or multiple criteria models as the structure for analyzing decision problems.

Modeling is one of two major approaches to decision support: analysis and advice. Analyzing systems, also called decision-modeling systems, are computer programs specifically designed to help nurses structure problems, explicitly consider risk and uncertainty, and make selections consistent with a set of objectives. Advising systems, on the other hand, recommend solutions to nursing problems, solutions that reflect the judgment of nurse experts regarding the most expedient response to nursing situations.

Modeling Concepts

Models and selected software packages to build models provide clinical practitioners with decision-support capabilities. Many nurses are already familiar with the concept of models. A nurse relies on a model of the renal system each time she/he interprets a patient's fluid balance for a specified period. Nurses employ Bowlby's model of loss as they attempt to understand why the 4-year-old patient cries when her parents leave her in the hospital. A model of political change guides actions in initiating a new way of assigning nurses to patients.

In these examples, the models employed serve:

- to represent a complex process (kidney function)
- as a template for categorizing and interpreting behavior (separation and loss)
- as a prescriptive pathway for action (change process).

A model is an observable structure that represents the essential components of some entity. Maps, formulae, and stick figures are all models. In modeling a nursing decision, the nurse uses familiar words and phrases to flesh out the skeleton of the model to produce a small replica of the problem she faces.

Following normative decision theory, mathematical functions are the skeletons on which the nurse builds the representation of a decision problem. Two mathematical representations form the core of computerized decision modeling systems: decision-analytic models and multiple criteria models.

Decision-Analytic Models

Decision-analysis trees provide structure to a decision problem in which the choice of a present course of action depends on the outcome of some future event. Decision trees have four components: actions, events, outcome states, and probabilities. For example, in a pain management decision, the nurse may consider two alternative courses of action (chemical analgesic or relaxation coaching) (Corcoran, 1986). The events include the occurrence of side effects and the relief of pain. The various levels of patient function comprise the outcome states for this problem. The nurse uses the tree to visually represent the likelihood, or probability, that a particular action leads to certain events. By attaching a numerical value to each outcome and following the laws of subjective probability, the nurse can compute the expected value of each action under consideration. Normative decision theory dictates that the most desirable action is the one with the highest expected value.

Multiple Criteria Models

Many nursing decisions require that choices simultaneously satisfy numerous values and objectives. Consider, for example, the problem of determining how to handle patient falls. The nurse could use cloth restraints, have a staff member seated with a patient at all times, or keep the lights on in the patient's room. An effective course of action must be legally appropriate, feasible within the nurse's budget, and respectful of the patient. No single alternative meets all these criteria.

Multiple criteria models reduce complex decisions such as these into their elemental parts, and help the nurse select the alternative that performs best on all criteria. Weighted sums are computed after determining how well a particular alternative meets each individual criterion and how important the criteria are to each other. Again, decision theory dictates that the best action will be that alternative with the highest score.

Capabilities

Decision analysis and multiple criteria are two types of mathematical models that can represent the decisions faced by nurses. By constructing these models, the nurse gains understanding and insight into the problem at hand. This modeling process, based on a problem description presented in the nurse's own words, results in a recommendation for action. Mathematical modeling of decisions is a specialized skill generally requiring the presence of a decision analyst. Recent developments in computer software permit many of the analyst's functions to be taken over by an English language interactive query. Three features distinguish these decision-modeling systems from other types of decision support:

- domain independence

- focus on analysis rather than advice

- intent to augment rather than replace the judgment of the nurse.

Software

Decision-modeling systems may serve as stand-alone decision-support tools, or may form the basis for the advising decision-support systems. In this section we describe only the stand-alone systems. Decision-modeling systems are domain independent, content-free decision aids (Brennan, 1986). The models can serve as a general purpose structure for analyzing a wide variety of problems. For example, a medical/surgical nurse may use a multiple criteria modeling package such as Lightyear to determine what type of aftercare is best for a 45-year-old patient with cancer. A pediatric nursing team may use the very same software package to select an exercise routine for a hospitalized adolescent.

Computerized decision-modeling systems are designed to reflect and structure the nurse's knowledge base. These systems are process oriented, with the emphasis on detailed understanding of the problem rather than on the recommendation of a solution. Decision-modeling systems show nurses the implications of their values and assumptions. Final recommendations result as a reflection of, rather than a replacement of, the nurse's judgments.

Types of Computerized Decision-Modeling Systems

Most decision-modeling software packages run on microcomputers. Here we describe software designed to support the two major categories of mathematical models: decision analysis and multiple criteria.

Decision Analysis

Decision-tree programs provide a visual display on the computer screen of the acts/events sequence encountered in a problem. The program computes the desirability of each action based on data entered by the nurse.

Developed by Jim Hollenberg in 1985, SMLTREE is a decision-analysis program that enables the nurse to construct a decision tree. Running on an IBM PC, SMLTREE helps the decision maker model the series of actions and events relevant to the decision problem. SMLTREE can handle the generic class of decision problems in which the uncertain future consequences must be considered when selecting a course of action.

Decision Maker 6.0, created by Stephen Pauker and running on the Apple Macintosh, specifically models diagnostic and treatment problems faced by clinical practitioners (Sonnenberg and Pauker, 1986). Decision Maker 6.0 helps the nurse to construct decision trees useful in selecting a course of treatment in which the outcome of the treatment and the state of the disease process are uncertain. Using Bayesian models and utility theory, Decision Maker 6.0 helps the nurse determine the intervention most likely to successfully bring a patient to a particular state of health.

Two analytical functions make Decision Maker 6.0 particularly useful for clinical judgment. One is the ability to determine how sensitive is the recommended action to imprecision in the nurse's estimates of disease status and efficacy of treatment. The second is that the preference for future outcomes (in this case, patient status) can be specified in terms of quality-adjusted life-years, a more familiar, understandable concept to both nurses and patients.

Multiple Criteria Models

Multiple criteria decision-modeling software helps nurses choose alternatives when the choice of action depends on satisfying many criteria simultaneously. Multiple criteria decision-modeling programs break down complex problems into smaller components that include the options under consideration, the criteria used to determine the best option, and the relative importance of the criteria. At the end of the modeling session, these programs provide a printed and/or screen display of the results, including a designation of the most desirable option.

Nurses have successfully used MAUD, a multiple criteria decision-modeling program, for clinical management decisions (Brennan, 1986). For example, a nurse may consider several approaches to treating a patient with chronic schizophrenia: hospitalization, day hospitalization, and individual treatment. Factors critical to this selection include the cost of the program, the patient's need for transportation to and from the site, and the likelihood of obtaining the needed treatment. MAUD asks the nurse to first type in the alternative sites, then the name of each factor. Once the nurse evaluates each site individually on each factor, MAUD then elicits the relative importance of each factor to the other factors. Finally, a list including all alternative treatment sites listed in rank order is printed.

Other multiple criteria programs and their vendors include Expert Choice (Decision Support Software), Policy (Executive Software), Decision Aide (Kepner-Tregoe), and Lightyear (Thoughtware). While the underlying models differ, each package is designed to help the decision maker select the best option in light of the complex factors to be considered.

Use of Decision-Modeling Systems

Selection of a course of action is only one reason for using decision-modeling software. Modeling systems can also help nurses aggregate signs and symptoms to produce diagnostic statements. Some modeling software (such as Confidence Factor, produced by Kepner-Tregoe) specifically focuses on helping the nurse identify new options for creative problem solving.

A nurse would consult a decision-modeling package when faced with an important, difficult decision. The software guides the nurse through the decision problem to arrive at a recommendation. Additionally, decision-modeling software helps with post hoc analysis of a decision to verify the nurse's judgment. Use of decision-modeling software requires sessions from 10 to 60 minutes (Brennan, 1986).

Many of the decisions faced by nurses must be made in group settings. These groups may include other nurses, or members of many disciplines. Computerized group decision-support systems (GDSS) facilitate group conferencing and communication. In addition to providing the benefits afforded individuals in decision making, GDSSs help members with some group process tasks. For example, in a multiple criteria analysis, the voting power can be divided proportionally to the extent of influence held by the various members. A discharge planning group may elect to use a GDSS to help a family resolve the issues surrounding after care placement of an ill family member.

Most decision-modeling packages are designed to replace the decision

Table 3-1
What Decision Model Should Be Used?

Decision problem	Model type	
If the problem involves ...	Then the decision model is a ...	And appropriate software is
Selecting one alternative from several	Multiple criteria model	Policy (Decision Techtronics) Lightyear (Thoughtware) Decision Aide (Kepner-Tregoe) Expert Choice (Decision Software)
Choosing an action now and the best choice depends on uncertain events in the future	Decision tree analysis	SMLTREE (Hollenberg) Decision Maker 6.0 (Pauker)

analyst and therefore can be used without extensive understanding of computers, mathematics, and decision analysis. English language directions guide the nurse through these programs. Printouts and graphical display screens show the results of the decision modeling.

To obtain the greatest benefit from decision-modeling software, the nurse should have a cursory knowledge of the underlying models. Some familiarity with the assumptions of utility theory and decision analysis will enable the nurse to select the correct decision aid and to interpret its results accurately. Several texts (*Decision Analysis and Behavioral Research* or *Clinical Decision Analysis*) provide basic introduction to some of the concepts underlying the packages described (Von Winterfeldt and Edwards, 1986; Weinstein and Fineberg, 1980). For full appreciation of the power of decision modeling, these texts should be consulted.

Conclusion

Where the nurse faces a problem of selection, multiple criteria models will serve the nurse best. When the nurse encounters a problem of great uncertainty with various pathways to resolution, the decision tree models provide the greatest assistance (Table 3-1).

Acknowledgment. Preparation of this manuscript was supported by a grant from the University Hospitals of Cleveland and the Cleveland Decision Analysis Group. The creative editorial assistance of Jane Ann Jewell is gratefully acknowledged.

Questions

1. What benefits can nurses expect when using decision support systems?

2. Compare and contrast multiple criteria modeling with decision-tree analysis in terms of problem types and solutions provided.

3. For what types of decision problems and in what circumstances are decision-modeling tools preferable to expert systems?

4. How can the nurse ensure that the analysis produced from a decision-modeling system is correct?

5. How could the nurse obtain the probability estimates required for using a decision-tree analysis package?

References Cited

Brennan PF: The effects of a computerized decision aid on the decision making of nurse managers. Doctoral dissertation. Madison: University of Wisconsin, 1986.

Corcoran S: Decision analysis: a step-by-step guide for making clinical decisions. *Nursing and Health Care* 1986; 7: 149–154.

Sonnenberg FA, Pauker SG: Decision Maker 6.0. In: Salamon R, Blum B, Jorgensen M, eds. *MEDINFO 86—Proceedings of the Fifth Conference on Medical Informatics*. Vol. 5. Amsterdam: North Holland, 1986; 1152.

Von Winterfeldt D, Edwards W: *Decision Analysis and Behavioral Research*. Cambridge: Cambridge University Press, 1986.

Weinstein M, Fineberg H: *Clinical Decision Analysis*. Philadelphia: WB Saunders, 1980.

Bibliography

Brennan PF: Decision support: beyond expert systems. *Health Matrix* 1987; 5: 3;s).

De Sanctis G, Gallupe B: Group decision support systems: a new frontier. *Database* 1985; 16: 3–10.

4—Knowledge-Based Systems for Supporting Clinical Nursing Decisions

Judy G. Ozbolt

Abstract

The development of decision-support systems for nursing has been limited by difficulties in defining and representing nursing's knowledge base and by a lack of knowledge about how nurses make decisions. Recent theoretical and empirical work offers solutions to these problems. The challenge now is to represent nursing knowledge in a way that is comprehensible to both nurse and computer, and to design decision-support modalities that are accurate, efficient, and appropriate for nurses with different levels of expertise. In this chapter are reviewed the issues and progress in developing knowledge-based systems for supporting clinical nursing decisions, critically evaluating the logic programming language Prolog as a tool for meeting the challenge.

System Development Efforts in Nursing

Accomplishments to Date

In contrast to medicine, in which researchers have been working to develop decision-support systems for the past two decades, nursing has given rise to only two programs of research and development aimed at supporting those decisions that are within its specific clinical domain. One of these led to the development of the COMMES system at Creighton University (Evans, 1984, 1985; Ryan, 1983). Originally designed to support education, the nursing component of COMMES has been extended and is currently marketed as an interactive consultative system wherein a nurse can enter data about a client, pose questions, and receive information derived from the stored knowledge base of the undergraduate nursing curriculum at Creighton, with bibliographic references for further reading. Programmed as a semantic network with the ability to learn from new information, COMMES can provide consultation at the generalist level on a wide variety of topics, and may be extended into some specialty areas.

Although it is innovative and ingenious in many ways, COMMES appears to have three significant limitations. First, because it is not designed to be part of a hospital information system, COMMES cannot draw on stored, client-specific data; the nurse posing a query must enter all the relevant data about the client. Second, a lengthy dialogue may be required to obtain information that may be obvious to some nurses and that could be easily retrieved by others from standard nursing textbooks or other readily available reference materials. (COMMES is marketed with an accompanying library of books and journals, and it is not clear that the computer is a necessary gateway to the paper library.) Third, because its knowledge base is highly specific to illness conditions and nursing procedures, keeping it up to date is expensive in both human and computer terms. Thus, although COMMES has been an important pioneer in the development of decision-support systems for nursing and may evolve into a more practical system, it is not yet a fully satisfactory response to nursing's needs for decision-support systems.

The other program of research and development in decision-support systems for nursing has been at the University of Michigan. Unlike the group at Creighton, we have not yet produced a system ready for implementation. Instead, we have explored problems of decision support in nursing through a series of prototypes. Rather than defining the domain of nursing knowledge as "whatever is included in the undergraduate curriculum plus whatever appears in the literature," we have looked for conceptual models and theories that would provide a logical structure for the elements and relationships in nursing's knowledge base. Using concepts from the literature (McCain, 1965; Orem, 1971, 1980), we wrote programs in FORTRAN IV, BASIC, and PASCAL that used production rules to prompt the nurse for client data, analyze the data, and propose nursing diagnoses; the last program included aids to formulating objectives and interventions as well (Goodwin and Edwards, 1975; Ozbolt, 1982; Ozbolt et al, 1984).

Although these programs demonstrated the feasibility of representing nursing knowledge and decision structures in a decision-support system, we have chosen not to develop them further because of some inherent shortcomings in the conceptual models that we used to define the nursing knowledge base. The available models (McCain, 1965; Orem, 1971, 1980, 1985) did not adequately reflect the full range of issues with which nurses assist their clients, nor does any provide an adequate basis for selecting objectives and interventions appropriate to an individual client's situation. Further, our programs shared a flaw with the COMMES system: the diagnoses, objectives, and interventions proposed were likely to be fairly obvious to the nurse, if not from the start, at least by the time the nurse had entered client data via a lengthy dialogue with the computer. Our recent efforts, therefore, have been directed toward answering the following questions:

Can nursing's knowledge base be represented comprehensively, concisely, and logically?
Can a decision-support system be designed that will be of practical use to nurses in the way they actually make clinical decisions?

Barriers to Development

Before nursing's knowledge base can be represented in a computer language, it must first be identified and defined in English or another natural language. That has been difficult for three reasons. First, nursing values a holistic approach to the client. The American Nurses' Association, for example, has said that nursing is "the diagnosis and treatment of human responses to actual or potential health problems" (American Nurses' Association, 1980, p. 9). What, then, in the universe of knowledge, can be ruled out as *not* nursing knowledge? Second, because nurses do have holistic concerns and because they have traditionally provided 24-hour coverage, they have often done whatever needs to be done, reinforcing the notion that nursing knowledge includes everything about human beings in health and illness. Finally, attempts to articulate what is and what is not nursing have resulted in not one conceptual model but many competing and incompatible ones. One researcher, referring to different kinds of conceptual models for nursing, noted that:

Clearly ... different classes of approaches to understanding the person who is a patient, not only call for differing forms of practice toward different objectives, but also point to different kinds of phenomena, suggest different kinds of questions, and lead eventually to dissimilar bodies of knowledge. (Johnson, 1974, p. 376)

Faced with disagreement about the nature of nursing and a broad and loose definition of the content of nursing, how can designers of a clinical decision-support system delineate a nursing knowledge base?

Even if an adequate knowledge base were available, there are no clear precedents as to how it should be used in a decision-support system to support the way nurses actually practice. In medicine there is an expectation that the physician will see and examine the patient, order diagnostic tests, and reflect on the results before diagnosing and prescribing. In this linear model of care, there is a built-in opportunity for time away from the patient during which the physician may consult a computer as well as colleagues and other references in order to arrive at appropriate decisions. The central activities of nursing, however, are carried on in the presence of the client, with the nurse simultaneously observing, diagnosing, and intervening in holistic psychologic, physiologic, social, and spiritual phenomena that evolve from moment to moment. While engaged in an intense diagnostic and therapeutic interaction with a client, the nurse cannot be turning away to consult a computer about how to interpret the client's condition and behavior and how to respond. In order to design an appropriate decision-support system for nursing, therefore, we must consider how to protect and promote what nurses already do well with clients and how to assist in those areas where they have difficulty.

Overcoming the Barriers

It is unlikely that nursing's conceptual models could be merged into one unified model, given their conceptual and philosophical incompatibility (Fawcett, 1984), and it will be some time, if ever, before one model of nursing emerges as empirically and theoretically superior. For the present, then, designers of decision-support systems who seek a conceptual framework on which to structure nursing's knowledge base must simply choose one of the existing models. The model selected should be one that meets criteria of internal and external criticism such as those proposed elsewhere in the literature (Stevens, 1979). If the knowledge base is comprehensive and if it helps nurses to make decisions leading to more effective care, users are not likely to be greatly concerned about which model is used.

One model that stands up well to the criteria of internal and external criticism is called modeling and role-modeling (Erickson et al, 1983). This paradigm is clear, consistent, and logically developed, and it provides theoretical bases for explaining and predicting client conditions and behaviors, including responses to specific nursing interventions. In offering a holistic view of the interactions of biophysic, psychologic, social, cognitive, and spiritual phenomena and showing how theoretical knowledge can be applied to increase the effectiveness of nursing care, it meets the criteria of adequacy, utility, significance, and discrimination of nursing from other health professions and from other helping actions. In terms of scope, it offers both a grand theory of nursing and more specific propositions giving rise to testable hypotheses. It is complex enough to address the full range of "human responses to actual or potential health problems" (American Nurses' Association, 1980). The complexity that makes it effective, however, also makes it difficult for any but expert nurses to practice within the framework of modeling and role-modeling. Because of this complexity and because of modeling and role-modeling's strength on the other criteria, a decision-support system that built its knowledge base on the modeling and role-modeling framework and helped nurses to practice in that context would be both adequate and useful. Because it deals with complex interrelationships of multiple factors it could help to organize data and make suggestions that were not obvious to the nurse. It would also have a practical advantage with regard to programming and maintenance: Its knowledge base would be sufficiently abstract and general to apply to clients throughout the life span and across all conditions of health and illness, making it relatively concise and in less frequent need of updating.

The question remains, however, *how* the system could help nurses to make decisions in practice. A series of studies of how nurses practice (Benner, 1982, 1984; Benner and Wrubel, 1982; Benner and Tanner, 1987) has differentiated between knowing *that*, or theoretical knowledge, and knowing *how*, or experiential knowledge involving intuition and insight (Polanyi, 1974). Benner (1982) has also described five levels of nursing proficiency, from novice to expert, as a continuum progressing from a minimum of experiential knowledge and a maximum reliance on theoretical knowledge to a high degree of experiential knowledge with a minimum need to rely on theoretical knowledge expressed as rules and maxims. As explained elsewhere:

> The beginner must rely on a deliberative analytical method to build the clinical picture from isolated bits and pieces of information. The expert has the skill and the option to grasp the situation rapidly, to see the whole, or the gestalt. (Benner and Wrubel, 1982, p. 13)

Other analyses (Dreyfus, 1972, 1979) held that intelligent activities involving perceptive guessing, insight, understanding in the context of use, and recognition of varied and distorted patterns—just the sort of activities included in experiential knowledge—represent an exclusively human capacity, one that computers are unlikely ever to mimic successfully. If we accept this premise, we cannot expect to create a computer-based system that will "think" like an expert nurse. What computers could be designed to do, however, is to "count out alternatives once (the human user) had zeroed in on an interesting area.... Likewise, in problem solving, once the problem is structured and an attack planned, a machine could take over to work out the details" (Dreyfus, 1979, p. 301).

Thus, a decision-support system could be designed to work with (not instead of) expert nurses in generating alternative hypotheses, goals, interventions, and consequences to consider in making a human judgment of what is most appropriate for a particular client. Such a function could help nurses to avoid the "error of tunnel vision, of the 'closed mind' or of 'projecting' the wrong set of data or their own fears into a situation," an error to which even expert clinicians are susceptible (Benner, 1987, p. 28). Similarly, once the nurse had decided on a course of action, the computer could generate detailed, individualized care plans and aids to documentation based on the stored knowledge base.

With its stored base of theoretical knowledge, the system could also help less expert nurses to think through a situation, posing questions to obtain information based on judgment, not rules (e.g., "Has Mr. Jones suffered a significant loss?"), and proposing inferences based on that information and on the theoretical knowledge base (e.g., "The information you provide suggests that Mr. Jones may be experiencing morbid grief"). The system could also provide the nurse with options to obtain more information about the hypothesized nursing diagnoses (e.g., common manifestations of morbid grief). Thus, less expert nurses could be assisted to make optimal use of a complex knowledge base, such as that represented by the modeling and role-modeling framework (Erickson et al, 1983).

A helpful decision-support system for nursing, then, would use a theoretical knowledge base (the specifiable or formalizable aspect of nursing knowledge), but would draw on the nurse's capacity to make human judgments (the nonspecifiable aspect of nursing knowledge). Less expert nurses might interact extensively with the theoretical knowledge base to arrive at decisions about client needs and nursing care. More expert nurses might use the theoretical knowledge base primarily to consider alternatives and to develop care plans and documentation quickly and efficiently. The union of the nurse's knowledge, experience, and judgment with the computer's capacity to store and process theoretical knowledge and data would lead to better clinical decisions than either nurse or computer could achieve alone.

Where and how would the nurse use this system? Because effective nursing depends on a therapeutic interaction between nurse and patient, it is important to avoid introducing the computer as an intrusive, competing presence. Therefore, while a bedside terminal might be used for brief entries of factual data such as vital signs, the more prolonged computer interaction necessary for diagnosing ongoing conditions (as opposed to transitory ones that are diagnosed and resolved during a single nurse-client interaction), planning, and documenting care should occur elsewhere, preferably in a quiet room where the nurse is subject to fewer distractions than in the typical nurses' station.

The Challenge

Efforts to date to develop decision-support systems for nursing have had only modest success because their knowledge bases were too limited or too unwieldy and because they provided little real assistance to nurses in making decisions about care. Now, however, we have the means to overcome these limitations. Within the context of modeling and role-modeling (Erickson et al, 1983), a knowledge base has been delineated for the nursing care of clients of all ages and conditions, although supplementary modules might be needed for some specialty settings. Further, we are beginning to understand how nurses use knowledge to make clinical decisions. The challenge now is to find the appropriate technologic tools and strategies to develop a system that can efficiently and accurately store and draw inferences from a theoretical knowledge base and a client data base, and that can communicate and interact effectively with nurses.

Prolog: A Tool to Meet the Challenge?

Representing Knowledge

At the heart of any decision-support system is its knowledge base. How this knowledge base is codified is a primary determinant of what the system will be able to do:

> The task of designing a knowledge representation scheme for any system that hopes to make use of artificial intelligence is one that has a critical importance. Ultimately, the style, format, and assumptions inherent in any knowledge representation scheme will have a pervasive impact on what can and cannot be encoded, processed, and ultimately accomplished in the system. (Brulé, 1986, pp. 38–39)

Two types of languages are available for codifying knowledge bases for decision-support systems: list processing languages such as LISP and Pop-II and logic programming languages such as Prolog. Of the two types, it may be that "Prolog is better suited to situations in which the knowledge to be processed consists of facts and relationships between the facts" (Brulé, 1986, p. 78). This is because logic programming is

> based on writing programs as sets of assertions. These assertions are viewed as having *declarative* meaning as descriptive statements about entities and their relations. In addition, the assertions derive a *procedural* meaning by virtue of being executable by an interpreter. Indeed, executing a logic program is much like performing a deduction on a set of facts. (Cohen and Feigenbaum, 1982, p. 120)

Because of these characteristics, Prolog would appear to be well suited for representing a nursing knowledge base structured within the modeling and role-modeling (Erickson et al, 1983) paradigm. The modeling and role-modeling knowledge base consists of statements of facts and relations. For example, the paradigm describes the relationships of basic need satisfaction to object attachment and loss, developmental growth, and adaptive potential (Erickson et al, 1983, pp. 86–92). The paradigm also relates theoretical principles to nursing aims and specific interventions. It thus provides a logical framework for deducing nursing diagnoses, objectives, and interventions. A program that could capture this knowledge base and exploit it to answer ad hoc questions about complex interrelationships would be useful indeed.

How might Prolog do this? Without going into the details of Prolog syntax, which can be found in the standard texts (e.g., Clocksin and Mellish, 1984), it can be noted that Prolog provides a means of stating relationships concisely. For example, the relation, "Need satisfaction promotes development" could be stated as

promotes(need_satisfaction, development).

A major advantage of Prolog is that, given a set of such statements, the system can perform deductions to find answers to ad hoc questions *without requiring procedural instructions in the program*. It would be possible to state all the relationships defined by modeling and role-modeling in the form of Prolog assertions, but a program consisting merely of a long list of such statements would probably be very inefficient to run. In searching for the answer to an inquiry, Prolog proceeds sequentially through the list of assertions, using exhaustive backtracking when necessary to try to satisfy all the conditions of the inquiry (Cohen and Feigenbaum, 1982). To increase efficiency, the knowledge needed to solve particular kinds of problems can be grouped in frames, with "slots" to be filled in with specific data and "procedural attachments" to pose English language questions to the user to obtain the data (or to get data from a data base) and to interpret the data so obtained (Marcus, 1986). Such an approach appears very promising to structure the knowledge base for a nursing decision-support system, particularly if the frames are linked hierarchically into taxonomies, "allowing the system to use the semantic richness of frames while being able to describe the relationships between those frames as in a semantic network" (Marcus, 1986, p. 162).

Supporting Decision Making

By using the theoretical knowledge base and a client data base to make logical inferences about nursing diagnoses, objectives, and interventions, a Prolog-based system could assist both expert and less expert nurses to make decisions about care. By organizing related information, generating alternatives, posing questions, and making suggestions, it could support both the formalized, theoretical, scientific aspects of nursing and the nonformalizable, intuitive, artful aspects of nursing. Would designing such a system, however, be as simple as Marcus would make it appear?

Probably not. Linking a client data base to a Prolog knowledge base would require innovative approaches to system design and programming. In Prolog, data base operations and other input/output functions are accomplished as side effects to the logic programming paradigm, making Prolog less than ideal for data base management systems (Brodie and Jarke, 1986). Nor can the problem of integrating a knowledge base and a data base be readily resolved by linking a Prolog system to a sophisticated data base management system, because of Prolog's difficulty in communicating with other languages. The best of some difficult alternatives may be the "tight integration" of a logic programming system with a data base management system. To achieve this, it would first be necessary to resolve certain problems by research and development, including deciding how to divide the inference functions between the data base management system and the knowledge-base system (Brodie and Jarke, 1986). Others support the "tight integration" approach, giving examples to show how it is possible to design a single integrated system combining inferencing and data retrieval (Sciore and Warren, 1986). They propose that this can be done by extending a Prolog system to include some components of a data base management system.

Assuming that the integration of the knowledge base and the client data base can be achieved, it will still be necessary to develop a user interface that will allow nurses to communicate with the system in a language that approaches English. Efforts have been made to develop a user-friendly, front-end translation program to aid children and other naive users to write programs using "an infix binary notation that closely resembles English" (Ennals et al, 1984, p. 378). In this and other approaches they describe, however, the emphasis is on helping users to write programs. Nurses seeking decision support in clinical settings are not interested in writing programs. They need to be able to communicate with the system in English to pose questions and to enter and receive information. Perhaps "procedural attachments" (Marcus, 1986) will resolve this issue, but their effect on program efficiency will have to be evaluated.

A final issue in decision support concerns uncertainty. "In order to be used responsibly, expert systems must be able to communicate a confidence factor so that the user can judge the system's findings" (Marcus, 1986, p. 153). Although the numerical values of confidence factors may be suspect, Marcus says, they have been found useful for ranking conclusions from best to worst. She describes three basic approaches to confidence factors, a "standard" approach, a "fuzzy logic" approach, and a Bayesian approach, and shows how each can be managed in Prolog. To have confidence factors associated with inferences would be an important enhancement to a nursing decision-support system. It will be necessary, however, to find a way to incorporate the rules for calculating confidence factors without detracting excessively from the speed or efficiency of the program.

Conclusions

Prolog appears to be a promising tool for programming decision-support systems for nursing. Its advantages over other approaches include conciseness and efficiency. The most important difference, however, is the capacity of logic programming to respond to ad hoc questions by drawing inferences from the knowledge base. Given a complex nursing knowledge base, a Prolog-based system could help nurses of varying expertise to consider relationships and alternatives and could facilitate care planning and documentation.

In order to achieve these objectives, however, several problems must be resolved. The nursing knowledge base must be represented in Prolog, the effects on system efficiency of including confidence factors must be determined, the ability of the system to draw on and manage the client data base must be developed, and a user-friendly interface must be designed. Each of these tasks is formidable. Prior accomplishments and current trends, however, suggest that all are achievable. The time has come to begin to develop practical, useful systems that will support the science and the art of nursing.

Acknowledgment. An earlier version of this chapter was published under the title "Prolog: A Practical Language for Decision Support Systems in Nursing?" in the *Proceedings of the Eleventh Annual Symposium on Computer Applications in Medical Care* (SCAMC, 1987).

Questions

1. Where was the COMMES system developed? How is the nursing knowledge base defined in this system? What difficulties arise from defining the knowledge base in this way? What is the major disadvantage of *not* linking COMMES to an integrated hospital information system?

2. How have Ozbolt and her group at The University of Michigan defined the nursing knowledge base for their prototype decision-support systems? Why have they chosen this approach? What are the major limitations of their previous prototype systems?

3. Why is it difficult to represent nursing's knowledge base comprehensively, concisely, and logically? Why does Ozbolt think this can best be done by deducing the knowledge base from a conceptual

model? What criteria must a conceptual model meet in order to be a suitable framework for a nursing knowledge base? What approach would you take to representing nursing's knowledge base comprehensively, concisely, and logically? Why?

4. Think about the decisions that you make easily and well as a nurse and those that you find more difficult. Think, too, about how you interact with your clients. What kind of help would you want from a computer? Where and how would you want to use the computer in order to enhance, not impede, your interactions with your clients and the efficiency of your performance?

5. Give two major reasons why a logic programming language such as Prolog may be better suited to supporting clinical decision making in nursing than a list processing language that depends on procedural rules to find the answers to questions?

6. Briefly describe four major problems that must be resolved when creating a decision-support system for nursing based on Prolog.

7. If an "ideal" support system for nursing existed, how might it enhance the art, as well as the science, of nursing?

References Cited

American Nurses' Association: *Nursing: A Social Policy Statement*. Kansas City: ANA, 1980.

Benner P: From novice to expert. *American Journal of Nursing* 1982; 82:402–407.

Benner P: *From Novice to Expert: Excellence and Power in Clinical Nursing Practice*. Menlo Park, CA: Addison-Wesley, 1984.

Benner P, Tanner C: Clinical judgment: how expert nurses use intuition. *American Journal of Nursing* 1987; 87:23–31.

Benner P, Wrubel J: Skilled clinical knowledge: the value of perceptual awareness. *Nurse Educator* 1982; 7:11–17.

Brodie ML, Jarke M: On integrating logic programming and databases. In: Kerschberg L, ed. *Expert Database Systems; Proceedings from the First International Workshop*. Menlo Park, CA: Benjamin-Cummings, 1986; 191–207.

Brulé JF: *Artificial Intelligence: Theory, Logic, and Application*. Blue Ridge Summit, PA: Tab Books, 1986.

Clocksin WF, Mellish CS: *Programming in Prolog*. 2d ed. Berlin: Springer-Verlag, 1984.

Cohen PR, Feigenbaum EA: *The Handbook of Artificial Intelligence*. Vol. 3. Menlo Park, CA: Addison-Wesley, 1982.

Dreyfus HL: *What Computers Can't Do*. New York: Harper & Row, 1972.

Dreyfus HL: *What Computers Can't Do*. Revised ed. New York: Harper Colophon, 1979.

Ennals R, Briggs J, Brough D: What the naive user wants from Prolog. In:

Campbell JA, ed. *Implementation of Prolog*. New York: Wiley, 1984; 376–386.

Erickson HC, Tomlin EM, Swain MAP: *Modeling and Role-Modeling: A Theory and Paradigm for Nursing*. Englewood Cliffs: Prentice-Hall, 1983.

Evans S: A computer-based nursing diagnosis consultant. In: Cohen GS, ed. *Proceedings of the Eighth Annual Symposium on Computer Applications in Medical Care*. Washington, DC: IEEE Computer Society, 1984; 658–661.

Evans S: Clinical and academic uses of COMMES: an implemented AI expert system. In: Ackerman MJ, ed. *Proceedings of the Ninth Annual Symposium on Computer Applications in Medical Care*. Washington, DC: IEEE Computer Society, 1985; 337.

Fawcett J: *Analysis and Evaluation of Conceptual Models of Nursing*. Philadelphia: Davis, 1984.

Goodwin JO, Edwards BS: Developing a computer program to assist the nursing process: Phase I—from systems analysis to an expandable program. *Nursing Research* 1975; 24:299–305.

Johnson DE: Development of theory: a requisite for nursing as a primary health profession. *Nursing Research* 1974; 23:372–377.

Marcus C: *Prolog Programming: Applications for Database Systems, Expert Systems, and Natural Language Systems*. Menlo Park, CA: Addison-Wesley, 1986.

McCain RF: Nursing by assessment—not intuition. *American Journal of Nursing* 1965; 65:82–84.

Orem DE: *Nursing: Concepts of Practice*. New York: McGraw-Hill, 1971.

Orem DE: *Nursing: Concepts of Practice*. 2d ed. New York: McGraw-Hill, 1980.

Orem DE: *Nursing: Concepts of Practice*. 3d ed. New York: McGraw-Hill, 1985.

Ozbolt JG: A prototype information system to aid nursing decisions. In: Blum BI, ed. *Proceedings of the Sixth Annual Symposium on Computer Applications in Medical Care*. New York: IEEE Computer Society, 1982; 653–657.

Ozbolt JG, Schultz S II, Swain MAP, et al: Developing expert systems for nursing practice. In: Cohen GS, ed. *Proceedings of the Eighth Annual Symposium on Computer Applications in Medical Care*. Washington, DC: IEEE Computer Society, 1984; 654–657.

Polanyi M: *Personal Knowledge: Towards a Post-Critical Philosophy*. Chicago: University of Chicago Press, 1974.

Ryan SA: Applications of a knowledge based system for nursing practice: inservice, continuing education, and standards of care. In: Dayhoff RE, ed. *Proceedings of the Seventh Annual Symposium on Computer Applications in Medical Care*. Silver Spring: IEEE Computer Society, 1983; 491–494.

Sciore E, Warren DS: Towards an integrated database-Prolog system. In: Kerschberg L, ed. *Expert Database Systems: Proceedings from the First International Workshop*. Menlo Park, CA: Benjamin-Cummings, 1986; 293–305.

Stevens B: *Nursing Theory: Analysis, Application, Evaluation*. Boston: Little, Brown, 1979.

Section 2—Where Caring and Technology Meet

Unit 4—Educational Innovations

Unit Introduction

The first unit of this book is intended to provide the gestalt and overview required for subsequent content. In the first chapter, Protti establishes the context by describing the evolution of information technology, its place in society generally and in health care specifically. This leads the reader to Chapter 2 in which Ball and Douglas provide the transition into specific consideration of nursing informatics and professional change. This discussion is followed by Daly's introduction to organizational change. In the final chapter of this unit, E. Ball and Hammon focus the reader's attention on the use of resource people to assist nursing professionals in operationalizing nursing informatics in their own local work environments.

1—Using Computers to Educate Nurses

Kathryn J. Hannah

Introduction

The purpose of nursing education is to prepare individuals for the practice of the profession of nursing. That preparation should encompass entry into the practice of nursing as it exists on the completion of training and, as far as can be anticipated, into the practice of nursing in the future. As the use of computers and information science in nursing practice, education, and administration increases, the need also increases for nurses who possess the skill and knowledge to use and manage information technology in nursing environments.

Our task as nursing educators is changing. Our new responsibility is to teach our students to become discriminating users of information. Our graduates will need to have expertise in the use of computer-based information systems in the health care organizations and agencies in which they are employed. They must also be taught to use the technology as a tool to practice their chosen profession rather than practicing their profession to suit the needs of technology. In the delivery of health care, nurses have traditionally provided the interface between the client and the health care system. They will fulfill this function in new ways in a technologically advanced environment.

There is consensus in the literature that knowledge about nursing uses of computers should be included in nursing education curricula. Unfortunately, these curriculum needs are most frequently identified by using the ambiguous term "computer literacy," for which "no definition ... has gained widespread acceptance" (Skiba, 1983).

Compounding this situation is the fact that virtually no nursing educator in practice today was educated with computers as part of either general or professional education (Hannah, 1983). Therefore, there are no generally accepted standards, and very few individuals who are either experientially or academically qualified to establish standards for the content of nursing informatics curricula. Finally, even when informatics content is incorporated into curricula and courses are mounted, there is only limited learning material available to support the teaching of these concepts (Ronald, 1979; Ball and Hannah, 1984).

Thus, before nursing can realize the benefits of information technology and bring nursing informatics to its full potential, we must address a number of fronts.

Faculty Development

Faculty development programs have been proposed as a method of coping with the problem of the lack of expertise among faculty members. Guidelines for faculty competence are followed by a warning to nurse educators:

> When faculty members have developed a degree of computer literacy, they will be able to make decisions with respect to what computer-related content should be integrated into the nursing curriculum, at what levels, and how it should be organized.... Until faculty have this knowledge, it is probable that most nursing curricula will not include computer concepts as they relate to nursing. (Ronald, 1983)

In the interim, a working conference sponsored by the International Medical Informatics Association (IMIA) has proposed model curricula for teaching informatics content to students in the health care professions (Pages et al, 1983). A curriculum based on the IMIA models has been implemented by the Faculty of Nursing at the University of Calgary (Hannah, 1983). Currently, the School of Nursing at the University of Maryland at Baltimore is developing a master's degree program in nursing informatics.

Today, more texts, videotapes, and CAL lessons are becoming available to assist in teaching nursing informatics content. At the same time, student learning needs in informatics are changing. With computer literacy soon to become a requirement for graduation from high school, an increasing number of students enter the nursing curriculum with advanced keyboarding skills and an understanding of computer terms, concepts, and history as well as computer applications in nursing.

The involvement of nurses in projects in instructional and educational uses of computers is long standing and diverse. Nurse educators have been in the forefront of projects on large mainframes and on microcomputers, developing and evaluating computer hardware and software. Applications range from patient education to professional education for nursing students and nurses in practice.

Nurse educators are using the computer in a number of ways to manage the educational environment:

- to instruct

- to evaluate

- to identify individual students' learning problems

- to gather data on how learning takes place

- to manipulate data for research purposes

- to direct continuing education.

In addition, nurse educators teach and interpret the jargon and basic tenets of modern nursing for the information specialists. They play an active role in preparing their professional colleagues through both basic and continuing education for the inevitable widespread implementation of automated information systems.

Developments in nursing informatics are beginning, and will continue, to have an impact on what and how nursing is taught at every level of nursing education. Nursing will manifest the effects of nursing informatics at the bedside, in professional practices, in curricula, and even in ergonomics. Ultimately, the impact of nursing informatics will be so profound as to change totally the nature of nursing education—and nursing itself.

Introducing Computers into Nursing Education

Initiating and Restraining Factors

Since the seminal work in the field, which demonstrated that nursing students taught using computer-assisted instruction learned the same material in one-third to one-half of the time, nursing educators have increasingly begun to use computers as an instructional methodology (Bitzer, 1963). In investigating the motives for use of computer-assisted instruction (CAI) in postsecondary education, similar findings were consistently identified (van Dijk et al, 1985; Murphy, 1984):

1. Compatibility with established learning theory including the provision of immediate, impartial, nonpunitive feedback

2. Stimulating multisensory learning environment supportive of teaching/learning strategies

3. Individualization of student learning

4. Stimulation and response to self-directed and self-motivated student learning behavior

5. Reduced student anxiety

6. Curriculum extension, including enrichment/remediation experiences as well as learning opportunities that could not be achieved in other ways without risking harm to the client

7. Initiation of students to learning about computers and students to basic computing skills

8. More time for faculty to provide individual attention to students and to pursue their own continuing education and research needs

9. Almost continual availability of the computer

10. Teaching efficacy and cost-effectiveness.

There are also restraining forces related to the implementation of CAI (Murphy, 1984):

1. Costs of acquiring and maintaining equipment as well as costs for developing software

2. Lack of transportability of software across hardware, operating systems, and programming languages

3. Lack of computer experience and expertise among educators

4. Potential change in the teacher's role

5. Lack of institutional recognition/reward toward promotion/tenure for development of CAI courseware

6. Concern regarding the potential of CAI to limit the socializing experiences provided by classroom learning

7. Seemingly less personalized education

8. Anticipated downtime of the computer system

9. Fears of invading student privacy

10. Concerns related to the possible reduction of faculty numbers.

Limitations

Based on these motivating forces, with little regard for restraining forces nursing educators have increasingly been purchasing hardware for educational computing, including computer-managed instruction (CMI) as well as computer-assisted instruction (CAI). Unfortunately, the technology has outdistanced our capacity to use it. One researcher maintains that the number of educational computers has doubled in the recent past "in spite of the fact that virtually no decent educational software existed for use with these machines" (Bork, 1984).

Generally, nursing educators lack awareness and understanding of computer-assisted learning (CAL) technology. They have limited knowledge of lesson design appropriate to CAL technology. Similarly, they have limited understanding of the physical and psychosocial aspects of ergonomics associated with learning. In addition, nursing educators generally do not use rational means for selecting appropriate topics for CAL lessons or for matching CAL instructional strategies to teaching/learning objectives and course content.

Before nursing educators can fully exploit the capabilities of advanced technology for instructional purposes, they must have access to such awareness, knowledge, and skills. Because they do not, much of the equipment purchased for instructional computing in nursing education remains underutilized.

Integrating Computers into Nursing Education

Only now, after 25 years, are we beginning to integrate CAL into the repertoire of teaching/learning strategies used in nursing education. In the interim, technologic advances in educational computing have continued. Innovations such as videotext, videodisk, fiber optics, programmer-less systems, and robotics are all available to supplement computer-assisted learning. These technologic advances have been used in nursing education in only peripheral fashion, primarily for purposes of demonstrating the technology. However, pioneering efforts to develop and promote nursing education use of the most sophisticated technology available are being conducted by R.O.I. Limited, Mirror Systems, in conjunction with Mosby Systems, IXION, and IVIS.

The Technological Innovations in Medical Education (TIME) project of the Lister Hill National Center for Biomedical Communications is exploring new educational designs and new theoretical approaches to medical education by developing a series of clinical simulations that utilize the combined technologies of microcomputer, videodisk, and voice recognition (Harless, 1984). These simulations will demonstrate the use of the new technology to implement problem-based, patient-related learning strategies in all phases of medical education. Models being developed in this project should prove readily transferable to nursing education.

Software Development

Instead of first determining the use, finding the software, and then buying the machine to run the software, nursing educators frequently rushed out to purchase computer hardware and then began to search for a purpose for which to use the hardware. Until recently, they discovered that there was very little instructional software commercially available for nursing. Thus, nursing educators began, with limited resources, to attempt to design their own software in order to justify the previous expenditure on hardware. These well-intentioned efforts were developed primarily with a view to using the hardware and minimizing developmental expenses. They produced some useful material, but most were amateur efforts undertaken without due regard for process and resulted in materials that were, at best, of dubious utility and value.

It behooves curriculum planners who elect to develop their own CAL software to be attentive to the process of development. Curriculum planners in nursing education choosing to develop their own computer-based instructional material would be well advised to give due regard for process. A formal development process has been used at the Educational Technology Center at the University of California, Irvine (Bork, 1984). A similar process is being implemented at the University of Calgary by the Institute for Computer Assisted Learning in conjunction with the Canadian Centre for Learning Systems.

Curriculum planning begins with defining clearly a set of instructional objectives and learning outcomes and ensuring that adequate funding is in place to complete the project. It uses a developmental team of experts, among them a content expert, lesson design expert, systems analyst, programmer, and graphics specialist. This process relies on careful attention to detail during software development and incorporates both formative and summative evaluation by the developmental team and by users. In short, nurse educators choosing to develop nursing CAL must accept the responsibility for ensuring that it is of high quality.

A less costly alternative than establishing a developmental team is that of purchasing an authoring system. An authoring system is a computer program designed to permit faculty members with limited programming skills to develop instructional computing materials with relative ease. The advantages of an authoring system are that it provides a simplified means of producing educational computing materials at modest cost. The disadvantage is that the faculty-member user is confined to those instructional designs and strategies that have been incorporated into the authoring system. Two different approaches to authoring systems have been developed (Pogue and Pogue, 1985; Grobe, 1985).

Evaluation of Software Solutions

Nurse educators electing to purchase software rather than produce their own need to become much more sophisticated and selective in evaluating software before purchase. On the basis of previous educational experiences, nurse educators have established personal criteria for evaluating instructional materials for use in the courses they teach.

However, virtually no nursing educator has experienced instructional computing as a part of either general or professional education. Therefore, they lack the experiential learning necessary to differentiate good CAL software from bad.

Educational Criteria

Consequently, nursing educators must make a conscious effort to acquire the necessary skills. In choosing among alternative CAL software or between CAL and other teaching/learning strategies, nurse educators must compare alternatives on the basis of effectiveness, quality, and cost. Each of these variables must be included in the evaluation of each alternative and the comparison among different alternatives. This will result in increasing pressure on the marketplace to improve the quality of their products.

The evaluation process must address a number of key considerations. To begin, the evaluation team must take into account the fact that not all content is equally well taught by different teaching methodologies. For example, group process terminology or concepts can be taught using instructional computing, but group process interaction skills cannot. At the present time, there are few criteria for discriminating among teaching strategies to identify that most appropriate for learning specific content.

The evaluation team must also make a concerted effort to determine the congruence between instructional objectives and the objectives of a particular CAL program. Although to some this may appear obvious, experience suggests that decisions to purchase instructional computing software are sometimes made without examining the objectives of that software and comparing them to the program, course, or learning unit objectives.

Quality

Even though more software for nursing education is now commercially available, quality remains questionable:

> The amount of software—particularly commercially produced programs—available for use at all grade levels and in all content areas has increased greatly. But the quality of this software has remained consistently low.... We know how to produce decent computer-based learning materials. But that knowledge has largely gone unused. Most of the programs now available are not the products of a careful design process, and very few of them have undergone careful evaluation. (Bork, 1984)

Numerous guides, checklists, and evaluation tools are available to assist the nurse educator in judging the worth of a particular CAL package for a specific instructional purpose (Alberta Education, 1984;

Table 1-1
Criteria Frequently Used for Evaluating
Instructional Computing Software for
Nursing Education

Content
    Accurate
    Relevant
    Current
Format
    Frames
    Graphics
    Ergonomics
    Psychosocial
    Physical
Documentation Style
    Scholarship
    Parsimony
    Use of humor
    Personalization
Strategies
    Predominant type
    Variety
    Remediation

Hudgings and Meehan, 1984; Komoski, 1984; Caissy, 1984; Bork, 1984; Sawyer, 1984). Table 1-1 lists the criteria most frequently used in evaluating the quality of instructional computing software.

Costs

When comparing commercial CAL software, usually only the purchase price is considered because all other costs are considered to be equal. In comparing commercially available CAL to locally developed CAL, usually only direct rather than full costs are considered. Direct costs are those costs related specifically to the alternative under consideration. Full costs are all costs associated with an alternative including direct costs as well as indirect overhead costs, such as a proportion of utilities or administration. However, remember that direct costs of locally developed CAL materials must include design, development, and operation of the CAL software program.

Comparison between CAL and other alternative teaching/learning strategies involves more elaborate and sophisticated calculations than when making comparisons between different CAL software programs. When comparing CAL with other teaching/learning strategies, the following categories of costs should be included:

Personnel salaries and benefits
Administrative fees or salaries and benefits

Services such as printing, postage, telephone, equipment rental
Hardware
Software
Facilities.

Evaluation Methodologies

The most useful method of comparison would permit comparison
among alternatives using all of the variables identified above, i.e.,
effectiveness, quality, and cost.

Cost-Benefit Analysis

Cost-benefit analysis involves the calculation of the monetary costs
and benefits of alternatives. The relative attractiveness of each alternative is then assessed by determining which alternative has the lowest
dollar cost and highest dollar benefit (Fig. 1-1).

$$B_1 - C_1 \geq B_2 - C_2$$

where B represents the Benefits in dollars, and C represents the Costs
in dollars.

Figure 1-1
Cost-benefit analysis model.

Cost-benefit analysis provides for the use of quantitative objective
data to compare two alternatives. Unfortunately, many benefits and
costs in nursing education are not quantitative; rather, they are qualitative. This model does not allow consideration of measures of either
the effectiveness or quality variables identified above. Therefore, in the
author's opinion this model is usually not useful for evaluating instructional computing software for nursing education.

Cost-Utility Analysis

Cost-utility analysis provides comparison of ratios between alternatives. The costs of an alternative are calculated. The decision makers
determine the utility or usefulness of the alternative. These two factors
are then compared to the same factors for other alternatives under
consideration (Fig. 1-2).

$$\frac{C_1}{U_1} \geq \frac{C_2}{U_2}$$

where C represents Costs in dollars, and U represents subjective
judgment by decision maker of the perceived Utility of the software.

Figure 1-2
Cost-utility analysis model.

The cost-utility analysis method relies on a combination of quantitative and qualitative data, but unfortunately only the quantitative data are objective. The utility (qualitative) data are based on the subjective judgment by the decision maker of their perception of the alternative's utility.

Cost-Effectiveness Analysis

Cost-effectiveness analysis also establishes a ratio. In this case, the ratio is between the measure of the extent to which an alternative is effective in achieving a predetermined goal and the cost of the alternative in dollars. Ratios for different alternatives are then compared (see Fig. 1-3).

$$\frac{GE_1}{C_1} \geq \frac{GE_2}{C_2}$$

where GE represents measures of *Goal Effectiveness*, and C represents *Costs* in dollars.

Figure 1-3
Cost-effectiveness analysis model.

In this method both quantitative (costs) and qualitative (goal effectiveness) data are considered and objective measures are gathered for both types of data. Finally, this method of comparison permits both the effectiveness and quality variables identified here to be considered as goals. Thus, cost-effectiveness analysis is the superior method for choosing among instructional alternatives.

With a conscious effort to develop experience through practice, nurse educators will become more sophisticated in judging the quality of CAL software. This will translate into increasing pressure on developers and distributors of nursing CAL software to improve the quality of their products.

Implications of Nursing Informatics

The implications of nursing informatics related to the hardware are clear for curriculum planners. They must acquire awareness and understanding of CAL technology. They must learn lesson design techniques appropriate to CAL technology. They must use rational means for selecting appropriate topics for CAL lessons or for matching CAL instructional strategies to teaching/learning objectives and course content. In addition, nursing educators also must monitor continually the new developments in technology.

Nursing educators must accept the responsibility of becoming knowledgeable about the use of computers in nursing practice and nursing education to make rational curriculum decisions about the integration of nursing informatics content into nursing curricula. In the meantime they can make use of the model curricula described in the literature. They should also expect guidance and advice from the professional organizations such as the International Medical Informatics Association, the Alberta Association of Registered Nurses, the National League for Nursing, the American Nurses' Association, the British Computer Society, and the Computer Applications in Nursing Special Interest Group of the Royal Australian Nursing Federation, all of which have active groups addressing the need for nursing informatics content in nursing education curricula. In addition, curriculum planners must locate instructional materials, evaluate their utility, and use them to support the teaching of nursing informatics. Finally they must accept the responsibility to be proactive in the anticipation of the need to prepare graduates who are discriminating users of information and not hampered by the technology.

Questions

1. What are the newly evolving competencies required of nurses graduating in the future?

2. Describe the problems affecting development and implementation of curriculum content related to nursing uses of computers.

3. Comment on the relevance to your setting of the general limitations discussed in this chapter relative to implementation of computer-assisted learning in nursing education.

4. Compare and contrast two methods of developing computer-assisted learning materials for use in nursing education.

5. Summarize the implications of nursing informatics for nursing education.

References Cited

Alberta Education: *Clearing House Evaluator's Guide for Microcomputer-based Courseware*. Edmonton: Alberta Education, 1984.

Ball MJ, Hannah KJ: *Using Computers in Nursing*. Reston: Reston Publishers, 1984; 111–112.

Bitzer MAD: *Self-Directed Inquiry in Clinical Nursing Instruction by Means of PLATO*. Simulated Laboratory, Co-Ordinated Science Laboratory, Report R-184. Urbana: University of Illinois, 1963.

Bork A: Computers in education today—and some possible futures. *Phi Delta Kappan* 1984; 65–66, 239–243.

Caissy G: Evaluating educational software: a practitioner's guide. *Phi Delta Kappan* 1984; 65–66, 249–250.

Grobe S: Effective use of nursing information systems: a nursing education perspective. In: Hannah KJ, Guillemin EJ, Conklin DN, eds. *Nursing Uses of Computers and Information Science.* Amsterdam: North Holland, 1985; 201–203.

Hannah KJ: The place of medical informatics in a baccalaureate nursing curriculum. In: Pages JC, Levy AH, Gremy F, et al, eds. *Meeting the Challenge: Informatics and Medical Education.* Amsterdam: North Holland, 1983; 67–78.

Harless WG: *The Time Project.* Washington, DC: U.S. Department of Health and Human Services, 1984.

Hudgings C, Meehan N: Software evaluation for nursing educators. *Computers in Nursing* 1984; 2:35–37.

Komoski K: Educational computing: the burden of ensuring quality. *Phi Delta Kappan* 1984; 65–66, 244–248.

Murphy MA: Computer-based education in nursing: factors influencing its utilization. *Computers in Nursing* 1984; 2:218–223.

Pages JC, Levy AH, Gremy F, et al, eds: *Meeting the Challenge: Informatics and Medical Education.* Amsterdam: North Holland, 1983; 317–330.

Pogue LM, Pogue RE: Authoring systems: a key to efficient production of computer-based nursing learning materials. In: Hannah KJ, Guillemin EJ, Conklin DN, eds. *Nursing Uses of Computers and Information Science.* Amsterdam: North Holland, 1985; 229–233.

Ronald JS: Computers and undergraduate nursing education. *Journal of Nursing Education* 1979; 18:4–9.

Ronald JA: Guidelines for computer literacy curriculums in a school of nursing. *Journal NYSNA* 1983; 14:12–18.

Sawyer T: Human factors considerations in computer-assisted instruction. *Journal of Computer-Based Instruction* 1984; 12:17–20.

Skiba DJ: Computer literacy: the challenge of the '80s. *Journal NYSNA* 1983; 14:6–11.

van Dijk TAM, Gastkemper F, Moonen J, et al: Motives for CAI in postsecondary education. *Journal of Computer-Based Instruction* 1985; 12:8–11.

Bibliography

Beilby A: Determining instructional costs through functional cost analysis. *Journal of Instructional Development* 1979; 3:29–34.

Edwards M: Cost analysis comparison of traditional and interactive videodisk CPR instruction. In: Hannah KJ, Guillemin EJ, Conklin DN, eds. *Nursing Uses of Computers and Information Science.* Amsterdam: North Holland, 1985; 201–203.

Jenkins TM: Cost-effectiveness of computer-based job training for nurses. In: Hannah KJ, Guillemin EJ, Conklin DN, eds. *Nursing Uses of Computers and Information Science.* Amsterdam: North Holland, 1985; 223–227.

Ronald JS: Guidelines for computer literacy curriculums in a school of nursing. *Journal NYSNA* 1983; 14:12–18.

2—Educational Software

Barbara S. Thomas

Instructional Computing: Where Are We?

A Brief Look at Beginnings

Computer-based education (CBE) and computer-assisted learning (CAL) are interchangeable terms that refer to computers as an instructional medium (Ball and Hannah, 1984). Both include computer-assisted instruction (CAI) and computer-managed instruction (CMI). While CAI is used to assist students in the teaching/learning process, CMI is used to manage components of instruction such as student testing, student rotations, use of instructional materials, and course scheduling. This chapter will focus primarily on computer-assisted instruction and its usefulness in nursing education.

CAI was developed more than 20 years ago on time-sharing computers (Deland, 1978). Several of these systems are still in wide use, for example, PLATO and the Health Education Network. Although there is a trend toward converting these programs for use with microcomputers, the use of instructional materials for mainframe or minicomputers is still fairly widespread. The primary advantages are simply that there are no limits on memory or possibilities to deal with in developing a CAI lesson; high-level, powerful computer languages such as FORTRAN or PL-1 can be used. Moreover, many students can access the lessons simultaneously, and the chances for user damage to the lesson are remote. The disadvantages are well known: lack of transportability and costs.

These disadvantages prevented the spread of CAI in nursing education until the advent of microcomputers, which ameliorated both situations and introduced a new era of instructional computing in nursing education. In 1970, the editors of *The American Journal of Nursing* published views of what nursing education would be like in the 1970s. One prediction was that computers would become commonplace in hospitals, classrooms, libraries, dormitories, and homes

Table 2-1
Factors Identified as Inhibiting Growth of Instructional Computing in Professional Nursing Programs, 1983–1985

Factor	Rank order	
	1983	1985
Faculty's lack of opportunity to learn	1	6
Faculty's lack of skills	2	2
Hardware costs	3	5
Software costs	4	4
Lack of useful software	5	3
Lack of information about software	6	9
Lack of faculty time/interest	7	1
Lack of information about hardware	8	10
Lack of evaluative evidence of worth	9	7
Transportability problems	10	8

(Bitzer, 1970). Her predictions, as we know, did not come true for a number of reasons. The slow process of accepting a new technology has been cited and described (Rogers and Shoemaker, 1971; Jenkins et al, 1983). More pragmatic reasons were given by deans and directors of baccalaureate and higher degree programs accredited by the National League for Nursing (NLN) (Table 2-1) (Thomas 1985, 1986). Two surveys were conducted, one in 1983 and one at the end of 1985. The rank order of barriers identified by respondents shows that faculty development issues, costs, and lack of information about the availability and usefulness of software were cited as most important.

There are several interesting changes over the 2-year period. Faculty's lack of opportunity to learn dropped from first to sixth place, reflecting the enormous number of conferences, workshops, and symposia on computing as well as substantial improvements in dissemination of information about computing in nursing through publications. Problems associated with the quality of available software are cited as more important in the more recent survey as opposed to lack of information about software, which lessened in importance.

There is wide agreement that microcomputers serve as unique learning tools in that they process software (or courseware) in ways that keep the learner actively involved. They personalize instruction, give the learner control of the route and pace of instruction, and provide immediate feedback. Because software is developed on floppy diskettes, it is readily available for many sites at reasonable cost. Thus, the issue of transportability has been replaced by compatibility, and even this issue is fading.

However, faculty development problems are likely to remain serious deterrents to software development for several reasons. Gaining faculty acceptance may be the biggest obstacle to the growth of instructional computing (Aiken and Braun, 1980). Faculty may fear the changes in their teaching styles which use of CAI may demand, and they may be reluctant to change their roles from being a primary source of knowledge to being a facilitator. Another reason that has been cited less often is the extremely low regard administrators have for production of software by faculty. In both surveys cited above, deans and directors were asked to rank the importance of selected faculty accomplishments in making promotion, tenure, and salary decisions. Of 12 types of accomplishments, development of CAI or interactive video was rated dead last, behind all sorts of publications including nonresearch articles in nonrefereed journals, development of programmed learning modules, and even service activities (Thomas, 1985, 1986).

Recent Growth of Instructional Computing in Nursing

Data from the two surveys indicate that use of microcomputers increased substantially over the 2-year period. In 1983, 62% of the faculty, 22% of the graduate students, and 31% of the undergraduate students were reported to be using microcomputers; the figures for 1985 were 94%, 80%, and 77% respectively. The number of microcomputer systems in nursing programs increased from 365 to 1440 in the sample. Numbers of available peripherals increased similarly. As might be expected because of cost considerations, videodisc equipment was least reported. Levels of faculty expertise in computing were shown to improve also. The percentages of unskilled faculty went from 77% in 1983 to 50% in 1985 (Thomas, 1985, 1986).

Information about applications used most on all types of computers shows that word processing was used most frequently by staff, whereas data analysis with statistical packages was most heavily used by faculty. Results remained consistent over both surveys. Data for graduate students were similar. However, undergraduate student use of computers in both surveys was primarily for instruction, followed by word processing, personal computing, retrieving patient data, and analyzing research data, in that order (Thomas, 1985, 1986). This is related to the availability of software for undergraduate instruction and the relative scarcity of it for graduate education in nursing.

In spite of all of the barriers to CAI development, there has been a remarkable increase in the availability of software and access to information about it. The appearance of a journal devoted exclusively to computing in nursing and the publication of a monthly Software Exchange in *Computers in Nursing* have had a substantial impact on the growth of CAI. More recently, software directories have made information about software readily accessible (Bolwell, 1984, 1985, 1987).

Types of CAI

There are six types of CAI in current use: drill and practice, tutorials, problem-solving, simulation, gaming, and testing. The diversity in both topics and quality is enormous. In many cases, the CAI is used with printed materials such as workbooks, or with visuals such as slides, and with interactive videotapes or videodiscs.

Drill and practice lessons allow users to learn facts or to review and sharpen their skills regarding prior learning of factual material. In the simplest programs of this type, the learners are presented with questions and choices and are simply given information about the correctness of their responses. They may spend as much time with the lesson as desired. More complex drill and practice programs give the learner more control over the practice session, provide remediation, and may prevent the user from leaving the lesson until all correct choices have been entered at least once. Although most drill and practice programs rely on textual materials, the use of graphics can make the learning experience more interesting and effective. One program on anatomy, *Body Language*, is totally made up of graphics, and is without doubt one of the best examples of drill and practice lessons available (Peters, 1986).

Tutorials are designed to give the user factual and conceptual information with active involvement of the user maintained to facilitate learning. When the learner is given questions to answer or choices to make, a variety of branching options can be used to tailor the lesson to the knowledge base and needs of each individual learner. The lesson may be organized on a deductive or inductive basis, with concepts, examples, and "non-examples" arranged according to the strategy employed. A careful sequence of lesson components is critical to the success of tutorials.

Problem-solving programs give the learner the initiative in the sequence of the learning process. The user is given a problem and then allowed to gather data and make choices in its solution. A score is often generated, based on the efficiency of the learner's inquiry. Most problem-solving programs are simulations.

Simulations present the user with models of reality in varying degrees of detail and complexity. The usefulness of CAI for simulating student–patient encounters was early described as follows:

> Students could initially become involved with a "hypothetical" patient through a computerized program, identify nursing problems, test solutions, and find out the results of their interventions without involving "real patients" with all the inherent dangers requiring close supervision and consequent loss of student experimentation and without the problems involved in clinical areas that are scarce in the community. (DeTornyay, 1970, pp. 34–35)

In 1972, predictions were made that simulations would become the most widespread modes of CAI in higher education. This prediction appears to be accurate in that the number and variety of simulations being produced for nursing education are growing at a very rapid rate. Currently, simulations are available based on both the nursing process and the research process.

Testing can take many forms in CAI. There may be pretests and posttests as parts of menus of drill and practice, tutorials, or simulation lessons. The tests may tap knowledge, skills, or attitudes. Generally, such tests are used for user guidance only, because security of a computer-based test can only be maintained if its use is totally supervised. An important use of the testing mode is for review before taking state board examinations. Depending on the type and amount of feedback given after each user response, the testing programs can serve real teaching functions.

Gaming may function as a stand-alone program or be incorporated into CAI menu-driven programs including drill and practice, tutorials, problem-solving lessons, or simulations. The game introduces students to questions or situations that are rewarded when correct responses are entered. Various strategies such as moving along a path toward a goal or accumulating points serve to motivate the player(s). Games can be played with two or more competing players using the program together or by one player against the computer. The best games are truly novel and fun, with learning value present but secondary.

Selecting Software

A few years ago, it was necessary to make software decisions before acquiring the hardware to run the programs. If initial software selections were made poorly, a school of nursing might find itself with a large investment in hardware and few applications for its use. It is still true that software reviews should precede hardware purchases. However, more and more, CAI programs are being distributed by publishers in more than one version, for example, both APPLE II and IBM PC versions. The focus in this section will be on delineating that elusive factor, quality. The CAI program, its documentation, and its user support must be appraised.

The central issue in evaluating software for possible purchase is how important the instructional objectives of the program are for the setting and how well those objectives are attained through use of the CAI lesson. Does the CAI program serve a useful purpose in the school, hospital, or clinic? Is it easy to incorporate with existing coursework? In short, does it fill identified needs? An evaluation form based on a semantic differential provides a great deal of information

Table 2-2
Using Semantic Differentials to Evaluate Software

The lesson objectives are	very clear	1	2	3	4	5	very unclear
The directions for use are	very clear	1	2	3	4	5	very unclear
The lesson content is	helpful	1	2	3	4	5	not helpful
The level of the lesson is	too low	1	2	3	4	5	too high
The learning value is	low	1	2	3	4	5	high
Using the program is	easy	1	2	3	4	5	hard
Interest in using program is	low	1	2	3	4	5	high

in a minimum of time. Table 2-2 illustrates the adjective pairs that have been found useful in this type of evaluation. CONDUIT (1970) has developed and refined comprehensive evaluation tools for software. These have served as models for other organizations and individuals. Copies of their evaluation tools are included in the Appendix.

If the intended user is a registered nurse instead of a nursing student, the evaluation must include data on whether the guidelines of the American Nurses' Association (ANA) for continuing education are met. Table 2-3 illustrates one approach to this issue—one section of a tool that was used in the University of Iowa Nursing Microcomputer Project (Division of Nursing Special Project #D10 NU27075). Here the focus is on the criteria adopted by the ANA and the Iowa Board of Nursing for continuing nursing education credits.

It is important that the focus for each evaluator be determined by that individual evaluator's expertise. Content experts, instructional designers, nursing faculty members, nursing students, and nurses all provide useful data about the quality of a CAI program. But it is the content expert, not the student, who can assess the quality of the information contained in the program, and it is the instructional designer who can judge the screen design for effectiveness and consistency. All can comment on the user-friendliness of the program and its accompanying documentation.

Developing Software

The Team Approach

Probably the most effective approach to the development of quality CAI is the team approach, using the competencies of a content expert, an instructional designer, and a programmer. It is rare that one individual possesses all of the necessary skills, although many authors serve as their own instructional designers. In the Iowa Nursing Project, all but two authors used the services of instructional designers. The advantages of such collaboration go beyond improving screen design

Table 2-3
Review Items for Continuing Nursing Education[a]

CONTENT: Please check the content areas below (quoted from ANA criteria that this program addresses). Please check (√) all that apply.
_____ nursing practice related to counseling, teaching, or care of clients in any setting
_____ sciences upon which nursing practice, nursing education, or nursing research are based, e.g., nursing theories and biological, physical, behavioral, computer, social, or basic sciences
_____ social, economic, and legal aspects of health care
_____ management or administration of health care
_____ education of patients or their significant others, students, or personnel in the health care field
_____ content is included in the form of a course description and detailed outline with time frames
_____ relates to and is consistent with the offering objectives
_____ content is current
_____ content reinforces basic knowledge or skills and includes advanced content to build on nurses' knowledge base
_____ content is appropriate for the time estimated as needed for completing the program
_____ content is appropriate for continuing nursing education

OBJECTIVES: Please check (√) all that apply.
_____ are stated in behavioral terms that define the expected outcomes for the learner
_____ are consistent with the time and continuing education units (CEU) estimates for completion of the program
_____ are consistent with the educational level of the target population(s)

TEACHING/LEARNING STRATEGIES: Please check (√) all that apply.
_____ use principles of adult learning
_____ provide learning experiences that are congruent with the program's objectives
_____ are consistent with the program content
_____ are appropriate for the target population(s)

EVALUATION: Please check (√) all that apply.
Participants are given an opportunity to evaluate
_____ teaching/learning effectiveness
_____ achievement of stated objectives
_____ content
_____ teaching strategies
_____ achievement of personal objectives

[a] Adapted from the Iowa Board of Nursing and ANA criteria.

and ensuring adequate user interaction. The instructional designer, to do the job well, must understand the content at least at a novice level. Thus the content expert is forced to clarify concepts using graphics or perhaps additional frames to break the content down into instructionally sound modules. The disadvantages are that the content expert's constant explanations to the designer are time consuming and sometimes frustrating. The best CAI authors are master teachers who have given a good deal of attention to how people learn in their teaching by means of lectures, seminars, and laboratories.

The first step is to develop objectives and a content outline. The storyboard follows, and sometimes requires changes in the outline as problems of sequence appear and are resolved. Review of the storyboard by content experts, instructional designers, and possibly prospective users follows to identify needed changes. At this stage, consideration of standards and conventions should take place if they have not already been established. Decisions must be made about such matters as the degrees of user direction and flexibility, the placement of prompts, and the forms of allowable responses. Once consistent approaches are established and the program is refined, the coding or programming begins.

If more than one version (such as APPLE II and IBM PC) is being developed, the Iowa protocols might be considered to save time. Briefly, the storyboard along with programming notes is entered via MUSE onto the PRIME, a minicomputer, by the editorial associate or a secretary. Hard copy is produced for review by the author and possibly other members of the team. Following this review and refinement, programming begins. Note that the programmers are using a minicomputer (with pseudocodes of BASIC) to avoid memory limitations, and they have no need to type in any of the text; they can concentrate their efforts on commands. Once the text is coded, the program is downloaded to a microcomputer where the machine-specific programming such as graphics is completed. Downloading to another brand of microcomputer follows the review and refinement of the first version (McClain and Wessels, 1985).

Extensive evaluation is part of the development process. Reviews by other content experts, instructional designers, nurse educators, and students must be completed. It is important to tailor the evaluation tools to the tasks that each reviewer will complete. When disagreements arise about format or content, which we found to be rare, the author makes the final decision.

Authoring Systems

Authoring systems are systems software that allow authors to develop CAI programs without the use of programming languages. The power or complexity of available authoring systems differs considerably. An example of one of the simplest is a user-distributed program called Author/Quiz (Martin and Jeffreys, 1984) distributed free by its authors. The documentation automatically prints out from the diskette, which has been copied from the authors' diskette. There is a message asking for a payment if the copy is used. This program provides prompts and options for developing multiple-choice or true-false tests. Another single purpose but very complex authoring system is called NEMAS. Based on a formal nursing process (Grobe, 1982), it is distributed by the Lippincott Company. NEMAS is complex in its ability to produce a wide variety of simulations; the system is actually quite easy to use. Nurse educators can use this system to design nurse–patient encounters in a variety of settings to teach protocols, decision making, and the consequences of one's decisions.

The general-purpose authoring systems are generally menu driven so that the user can select from several options for developing the lesson. An example that was converted from minicomputer for microcomputers is MICROINSTRUCTOR (Pogue, 1985). It is distributed in both IBM PC and APPLE II versions. Its documentation includes the following statement:

> All commercial rights reserved. The sale or distribution of any software developed by the MICROINSTRUCTOR system is prohibited without the express written permission of the C.V. Mosby Company. Any lesson created with the MICROINSTRUCTOR is for the exclusive use of the purchaser.

Other packages carry similar restrictions. Before using an authoring system, these sorts of constraints must be considered carefully.

Instructional Computing: Where Are We Going?

In the early 1970s, there was a spurt of activity in CAI that produced some useful software and demonstrated the possible effectiveness of CAI. However, the cost-effectiveness was not established, nor were evaluative studies completed to support CAI as either improving learning or saving time. The early efforts faded, and it was not until the end of the decade that renewed interest emerged.

It appears that sufficient evidence of the worth of CAI has been demonstrated to sustain its growth, however slow. Learning outcomes are at least as good as alternative teaching/learning strategies, and a saving of time has been shown. These factors plus the appearance and refinement of authoring systems provide nurses with incentives for putting forth the effort to develop CAI in new content areas. Simulations appear particularly valuable and will probably dominate the new software produced in the next few years.

310   Barbara S. Thomas

The trend toward increased acquisition of hardware and software by nursing programs should continue at least through the 1980s. Faculty comfort with computer technology will continue to grow as well. Self-directed learning by nursing students will expand. CAI will be used to augment instruction, replace certain repetitive tasks, simulate nursing experiences in safe environments, and enrich nursing curricula by providing instruction on selected topics in greater depth than is currently possible in crowded nursing curricula.

Perhaps, as CAI becomes more widespread in nursing education, the task of developing it will take its place as a scholarly endeavor alongside research publications. When this happens, the true incentives for nurse educators to turn their attention to CAI development will be present and the growth of CAI will accelerate.

Questions

1. Why was there a surge of growth in instructional computing with the introduction of microcomputers?

2. Identify at least five reasons that growth of instructional computing in nursing has been rather slow.

3. What incentives are there for nursing faculty to spend time and effort developing software? What changes are needed in the reward system?

4. Describe the process of developing a simulation for nursing education.

5. Describe the process and the participants in evaluation of software for nursing.

References Cited

Aiken R, Braun L: Into the 80's with microcomputer-based learning. *Computer* 1980; 13:11–16.

Ball M, Hannah K: *Using Computers in Nursing*. Reston: Reston Publishing Company, 1984.

Bitzer MA: Nursing in the decade ahead. *American Journal of Nursing* 1970; 70:2117–2118.

Bolwell C: *Directory of Software for Nursing*. San Francisco: Diskovery, 1984.

Bolwell C: Identification of the unique educational attributes of CAI for the microcomputer. In: Levy AH, Williams BT, eds. *Proceedings of the AAMSI Congress 1985*. Washington, DC: AAMSI, 1985; 99–102.

Bolwell C: *Directory of Software for Nursing*. Washington, DC: National League for Nursing, 1987.

CONDUIT: *CONDUIT Evaluation Form for Microcomputer Based Instructional Materials*. Iowa City: CONDUIT, 1970.

Deland EC: *Information Technology in Health Science Education*. New York: Plenum Press, 1978.

DeTornyay R: Instructional technology and nursing education. *Journal of Nursing Education* 1970; 9:3–8, 34–35.

Grobe S: An authoring system based on the nursing process. In: Attala E, ed. *Proceedings: 1982 ADCIS Conference*. Vancouver, BC: ADCIS, 1982; 348.

Jenkins TM, Ball MJ, Bruns BM: The state of the art in technology-assisted learning. In: Lindberg DAB, Van Brunt EE, Jenkin MA, eds. *Proceedings: AAMSI Congress 83*. Bethesda: AAMSI, 1983; 279–283.

Martin L, Jeffreys J: *AUTHOR/QUIZ Users' Manual*. Cleveland: Mount Sinai Medical Center, 1984.

McClain D, Wessels S: One software development process at the University of Iowa. In: Thomas BS, ed. *Proceedings of Instructional Computing in Nursing Education*. Iowa City: University of Iowa Press, 1985; 163–168.

Peters H: *Body Language*. Iowa City: Educational Software Products, 1986.

Pogue R: *The MICROINSTRUCTOR*. St. Louis: CV Mosby, 1985.

Rogers E, Shoemaker F: *Communication of Innovations*. New York: Free Press, 1971.

Thomas BS: A survey study of computers in nursing education. *Computers in Nursing* 1985; 3:173–179.

Thomas BS: *Final Report: The Use of Microcomputer and Videodisc Technology in Continuing Nursing Education*. Iowa City: University of Iowa, 1986.

3—Video Disk Technology in Nursing Education

James F. Craig

Abstract

Nurses and nursing educators alike rely heavily on the use of visuals, usually 2 × 2 color slides, in the process of communicating with a variety of audiences ranging from other practitioners and office staff to patients, community organizations, or student groups. The diversity of these audiences requires that the person preparing the material tailor it to the audience to communicate effectively, which can be very time consuming and costly in terms of both material and human resources. Optical disks and computer technology offer a means of cataloging, storing, and retrieving thousands of visuals to accommodate the needs of these diverse audiences. These technologic innovations offer tremendous potential for nursing education and create a more cost-efficient and effective means of handling large quantities of visual material.

Introduction

In the past decade, new technologic developments, coupled with significant support aimed at increasing the number of health professionals, served as the impetus for encouraging the use of innovative teaching strategies and methods. During this time, health science institutions developed and utilized independent learning programs such as slide/tapes, videocassettes, instructional manuals, and case documentations as a primary method of teaching (Craig and Moreland, 1985). While these materials and methods are still used, computer and optical disk technology offer many unique options that are not readily available with these other forms. Of particular importance is the relative ease with which computers and optical disks store and retrieve visuals and information, provide immediate feedback, accumulate data, or enable an individual to update or modify a given program.

In this day and age, there is so much information available at the touch of a button that the present era is universally known as the Information Age. A recent article in TIME magazine indicated "The label fits. Information is the basis and driving force for almost every form of human activity." Continuing, TIME argued

> Even if there is an overload in some areas today, the Information Age, born of the computer, nurtured by the laser and the satellite, exemplifies a revolution from which there is no turning back, just as there was none after the invention of movable type or the cathode ray tube. (TIME Magazine, 1985)

In bringing the Information Age home to nursing education, it is estimated that of the more than 450 schools associated with nursing education in the country, at least 100 produce a significant number of slides each year in support of their academic and research programs. Dr. Elizabeth Lenz, Professor at the University of Maryland School of Nursing, indicated in conversation that "of these 100 institutions, it is realistic to assume that each produces approximately 1,000 slides a year in support of their academic and research programs." This represents more than 100,000 slides a year.

Assuming that the labor and material costs associated with the production of each of these slides were a modest $4.00, this is an annual expenditure of $400,000, a considerable sum just for the production of slides. Clearly, one of the primary reasons for such a large number of slides covering the same content area is the difficulty involved in sharing this material within a single school, let alone among institutions spanning the country. Dr. Lenz went on to say that, "nursing schools would and could use more slides for their programs, but unfortunately, many cannot afford to produce their own or pay for the cost of duplicating large quantities of material—regardless of how much they are needed."

A Novel Approach to an Important Educational Problem

It is safe to assume that of the slides produced by the nursing schools in 1 year a significant amount of duplication in visual information occurs, because these institutions are covering the same basic subject matter. If we had an opportunity to select the best and most comprehensive collection of slides from the 100,000 produced annually, and avoided duplicating the same content depicted in any given slide, how many unique items would be represented? Should we assume 10,000 or 15,000 or 25,000? Taking advantage of today's technology, we could place 54,000 images on just one side of an optical disk (Fig. 3-1) and access any one of them in less than a second. The total production

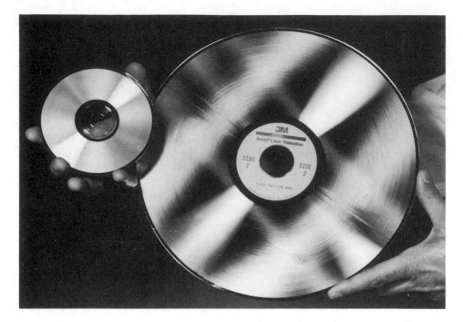

Figure 3-1
Videodisk.

costs involved in creating a "master" disk with this many images would be approximately $60,000, with copies costing approximately $10 to $15. Recent advances in the emerging compact disk technology have made it possible to place 5 minutes of motion or 9,000 still images on a compact disk, referred to as CD-V (compact disk-video).

To help you comprehend the magnitude of this visual data base, if you were to put 54 slides into each of 1,000 carousel trays and stack them on top of each other the stack would be 21 stories tall (Fig. 3-2). Having this many items to choose from would place a tremendous wealth of visual information at your disposal. By interfacing an optical disk system with a computer, the unique characteristics of each technology create a powerful vehicle for academic and research applications. For example, can you imagine the logistics involved in storing, sorting, selecting, cataloging, and (worst of all) retrieving any of the 54,000 slides from 1,000 carousel trays? Combining the two technologies enables you to do all of these tasks easily and efficiently, and provides the added dimension of digitized audio, full color graphics, and "touch-screen" interactive applications.

One other problem eliminated by optical disk technology is one that even the most skilled presenter has endured, having a carousel tray overturn and watching an entire presentation fall all over the floor.

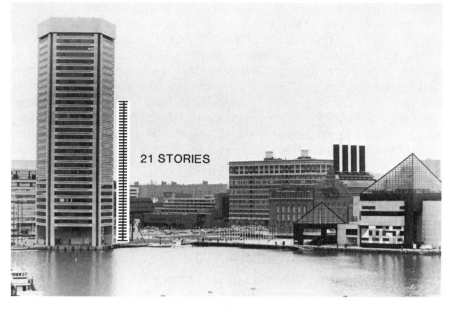

Figure 3-2
Storage requirements.

Optical disks store and retrieve visuals using laser technology, which eliminates the potential for having your slides fall out. Thomas Held, President of METAMEDIA SYSTEMS, INC., a firm that specializes in the development of optical disks for educational purposes, indicated he had made a discovery he refers to as "Held's Law of Diminishing Astonishment." In describing this law, Mr. Held said, "You can turn an optical disk with 54,000 images on it upside down and shake it and nothing happens. Try that with a carousel tray missing its locking ring and see what happens."

Optical Disk Technology

As early as 1927, John Logie Gaird had developed a means of storing visual images on a phonograph record. In 1935, Selfridges Department Store in London actually marketed such a device and sold the first "phonovision" disk (Bosco, 1984). Realizing the formative state of television at this time leaves little wonder why this invention lay dormant for so long.

As video technology became easier and less expensive to use, educators initially attempted interfacing a microcomputer with a videocassette player. The drawbacks to this interface were the difficulties encountered in accessing an individual frame quickly and accurately, for the video unit literally had to fast forward or rewind in order to find the frame. If the video unit did find the right image, maintaining a clear and steady picture often presented a problem. Additionally, if the frame were held in place for a considerable length of time, the tape was frequently damaged, for the reading mechanism for videocassette units involves a rapidly moving video "head" contacting the videotape.

Optical disks are made by etching single frames of video information into the metallic surface of the disk using laser technology. To view this information, a copy is made from the master disk and installed in a disk player. A player reads the information from the etched surface using a laser beam, translating the reflected light from the beam into an image. The disk rotates at a speed of 1,800 revolutions per minute. The significance of this process is that all 54,000 images can be accessed in a second or less with perfect accuracy. Because the image is merely reflected light, it provides a very stable image that can be held in one position for hours without damaging the image or the reading mechanism. The picture is viewed on a video monitor.

Disk systems are generally categorized as level I, II, or III based on the amount of interactivity they provide. A recent thrust has been toward a level IV system, which is still in the developmental stage. A level I system consists of a disk player and a monitor and allows the user a limited number of functions such as still frame, play (for full motion), fast forward, rewind, and search. In the latter case, the actual frame number may be brought up on the screen of the monitor as a reference for searching for specific images contained on the disk. These systems are commercially available for consumers and usually cost several hundred dollars. They are usually used for visual data bases or frequently played motion sequences.

A level II system consists of an industrial-grade disk player and a monitor. The player differs from the consumer unit in that it has a built-in microprocessor capable of storing up to 7 kbytes of memory. The disks used on this system usually contain programmed information that has actually been placed on the disk itself. As the user interacts with the system by responding to questions or choices, the microprocessor "reads" the programmed information from the disk and responds accordingly. These systems usually cost a few thousand dollars and are typically used by business and industry for commercial, educational, or training purposes. You may have seen such systems in hotels or shopping malls.

A level III system consists of an industrial-grade disk player, a microcomputer, and a monitor. These systems combine the power of the microcomputer with the image storage and retrieval capability of the optical disk player and are highly interactive. They typically in-

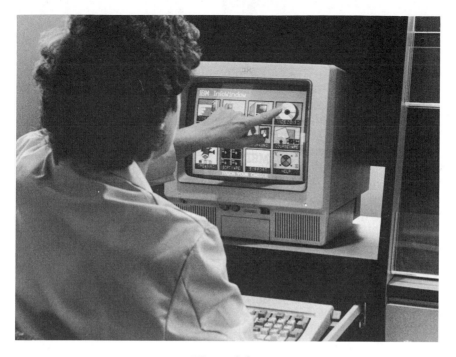

Figure 3-3
Infowindow screen.

clude high-resolution graphics, motion or still images, audio, and may
also include "touch screen" technology, a light pen, mouse, bit pad,
or bar code reader in order to further facilitate interactivity with the
user (Fig. 3-3). Such systems can be either stand alone, networked, or
both depending on the users' needs. They are most frequently used in
business and industry, and like the level II systems typically are used
for commercial, educational, or training purposes. A level III system
usually costs several to many thousand dollars depending on the
number of systems used and how they are configured.

Level IV systems are still in the developmental stage but offer the
greatest potential for a multiplicity of applications. They will provide
digitized video, graphics, and audio, and through a variety of compres-
sion techniques, do all of these through the use of compact disk
technology. The systems are generally referred to as CD-I or Compact
Disk-Interactive. They include a microcomputer, monitor, and compact disk system. The cost should range from a few to several thousand
dollars and like the level III systems can be either stand alone or
networked.

The Potential for Computer and Optical Disk Technology

Although its educational potential is widely acknowledged, educational institutions have yet to make widespread use of this innovative instructional methodology. Several reasons typically cited include the lack of good educational disks and the cost of the technology. "It appears as though interactive video is experiencing a chicken-and-egg type of problem," indicated Dean LaCoe, manager of Visage, Incorporated, a manufacturer of several IBM PC-compatible interactive videodisks. "People aren't developing software because there aren't enough systems out there, and people won't buy systems because there aren't enough programs available" (Jones, 1985).

Evidence indicates things are starting to change. The 1985 September issue of *T.H.E. Journal* listed 17 firms involved in the development and circulation of interactive videodisks (Jones, 1985). Additionally, METAMEDIA SYSTEMS and ON-LINE COMPUTER SYSTEMS, INC., two firms working together in Germantown, Maryland, have produced more than a hundred interactive disks for education and training purposes with many more presently under development.

Of particular importance to health professionals is the development of a prototype generic dental disk. This project is being undertaken by the Division of Information Resources Management and the Dental School at the University of Maryland at Baltimore. The estimated costs for placing 12,000 color slides on a master optical disk is approximately $15,000. Copies of this disk, depending on the total number made, could run as little as $10.00 to $15.00 each. The innovative aspects of this project include

1. Creating challenging clinical simulation exercises using a wide range of clinical situations while achieving a saving of time for students and minimizing a risk for the patients.

2. Providing a format that enables health professionals to develop software packages that can be shared nationally and internationally.

3. Creating a single audiovisual format accommodating most instructional situations ranging from individualized instruction through large group lectures and providing everything from full-color motion, still frame, color graphics, audio, image and data storage and retrieval, and rapid response to given commands.

4. Creating a method that enables health professionals to easily and inexpensively update, rearrange, and restructure instructional materials to allow for changes in educational philosophies, office practice procedures, methods or materials, or legal and ethical policies governing office practice.

5. Creating software for patient and continuing education that can be used in environments other than academic institutions.

It is anticipated that this project will encourage the use of optical disk and computer technology in a broad range of health-related applications and facilitate sharing and communicating information on a national and international basis. The biggest challenge before us is to take advantage of this technologic potential, for as Fredrick Williams indicates in *The Communications Revolution*:

> New communications and computing technologies allow us to manipulate and distribute as never before our knowledge and information resources. At the same time, many in our population spend up to a quarter of their waking hours mesmerized by a medium inundated by programmed mediocrity. These same communications as well as computing technologies could raise the educational level of every U.S. schoolchild and adult, yet our classrooms are administered in ways not unlike our own or even our parents' days in school. Education, which is our most valuable strategy for preparing a new generation for change, is the last to adopt the techniques of change. (Williams, 1982, p. 24)

Questions

1. How many images can be stored on one side of an optical disk?
   Answer: 54,000

2. How many images can be stored on a compact disk?
   Answer: 9,000

3. Optical disks store and retrieve visuals using _____ technology.
   Answer: Laser

4. A level III system consists of what three components?
   Answer: (1) Industrial-grade disk player
   　　　　　(2) Microcomputer
   　　　　　(3) Monitor

5. Level IV systems (still in the developmental stage) are referred to as _____ systems.
   Answer: CD-I or Compact Disk-Interactive

References Cited

Anonymous. A revolution for which there is no turning back. *TIME Magazine*, special advertising section, November 18, 1985 (no page numbers).
Bosco JJ: Interactive video: educational tool or toy. *Educational Technology* 1984; 24:13–19.

Craig JF, Moreland EF: An independent learning center in dental and dental hygiene education. *National Dental Association Journal* 1985; 42:17–18.

Jones P: Technology update. *T.H.E. Journal* 1985; 13:12–20.

Williams F: *The Communications Revolution*. Beverly Hills: Sage Publishing, 1982.

4—Computers and Staff Development

Kathryn J. Hannah and Maureen Osis

Introduction

Nursing is evolving in response to society (Romano, 1984), and part of that evolution involves the concept of lifelong learning (Buckholz, 1979). Information is being generated at explosive rates. Between 6000 and 7000 scientific papers are written each day, and knowledge is expected to double every 20 months in the decade ahead. Therefore, 5 years after a nursing student graduates from school, more than 50% of the knowledge acquired will be obsolete (McCormick, 1984).

Staff development and continuous learning are a major responsibility of nursing management. Staff development can be viewed as synonymous with continuing nursing education. Continuing nursing education can be defined as all those learning activities that registered nurses undertake following basic nursing education that enhance their nursing competence. The main goal of this ongoing professional educational process is to maintain and improve the quality of health care by providing educational opportunities directed toward the personal and professional growth of the individual nurse.

Staff development includes, but is not limited to, those activities directed at orientation of new staff to a facility, updating technical competency, progress toward professional and career goals (including development of leadership potential and of decision-making and problem-solving skills), and enhancing professional roles and accountability. A minisurvey of leaders in the field described the current status of continuing nursing education as:

- Deficient in the education and experience of continuing education personnel

- Disjointed, inadequately funded, haphazardly planned, and marked by poorly executed programs

- Failing to meet defined nursing needs (Ball and Hannah, 1984).

The resulting diagnosis was of an "acute need for instituting new teaching methods" (Ball and Hannah, 1984, p. 86).

Instructional Computing Applications

One new and promising teaching method involves the application of computers in staff development and continuing education programs. The text that follows describes the general advantages and disadvantages of instructional computing applications and provides examples of programs from the literature. It also offers practical suggestions for analyzing the costs and benefits of computer applications and argues for a collaborative approach in planning.

Terminology

A variety of terms has been used in referring to the use of computers in education. For the purposes of this discussion, we will rely upon the terminology, as clarified by Hannah. Computer-assisted learning (CAL) "refers to any of the wide range of educational techniques that rely on a computer to facilitate learning" (Hannah, 1983). CAL also appears in the literature as CATS, computer-assisted teaching system (Pazdernik and Walszed, 1983).

There are two distinct subdivisions of CAL. The first, computer-assisted instruction (CAI), is a "tutorial approach in which the information to be learned is stored in a computer and programmed for presentation and adaptation to each individual learner's needs" (Collart, 1973). The second, computer-managed instruction (CMI), also known as computer-managed learning (CML), refers to "an overall system for educational management in which detailed student records, complete curriculum data including schedules and timetables, and information on available learning resources are stored in the computer and integrated to develop unique programs of instruction" (Hannah, 1983). Finally, one of the latest technologic advances is computer-assisted video instruction (CAVI). An individualized learning system that combines the on-screen information and storage capabilities of the computer with the sound and motion of a video, it converts a passive learner into an active participant because it is interactive, user-paced, and user-controlled (Fishma, 1984).

Merits of Computer-Assisted Learning

Why use computers, either CMI or CAI or CAVI? According to one study, CMI can provide comprehensive documentation of all educational activities for all personnel whether inhouse or outside (Dixon et al, 1980). These records provide valuable information useful in reporting, for accreditation, maintaining individual files for performance evaluation, and planning new programs. The use of CAL has been more commonly studied in elementary or university education than in continuing professional education.

There is, however, growing evidence of its potential value in staff development. Twenty years of school-oriented research in CAI have substantiated its value, particularly when combined with other teaching strategies (Manning, 1984, p. 214). A review of the literature produced ample evidence that CAI demands active participation in the learning process, increases performance, and reduces total learning time (Fishma, 1984, p. 17).

Perhaps a more compelling argument relates to the application of principles of adult learning. "Many learners probably never reach their potential level of achievement because our usual teaching system does not allow them to discover or use their optimal learning approach" (Bitzer and Boudreaux, 1969). Computer-assisted video instruction (CAVI) presents a technology that can provide the diversity to help learners achieve optimal learning. Computer applications offer several advantages for the individual learner. Computer programs offer a variety of instructional processes: drill and practice, simulation, tutorial, decision-making. This variety, greater than that offered by lectures alone, can be more effective in achieving specific learning outcomes.

Computer technology also provides for individualization that is more suitable for adult learning needs and various learning styles. The computer can be a tool and tutor to enhance learning. Educational theory indicates that learning is increased when factual information is presented with examples. An individual lecturer has a limited number of examples to draw on constantly. Computer programs can compile the knowledge of many experts and increase the data base for the learner (Grobe, 1984).

Use of instructional computing applications offers one approach to solving the "deficiencies in education personnel" (Ball and Hannah, 1984). Currently, programs in a specific agency are dependent on the availability of resources and qualified instructors as well as the accessibility of the staff to these resources; e.g., staff working permanent shift or weekend duty may not attend in-service programs regularly. CAI is not dependent on the availability or accessibility of qualified instructors and can, in fact, facilitate an interagency sharing of resources and provide flexibility in scheduling to reach all personnel. Educational technology can also "extend the capabilities of ... qualified teachers" (Porter, 1978, p. 8). Initially, educators may feel threatened as they move from being "dispensers of knowledge" to moderators, facilitators, and coordinators of learning (Bitzer and Boudreaux, 1969; Porter, 1978). "CAI will not replace the teacher, but will "re-place the teacher" (Dale, quoted in Collart, 1973, p. 532). Authoring of programs encourages nurse educators to clarify the domain of nursing, essential nursing knowledge, in order to describe the what, why, and when of learning (Grobe, 1984).

Computerized instruction can be cost and time efficient. Computers can be timesavers. The average time spent learning on the computer was about one-third of the time required to attend lectures on the same material (Bitzer and Boudreaux, 1969). This approach can be used with a limited number of resource personnel; programs are easily updated. These are important factors considering that "training and education departments are frequently viewed as the most expendable units in an agency when budget cutbacks are necessary" (Porter, 1978, p. 6).

Disadvantages of Computer Applications in Staff Development

The purchase, installation, and maintenance of hardware (computer, monitor, keyboard/mouse) require an initial outlay, not only of money but also of the time of nurse managers who have the energy and expertise to select the most suitable products. Physical space for the computer may have to be provided or altered. An initial in-service program to overcome the "technophobia" of the users will demand time and effort.

Similar statements can be made regarding the choice of software, the programs that will be used for continuing education. If suitable programs are not available, the agency may require content and computer experts to write the programs. This is a costly venture, although the potential of marketing the programs out of house may offset the development costs (Hodson and Worrell, 1985; Joseph and Joseph, 1985).

Unfortunately, the technology has outdistanced our capacity to use it. One critic maintains that the number of educational computers has doubled in the recent past "in spite of the fact that virtually no decent educational software existed for use with these machines (Bork, 1984). Generally, nurse managers and nursing educators in staff development lack awareness and understanding of CAL technology. They have limited knowledge of appropriate lesson design. Similarly, they have limited understanding of the physical and psychosocial aspects of ergonomics associated with learning. Moreover, nursing educators in staff development generally do not use rational means for selecting appropriate topics for CAL lessons or for matching CAL instructional strategies to teaching/learning objectives and course content. Access to such awareness, knowledge, and skills is imperative before nurse managers can fully exploit the capabilities of advanced technology for staff development purposes.

Consequently, we are only now after 25 years beginning to integrate CAL into the repertoire of teaching/learning strategies used in staff development. In the interim, technologic advances in educational computing have continued. Innovations such as videotext, videodisk, fiber optics, programmer-less systems, and robotics are available to supplement computer-assisted learning. Regrettably these technologies have been used in nursing education generally and in staff development specifically in only a peripheral and rudimentary fashion.

Examples of CAL in Staff Development

An innovative collaborative project, called CoVenture, was designed to address the costly dilemma of retaining professional nurses (Krusa et al, 1985). A preliminary study revealed that, in a 1-year period, 40% of new graduates that resigned might have been retained if efforts had been made to resolve their conflicts. These conflicts include:

- lack of an effective orientation to the agency

- lack of congruence between education and practice

- lack of career advancement for clinical competence.

Following an assessment of needs, two schools of nursing and a county hospital designed a nurse transition program to assist new graduates to adjust to the work environment and to acquire the competencies needed within the practice setting. CAI was chosen because of its flexibility and individualized instruction capabilities. Following the initial CAI project, CoVenture explored the development of interactive videodisk for an orientation and retention program. Initial results of the project are encouraging in that retention of new graduates has increased. However, as the authors correctly point out, many other factors may have contributed to this outcome.

One example of repetitive but necessary staff training is basic life support through cardiopulmonary resuscitation. A study of the efficacy of an interactive videodisk CPR learning system as a training method found that the system required one-third less time than the traditional instruction (Edwards and Hannah, 1985). This finding was substantiated, but should be interpreted with caution since the population was the lay community rather than health professionals (Edwards, 1986). However, the timesaving possibilities for both participant and instructor warrant further investigation in clinical settings where basic cardiac life-support certification and recertification occur so frequently.

Analyzing the Costs and Benefits

In making decisions about the feasibility of implementing CAL into staff development, managers may use three models of cost comparison to determine the costs and analyze the potential benefits (Edwards, 1985; Hannah and Edwards, 1986). Cost-benefit analysis requires the calculation of costs and outcomes of two or more alternative programs using monetary values. The difficulty in stating the monetary value of orientation, in-service education, or professional development of staff is immediately obvious and limits the appropriateness of this model. A second approach, cost-utility analysis, relies heavily on subjective judgment. Managers who are personally familiar with and friendly toward computers may opt for CAL without concrete analysis of costs and outcomes. Similarly, those without any experience may negate the potential value of computer applications. The final model, called cost-effectiveness, requires the evaluator to examine the effectiveness of a particular program in achieving specific goals without assigning monetary units to those goals (Warner and Luce, 1982). Valuing the outcomes of computer approaches in staff development bears a direct relationship to the value management places on staff development per se by any method.

Analysis of the cost-effectiveness of educational computing must address the hardware, software, degree of usage, life span of both hardware and programs, and the effectiveness of instruction, i.e., achieving the desired goals of staff development (Larson, 1985). Hardware costs have dramatically reduced over the past decade, and the same trend is affecting software costs as competition increases. Other than cost, the criteria for judging the effectiveness of computer-assisted instructional programs focus on several key areas, including:

- Content
- Learning strategies
- Format, including ergonomics
- Style
- Documentation.

Although in-house software development has the advantage of producing programs specifically designed for the institution, it also carries a significant disadvantage in actual costs. Producing a single hour of instruction can require from 100 to 400 hours of development time (Kearsley, 1982). For hardware, a reasonable life span is probably 3 to 5 years, whereas for software it varies depending on content. Potential usage and life span must be subjectively determined and applied in the cost-effective analysis. The cost of software installation and maintenance for educational applications is generally minimal. To obtain an accurate analysis, hardware costs should be computed to include a maintenance contract and other associated items, such as surge protectors, dust covers, antistatic floor mats, and so on.

Nursing research substantiates the effectiveness and efficiency of computer-assisted instruction for nursing students (Huckabay et al, 1979; Yoder and Heilman, 1985). Unfortunately, there is a gap in research on staff development in the clinical setting. One might assume that the reduced learning time observed in nursing students and lay people would also occur in staff nurses. Time savings are not only highly valued by adult learners but also result in increased productivity through saving staff and instructor time. CAI requires staff to be absent from their positions for shorter periods of time, and does not require ongoing instructor time. One study demonstrating these savings compared laboratory and CAI simulation for teaching calculation and regulation of intravenous flow rates. The CAI cost was found to be $1.44 per student, whereas the cost of laboratory instruction was $2.01 per student (Larson, 1985).

A final word on cost analysis. Too often value, costs, and payoffs are compared but the impact of time is neglected (Jenkins, 1985). Generally speaking, when a new program is implemented the costs are initially higher because of inexperience with the new situation. At either end of technology—the obsolete or the cutting edge—we are inefficient.

In addition to evaluating hardware, software, and effectiveness in outcomes, it is also important to explore ergonomics (Armstrong, 1984). Derived from the Greek words "ergon," or work, and "nomos," or law, ergonomics refers to the "design of equipment and environment to account for the construction of the human body" (Armstrong, 1984, p. 121). The physical environment should be evaluated for individual comfort and safety. In planning a computer program for staff, nursing managers should look at location (including potential distractions), lighting, temperature, noise, electronic interference, power sources, and furniture. A collaborative approach involving both the engineering and maintenance departments in the planning is needed, or the equipment may be available and staff prepared only to find there is no way to plug in the terminal (Harper, 1985, p. 138).

One of the authors (Osis) experienced a situation that substantiates this advice. In a pharmacology update project, the computer was used to provide testing for self-assessment and group evaluation after the lectures and discussion group sessions. The terminal, keyboard, and modem were available, but there was no telephone jack. The usual 6-week waiting list with the local telephone company was fortunately overcome!

Conclusion

It behooves nurse managers to familiarize themselves with the concepts of computer-assisted learning as a means of maximizing the resources available for staff development. Nurse managers must acquire sufficient understanding of the technology to make rational decisions about selection and implementation of such a learning system for use in staff development. In a period of economic constraints, relatively modest expenditures have the potential to create significant benefits. With CAL these benefits range from the availability of learning materials, to productivity increases and savings resulting from reduced learning time and hence less time away from assigned duties, to improved staff morale associated with maintaining the commitment to staff development.

Questions

1. What is staff development?

2. Differentiate among computer-assisted learning (CAL), computer-assisted instruction (CAI), computer-managed instruction (CMI), and computer-assisted video instruction (CAVI).

3. Describe the merits of computer-assisted instruction for staff education.

4. Discuss the disadvantages of computer applications for staff education.

5. Develop a personal checklist for evaluation of computer-assisted learning materials before purchase.

References Cited

Armstrong M: Ergonomic considerations in computer implementation: a primer. *Computers in Nursing* 1984; 2:121–124.

Ball MJ, Hannah KJ: *Using Computers in Nursing*. Reston: Reston Publishing, 1984.

Bitzer MD, Boudreaux MC: Using a computer to teach nursing. *Nursing Forum* 1969; 8:234–254.

Bork A: Computers in education today—and some possible futures. *Phi Delta Kappan* 1984; 66:239–243.

Buckholz L: Computer-assisted instruction for the self-directed professional learner? *Journal of Continuing Education in Nursing* 1979; 10:12–14.

Collart M: Computer-assisted instruction and the teaching-learning process. *Nursing Outlook* 1973; 21:527–532.

Dixon JM, Gouyd N, Varricchio DT: A computerized education and training record. In: Zielstorff RD, ed. *Computers in Nursing*. Rockville, MD: Aspen, 1980; 59–62.

Edwards M: A cost analysis comparison of traditional and interactive videodisc CPR instruction. In: Hannah K, Guillemin E, Conklin D, eds. *Nursing Uses of Computers and Information Science*. Amsterdam: North Holland, 1985; 201–204.

Edwards M: A program evaluation utilizing Cronbach's framework of an interactive videodisc CPR learning system. Doctoral dissertation. Alberta: University of Calgary, 1986.

Edwards M, Hannah KJ: An examination of the use of interactive videodisc cardiopulmonary resuscitation instruction for the lay community. *Computers in Nursing* 1985; 3:250–252.

Fishma D: Development and evaluation of a computer-assisted video module for teaching cancer chemotherapy to nurses. *Computers in Nursing* 1984; 2:16–23.

Grobe S: Computer assisted instruction: an alternative. *Computers in Nursing* 1984; 2:92–97.

Hannah KJ: Computer-assisted learning in nursing education: a macroscopic analysis. In: Scholes M, Bryant Y, Barber B, eds. *The Impact of Computers on Nursing*. Amsterdam: North Holland, 1983; 280–287.

Hannah KJ, Edwards M: Cost comparison models for use in evaluating instructional computing in nursing education. In: Salamon R, Blum B, Jorgensen M, eds. *MEDINFO 86—Proceedings of the Fifth Conference on Medical Informatics*. Vol. 5. Amsterdam: North Holland, 1986; 966–969.

Harper W: Computers and change: effective implementation. In: Hannah K, Guillemin E, Conklin D, eds. *Nursing Uses of Computers and Information Science*. Amsterdam: North Holland, 1985; 135–140.

Hodson K, Worrell P: Experiences in publishing nursing computer software. *Computers in Nursing* 1985; 3:122–127.

Huckabay L, Anderson N, Holm D, et al: Cognitive, affective, and transfer of learning consequences of computer-assisted instruction. *Nursing Research* 1979; 28:228–233.

Jenkins T: Cost-effectiveness of computer-based job (training) aids for nurses. In: Hannah K, Guillemin E, Conklin D, eds. *Nursing Uses of Computers and Information Science*. Amsterdam: North Holland, 1985; 223–228.

Joseph LS, Joseph AF: Developing educational software for publishing vendors. *Nursing Clinics of North America* 1985; 20:529–548.

Kearsley G: *Costs, Benefits, and Productivity in Training Systems*. Reading, MA: Addison-Wesley, 1982.

Krusa KS, Brinson H, Henning E, et al: Development of computer based instruction to facilitate hospital retention of new graduate nurses. *Computers in Nursing* 1985; 3:203–206.

Larson DE: Cost-effectiveness of educational computing in nursing environments. In: Hannah K, Guillemin E, Conklin D, eds. *Nursing Uses of Computers and Information Science*. Amsterdam: North Holland, 1985; 217–222.

McCormick KA: Nursing in the computer revolution. *Computers in Nursing* 1984; 2:4, 30.

Manning T: Computer assisted instruction: the right stuff but does it work and should you buy it? *Computers in Nursing* 1984; 2:214, 223.

Pazdernik RTL, Walszed FJ: A computer-assisted teaching system in pharmacology for health professionals. *Journal of Medical Education* 1983; 58:341–348.

Porter S: Application of computer-assisted instruction to continuing education in nursing: review of the literature. In: Zielstorff RD, ed. *Computers in Nursing*. Rockville, MD: Aspen, 1978.

Romano C: Computer technology and emerging roles: the challenge to nursing administration. *Computers in Nursing* 1984; 2:80–84.

Warner KE, Luce BR: *Cost-Benefit and Cost-Effectiveness Analysis in Health Care*. Ann Arbor: Health Administration Press, 1982.

Yoder ME, Heilman T: The use of computer-assisted instruction to teach nursing diagnosis. *Computers in Nursing* 1985; 3:262–265.

Bibliography

Billings DM: *Computer Assisted Instruction for Health Professionals*. East Norwalk, CT: Appleton-Century-Crofts, 1986.

Cobin J: Combining computers with caring. *Nursing Times* 1983; 79:24–26.

Cook M: Using computers to enhance professional practice. *Nursing Times* 1982; 78:1542–1544.

Fishman R, Dusbabek C: Computers in nursing administration and practice. *Computer Nurse* 1983; 1:1–3.

Hannah KJ: The computer and nursing practice. *Nursing Outlook* 1976; 24:555–558.

Hills P: Computers in hospitals: the first ten years. *Health and Social Services Journal* 1981; 91:986–987.

Lee ER: The computer's place in nursing education. *NLN Publication* 1981; 41:212–223.

Mullen E, Love R: An evaluation of the use of minicomputers for computer-assisted instruction in allied health curricula. *Journal of Allied Health* 1980; 9:33–40.

Valish A: The role of computer assisted instruction in continuing education for registered nurses: an experimental study. *Journal of Continuing Education in Nursing* 1975; 6:13–31.

Walker MB, Schwartz C: *What Every Nurse Should Know About Computers*. Philadelphia: Lippincott, 1984.

5—The Need for an Educational Program in Nursing Informatics

*Barbara R. Heller, Carol A. Romano,
Shirley P. Damrosch, and Mary R. McCarthy*

Introduction

Nursing informatics is defined as the use of information technologies in relation to the functions that are within the purview of nursing and are carried out by the nurse in the care of patients or in the educational preparation of individuals to practice the discipline (Hannah et al, 1985). It encompasses the wide range of activities relating to use of information management technologies to facilitate the conduct of nursing practice, education, administration, and research (Schwirian, 1986). According to Schwirian, the development of nursing informatics as a critical specialized professional focus is appropriate because the field of informatics

- contributes to the development of knowledge in the discipline of nursing
- enhances the communication of knowledge to present and new generations of nurses
- enhances use of knowledge in nursing practice.

Schwirian's model for nursing research in the field of nursing informatics defines fertile areas for research. She notes that information, computer technology, and nursing form an interactive, interdependent relationship that typifies nursing informatics activity.

Nursing practice is described as an information-intensive process; it concerns a body of knowledge dependent on skill in acquiring and using information. The field of nursing informatics, then, is not a focus on computer technology, but rather a field of concern with the nature of information, its access, the identification and formulation of problems based on it, and decision making dependent on appropriate arts and forms of information (Nelson, 1984). The framework for nursing informatics carefully considers the nature of nursing, how nursing information is acquired, manipulated, and used.

As suggested by Clinton at the National Nursing Minimum Data Set Conference held in the United States of America in Milwaukee, Wisconsin in 1985, the use and control of information technologies and nursing data sets would enable nursing to

- document an infinite volume of nursing information in a standardized, cost-effective, and time-efficient manner

- rapidly transfer information to other users

- conduct updated, multipurpose electronic analysis of nursing information whenever and wherever needed

- establish a national and international norm for nursing phenomena and other information relevant to nursing that is not generated or electronically disseminated by other sources.

Information technology and computer systems can play a unique and promising role in nursing if managed and developed appropriately. That role is analogous to that of a breakthrough tool—one enabling us to explore and better understand the informational and cognitive foundations of nursing. Applications in classification, retrieval of data, and the management of information will result in a deeper insight into the structure of nursing information and of knowledge itself. It has been noted that computers provide us with a general means for enhancing the effectiveness of human inference and judgment and have an increasing use in both the clinic and the research laboratory (Blois, 1986).

The Social Policy Statement of the American Nurses' Association asserts that nursing, as an essential part of society, must evolve with, and in response to, the society out of which it grew (American Nurses' Association, 1980). Computer-related technology has become a dominant force in the health care delivery system; therefore, the application and management of computerization and information technology in nursing is seen as essential for today's and tomorrow's nurse (Ball and Hannah, 1984; Grobe, 1984; Zielstorff, 1980; Andreoli and Musser, 1985; Heller et al, 1985).

In the 25 years since the first major scientific meeting devoted to the potential uses of the computer in medical care, computers have come into use in virtually every aspect of modern health care (Andreoli and Musser, 1985). It is projected that information technology will increasingly be employed to do more of the routine mental work that supports the judgments of all health professionals (Brannigan and Dayhoff, 1982). It has also been predicted that the use of computer-based information systems in health care institutions will continue to expand as a result of the growing pressures for greater economy and more detailed documentation of services provided (Zielstorff, 1980).

Because of the complexities specific to health care delivery systems and the uniqueness of nursing, the adaptation of the computer scientist to this environment is less than straightforward (Duncan et al, 1981). There is general agreement that nursing needs to be more involved in directing the development of computer and information technologies. Medicine and dentistry have already moved toward involvement with specializations in medical and dental informatics (Blois, 1986; Zimmerman et al, 1986). The lack of nursing leadership in this newly developing specialty invites others to address nursing information problems from a nonnursing perspective and allows other disciplines to design systems that may dictate nursing activities. Not only does this not contribute to nursing, it also subtly undermines the role of the nurse (Zielstorff, 1980).

Indicators of Need for an Educational Program in Nursing Informatics

One of the reasons for nursing's failure to capitalize on the potential of computer technology is the lack of specialized education (Zielstorff, 1980; Heller et al, 1985; Hardin and Skiba, 1982; Parks et al, 1986a). Major gaps exist among the information-processing power of the computer as a tool, its current use by nursing practice, administration, education, and research, and the availability of nursing leaders to direct technology toward the enhancement of nursing (Zielstorff, 1982; Ronald, 1981; Hardin and Skiba, 1982).

In the early 1970s, a study to identify the needs of health professionals for education in medical computing was conducted under the auspices of the International Federation of Information Processing. This survey of Western developed countries concluded that not only should nurses have a general knowledge of the computer and data processing, but also that a large number of nurses be specially educated to contribute effectively to the development of automated systems for information handling (Anderson et al, 1974). Despite these recommendations, little has been done to prepare nurses for such roles. Those without computer skills in the near future will be "among the educationally disadvantaged portion of the population" (Gattis, 1982, p. 47). In order to improve nursing's strategic position in health care, computing and the new information technology must be viewed as central to one's thinking, and systematic plans to integrate them into nursing education and service need to be developed (Grobe, 1985).

Recognizing that nurses need knowledge and skills to maximize the use of computers in health care and nursing, a number of academic institutions and organizations have developed workshops, continuing education programs, and national conferences related to computer applications in nursing. For example, in 1985, the Southern Regional Education Board received a special project grant from the Division of Nursing, Health Resources and Service Administration, of the Public Health Service, U.S. Department of Health and Human Services. Activities funded by this 3-year grant are designed to support continuing nursing education in computer technology and to promote the systematic implementation of computer-supported nursing education.

Concomitantly, the National Institutes of Health has cosponsored, with the Division of Nursing, U.S. Public Health Service, a series of conferences on Computer Technology and Nursing. The multisponsored Symposium on Computer Applications in Medical Care (SCAMC) has endorsed active nursing sessions since 1981, and Ohio State University has sponsored its fifth national conference designed to address the issues in nursing informatics. The International Medical Informatics Association has fostered international collaborative nursing working groups to address computers and information science in nursing (Hannah et al, 1985). An education working group convened in Sweden in June 1987 has also been commissioned to address, on an international level, the educational needs of nurses for leadership roles in this field.

The professional nursing associations have also responded in identifying nursing informatics as an important area of educational concern for nursing. In 1986, the American Nurses' Association (ANA) gave special mention to informatics, and has initiated an active council on computer applications in nursing with a focus on practice and research. The National League for Nursing has instituted a national forum on computer applications in health care and nursing with an emphasis on education and administration (Grobe, 1987). Nursing leaders in both organizations have heralded the need for nurses with the capability and background to provide leadership in the design and implementation of computer-based information systems in nursing and health care. In addition, Sigma Theta Tau, the International Honor Society of Nursing, has recently introduced information resources awards to recognize and honor outstanding individuals who have created and implemented the use of information technology to further the nursing profession in the health of the public.

Other indicators of the increasing interest and need for specialized education for nurses in the field of informatics include the recent publication of six texts, authored by nurses, on the subject of information technology and nursing. One such text received the 1985 Book of the Year award from the *American Journal of Nursing. Computers in Nursing*, the first professional refereed journal dedicated to this specialized area, has a documented readership of over 18,000. In addition, other nursing literature abounds with publications on computer applications. Research on learning needs of nurses also acknowledges the necessity of an academic curriculum response (Ronald, 1981; Heller et al, 1985; Walker, 1981; Parks et al, 1986b). The increasing number of advertised positions for nursing information systems (NIS) specialists also evidences the reality of this new role for nurses; the fact remains, however, that no nursing educational program currently addresses the specialized preparation of nurses that is required (Hersher, 1985).

Although it is recognized that all nurse clinicians and administrators will be involved in using computer applications in their working environment, the International Federation for Information Processing proposed that education be leveled depending on the degree of involvement of the health care professional (Anderson et al, 1974). Few nurses may have the knowledge or skills to initiate and/or design systems to enhance nursing functions. Even though a number of schools of nursing currently provide some sort of computer education to students by offering electives or by integrating content into required coursework either at the undergraduate or graduate levels to date, specialization in nursing informatics has not been systematically addressed in the curriculum (Heller et al, 1985). Given that information in and of itself has become a vital commodity in a technologic society and has been recognized as a phenomenon for scholarly study, an educational program is merely an acknowledgment of the need for trained information specialists and for scholars to continue the exploration of the synergism that is evolving among the computer, information systems, and humans. Education in nursing informatics would endeavor to meet these needs by providing both trained professionals and contributing scholars.

Rationale for the Development of an Educational Program in Nursing Informatics at the University of Maryland

Over the past few years, the University of Maryland at Baltimore has made a major commitment to informatics. Having recruited Dr. Marion Ball to head the Information Resources Management Division, the University has integrated the activities of that division with those of the Health Sciences Library as well as other academic units. Through collaborative efforts, a Dental Informatics Department, the first in the world, has been established as well as a similar program in the School of Medicine. The opportunity to put together a high-quality program in Nursing Informatics could hardly be better given the resources available.

The School of Nursing at the University of Maryland is one of the largest nursing schools in the country, and was recently ranked sixth among the nearly 200 public nursing schools in the nation. A dynamic and qualified faculty with curriculum and research expertise and experience in computer applications in nursing contributes to ensuring success of a new specialization in nursing informatics.

Feasibility Study

Following a review of the literature and an appraisal of currently circulating position descriptions and advertisements for nursing information systems (NIS) specialists, the faculty of the University of Maryland School of Nursing became convinced of the need for development of a specialized educational program in nursing informatics. A steering committee was formed and a proposal put forth within the University. Input was sought from experts in the field and from the professional nursing community at large regarding the appropriateness of the content for master's level education in nursing and career opportunities for graduates. Letters of endorsement were received from nursing service administrators and academicians alike, all enthusiastically supportive of the proposal to offer a graduate level program in nursing informatics.

An advisory committee comprised of internationally known experts in the field of nursing informatics was constituted and convened to validate the need for this area of specialization and to provide guidance in program development. To further test the feasibility of such a program in terms of job market for graduates and potential student applicant pool, a feasibility study was carried out by the University of Maryland in the spring of 1987. This feasibility study was conducted specifically to identify employer responses as well as the potential applicant pool for such a program. Questionnaires were distributed to a sample of employers and a sample of employed RNs. Questionnaires were also administered to generic and RN students currently enrolled in the baccalaureate program in the School of Nursing, University of Maryland. A summary of results is reported here.

Job Market

A mail survey was conducted of nursing directors of JCAH-accredited hospitals of 200 beds or more located in Maryland, Washington, D.C., Virginia, and other selected locations across the country. A participation rate of 76% was achieved. Questionnaires from the 128 respondents indicated that most (84%) of these institutions currently use computer technology in nursing practice and/or administration; virtually all remaining hospitals had plans to adopt such technology. Almost half of the 128 hospitals (49%) already allocate one or more budgeted positions for nurse managers of computer/information systems. (The median salary range reported for these positions was $26,000 to $30,000.) An additional 20% of the respondents foresaw a need for such positions in their institutions within the next year or two.

The nursing directors were enthusiastic in their evaluation of the proposed nursing informatics program. Virtually all respondents saw some need for such a graduate program, with 106 selecting a response in the upper end of the evaluation scale and 28 endorsing the maximum response. Moreover, these respondents expressed a high degree of willingness to employ nursing informatics specialists. The overwhelming majority showed at least some willingness, with 80 selecting a response in the upper end of the evaluation scale and 22 endorsing the maximum response.

These nursing directors also indicated a willingness to provide support (such as tuition reimbursement) to staff enrolling in the proposed program. Many of these respondents were also willing to cooperate with the University of Maryland by furnishing other resources to promote this educational endeavor.

Summary of Job Market Results

Questionnaires from 128 nursing directors yielded compelling evidence of their high level of interest in recruiting graduates of the proposed nursing informatics program as well as their willingness to encourage staff enrollment through tuition reimbursement incentives and other forms of support.

Potential Applicant Pool

Surveys were also undertaken of large samples of graduating baccalaureate nursing students as well as of locally employed nurses.

Baccalaureate Nursing Seniors

The spring 1987 survey of 188 generic and 74 RN University of Maryland graduating seniors produced cogent evidence of interest in the proposed nursing informatics program. These student numbers represent 82% of all baccalaureate nursing students graduated from the University of Maryland in the 1986–1987 academic year. An overwhelming majority (95%) were interested in pursuing a master's degree, and sizable majorities of the RN and generic students expressed at least some degree of interest in the nursing informatics program. Moreover, a total of 101 students in the combined RN–generic group selected responses in the upper end of the scale evaluating degree of interest and 15 endorsed the maximum response.

In terms of likelihood of enrolling in the proposed nursing informatics program at the University of Maryland, 77 of the combined group selected responses in the upper end of the scale, with 10 endorsing the maximum likelihood. Projecting these figures to represent the entire 1986–1987 University of Maryland graduating class yields an estimated 94 students responding in the upper end of the scale and 12 endorsing the maximum likelihood of enrollment. Also noteworthy is the fact that 83 seniors took the time and trouble to furnish their names and addresses so they might be kept informed of progress in the development of the proposed program.

Locally Employed Nurses

A total of 176 nurses employed by NIH and 139 working at the University of Maryland Hospital (UMH) was also surveyed. A sizable majority in each group indicated interest in pursuing a master's degree. In the combined NIH–UMH total group, 174 nurses expressed at least some degree of interest in nursing informatics, with 104 responding in the upper end of the evaluation scale and 20 endorsing the maximum evaluation.

In terms of likelihood of enrolling in the proposed University of Maryland program, 66 of the combined group responded in the upper end of the scale and 14 endorsed the maximum likelihood. Moreover, 80 of these nurses gave us their names and addresses so they might be kept abreast of latest developments concerning the proposed program.

Summary of Potential Applicant Pool Results

Surveys of large samples of University of Maryland baccalaureate nursing seniors and of NIH and UMH nurses indicated a high degree of interest and likelihood of enrolling in the proposed nursing informatics program. It should be noted that these samples constitute only part of the potential enrollees in this region. Thus, the results of this feasibility study provide most encouraging evidence that a more than adequate pool of applicants exists for the proposed nursing informatics program at the University of Maryland.

In sum, these data collectively indicated a high level of interest in and enthusiastic support for the development of the nursing informatics program at the University of Maryland. Findings affirm the need for such a program, a ready job market for the graduates and a sizable applicant pool. Overall, supporting resources for the nursing informatics track at the University of Maryland are unsurpassed. The program will be housed in the School of Nursing, Department of Nursing Education, Administration and Health Policy.

Graduate Specialization in Nursing Informatics

The University of Maryland School of Nursing intends to expand its existing master's program concentration in nursing administration to include the new specialty in nursing informatics by September 1988.

The ultimate goal of this prototype curriculum is to prepare nurses to manage the challenges of modern health care with the new tools of this era and to take advantage of the growing opportunities provided by the appropriate administration of information technology. As the first of its kind, the educational program in nursing informatics will be designed to provide the skills and knowledge necessary for the effective and efficient development and management of information technologies in nursing and health care. The graduate will be prepared to analyze nursing information requirements, define system design alternatives, develop implementation methodologies, identify and implement user training strategies, and evaluate effectiveness of clinical and management information systems in patient care.

On completion of the program of study, the graduate will be able to:

1. Analyze nursing information requirements for clinical and management information systems.

2. Analyze information needs and technologic issues related to productivity and quality assurance programs in nursing.

3. Develop strategies to manage technological and organizational change and innovation.

4. Apply management and nursing theories and information science to the planning, development, implementation, and administration of nursing information systems.

5. Evaluate the effectiveness of nursing information systems in patient care delivery.

6. Define methodologies related to technology and engineering planning for information systems in health care and nursing.

7. Apply concepts of budget, staffing, and financial management to the design of management information systems.

8. Apply concepts of nursing theory to the design of health care and clinical information systems.

9. Develop and implement user training programs to support the utilization of clinical and management information systems.

10. Analyze the contribution of information technology to nursing education, administration, clinical practice, and research.

11. Examine the political, social, ethical, and influential forces in health care as they relate to the use of information technology and management.

12. Evaluate hardware, software, and vendor support for technologies that underpin clinical and management decisions in nursing.

13. Examine data base management principles in relation to nursing information system file structures.

14. Apply concepts of programming logic to the analysis of a simple computer program.

The curriculum will consist of 42 credit hours, and coursework will combine detailed study of the discipline of nursing with theoretical and practical applications of management and information science. An interdisciplinary approach will be utilized.

Educational preparation will focus on the essential functions, processes, and system requirements to plan, develop, implement, finance, control, market, and evaluate clinical and management information technologies. Subject matter treated in the specialized nursing informatics courses will include the following:

nursing
information
communication and organizational theories
technology assessment and planning
operations analysis
research design and statistics
issues in clinical and management information systems
quality assurance
management of the innovation process
programming logic
decision analysis
information needs related to advanced clinical practice
influential forces in health care.

Program completion will lead to career opportunities as nursing information systems (NIS) specialists in every commercial, governmental, and service organization of the nation that employs computer-based information services related to health care. The program will provide instruction in those competencies needed for entry as well as for acquiring increased responsibility in a very wide range of occupations in the private and the public sectors. The nursing informatics track at the University of Maryland will serve as a model for the development of other such programs in the future.

Graduates of this interdisciplinary program will speak the language common to all health care administrators in a manner that best serves the interests of quality patient care and professional nursing. Because of their familiarity and interaction with almost all aspects of operation and systems design, graduates will be able to contribute to management decisions that impact beyond nursing services. Enhanced collaborative efforts in research in nursing administration and informatics with appropriate dissemination of research findings are also anticipated as outcomes of the program.

Conclusion

It is imperative that nurses be prepared with a firm knowledge base for the use of automated systems for both nursing management and the delivery of patient care. The health care field requires nursing personnel with this expertise to stay abreast of, and in control of, the technology that it uses. There is an urgent need to develop the role of nursing information systems (NIS) specialists who will influence practice, administration, education, and research. These specialists will be able to fill the void of qualified personnel needed for hospitals, community, and other health care facilities, industry, educational settings, and research centers where computer systems and information technologies are being implemented. The current gap in preparation of qualified nurses in this important arena definitely places systems design in health care settings in jeopardy and invites others to address nursing information problems from a nonnursing perspective.

Within the past few years, there has been a significant increase in the numbers of graduate students wishing to pursue advanced study in the field of nursing informatics. Currently, no other school of nursing either in the United States or abroad offers such specialized education and consequently students have had no way to fulfill their goals. The University of Maryland proposes the development of a prototype master's level program for role preparation of the nursing information systems (NIS) specialist. This educational program, as the first of its kind, will not only fill the void in nursing education but will also serve as a model for the development of other such educational initiatives. All evidence points to both the immediate and future need for master's-prepared nurses for positions in the new and emerging field of nursing informatics.

The ultimate impact of this program will be to improve the quality of nursing services through the preparation of nursing information systems (NIS) specialists who are qualified and competent to practice in acute care, long-term care, or community-based health care delivery settings. A more immediate visible contribution will be to meeting regional, national, and international manpower needs through increasing the availability of adequately prepared specialists in the field of nursing informatics. The lack of such specialists is viewed as a basic impediment to strengthening the organization and management of nursing services within the health care system.

Questions

1. What are the indicators of need for a specialized educational program in nursing informatics?

2. What are the key areas of study in a nursing informatics program?

3. What factors must be considered in determining the feasibility of an educational program in nursing informatics?

4. What resources need to be in place to support an educational program in nursing informatics?

5. Why is it more desirable to develop a new role in nursing informatics than to adapt the computer scientist to this field?

References Cited

American Nurses' Association: *Nursing—A Social Policy Statement.* Kansas City: ANA, 1980.

American Nurses' Association: *Development of Computerized Nursing Information Systems in Nursing Services, 1986 Resolution.* Kansas City: ANA, 1986.

Anderson J, Gremy F, Pages JC: *Education in Informatics of Health Personnel.* New York: American Elsevier, 1974.

Andreoli K, Musser LA: Computers in nursing care: the state of the art. *Nursing Outlook* 1985; 33:16–21.

Ball MJ, Hannah KJ: *Using Computers in Nursing.* Reston: Reston Publishing, 1984.

Blois MS: What is medical informatics? *Western Journal of Medicine* 1986; 145:776–777.

Brannigan VM, Dayhoff RE: Liability for personal injuries caused by defective medical computer programs. *American Journal Law Medicine* 1982; 7:123–144.

Duncan KA, Austing RH, Katz S, et al: *A Model Curriculum for Doctoral Level Programs in Health Computing: Report of the ACM Commission on Curriculum for Health Computing Education.* New York: Association for Computing Machinery, 1981.

Gattis WD: Corporate viewpoints on computers in education. *Educational Technology* 1982; 22:47–50.

Grobe S: *Computer Primer and Resource Guide for Nurses.* Philadelphia: JB Lippincott, 1984.

Grobe S: Computers: an information technology imperative for nursing. *Nursing and Health Care* 1985; 5:515.

Grobe S: Chairperson's message. *Member Update—Newsletter of the Forum on Computers in Health Care and Nursing* 1987; 2:2.

Hannah KJ, Guillemin EJ, Conklin DN, eds. *Nursing Uses of Computers and Information Sciences.* Amsterdam: Elsevier, 1985.

Hardin RC, Skiba DJ: A comparative analysis of computer literacy education for nurses. In: Blum BI, ed. *Proceedings of the Sixth Annual Symposium on Computer Applications in Medical Care.* New York: IEEE Computer Society, 1982; 525–532.

Heller B, Romano C, Damrosch S, et al: Computer applications in nursing: implications for the curriculum. *Computers in Nursing* 1985; 3:14–21.

Hersher BS: The job search and information systems opportunities for nurses. *Nursing Clinics of North America* 1985; 20:585–594.

Nelson S: Education and research in medical information science. *Medical Informatics* 1984; 9:265–267.

Parks P, Damrosch S, Heller B, Romano C: Faculty and student perceptions of computer applications in nursing. *Journal of Professional Nursing* 1986a; 2:21–31.

Parks P, Damrosch S, Heller B, et al: Comparison of nursing faculty and student definitions of computer learning needs. In: Salamon R, Blum B, Jorgensen M, eds. *MEDINFO 86—Proceedings of the Fifth Conference on Medical Informatics*. Vol. 5. Amsterdam: North Holland, 1986b; 950–954.

Ronald JS: Introducing baccalaureate students to the use of computers in health care. In: Heffernan HG, ed. *Proceedings of the Fifth Annual Symposium on Computer Applications in Medical Care*. New York: IEEE Computer Society, 1981; 771–775.

Schwirian P: The NI pyramid—a model for research in nursing informatics. *Computers in Nursing* 1986; 4:134–136.

Walker JA: Determining educational needs of professional nurses pertaining to computerization in nursing practice. Doctoral dissertation. Texas: University of Houston, 1981.

Zielstorff RD, ed. *Computers in Nursing*. Wakefield, MA: Nursing Resources, 1980.

Zielstorff RD: Computers for planning and evaluating nursing service. In: Marringer A, ed. *Contemporary Nursing Management: Issues and Practice*. St. Louis: CV Mosby, 1982.

Zimmerman JL, Landesman HM, Bilan JP, et al: Study of computer applications in dental practice. In: Zimmerman JL, ed. *The Dental Clinics of North America*. Vol. 30. Philadelphia: WB Saunders, 1986; 731–738.

6—Computers and Continuing Education

Gary D. Hales

Introduction

Over the last year, both higher education and the for-profit sector have sponsored seminars on nursing informatics. The topic is one of great concern as nursing begins to exploit the potential of computing and the new technologies. In focusing on educating nurses in the use of computers, we now address both professional and continuing nursing education. However, especially in the area of professional nursing education, this issue is rapidly approaching resolution: Ten years from now, discussing education directed at the use of computers in nursing will be as controversial as discussing how to use digital readout disposable thermometers.

Ten years from now, the high school or junior college student considering a nursing program will come from a primary/secondary education setting in which the understanding, use, and exploitation of computers is accepted practice. One danger to a nursing school's enrollment is lack of recognition of this fact; given the decrease in enrollment in many nursing schools, the faculty should remember what criteria a student will use to choose a school. Any school that does not have computers firmly integrated into the curriculum is less likely to be selected by top students. The question will soon be, "How can I be expected to do my work without a computer?" rather than "Should we integrate computers into this course?" The young men and women entering nursing will be as comfortable with computers as their predecessors are with stethoscopes and blood pressure cuffs. Simply put, the "magic" will be gone.

Thus, for one group of nurses, those newly entering the profession, introduction to computer use will become unnecessary. But this certainly does not imply that future continuing education will be exempt from addressing computer use for nurses already practicing. Computers should have a major impact on continuing education in nursing in two areas in particular.

Continuing Education, Computers, and Nursing Staff

Technologic Implications for Current Staff

The nurses who enter the profession in a few years will need no introduction or comforting in regard to computers, but this is not true for those who are already practicing. In almost all cases, the nurse in a hospital, clinic, or physician's office comes from an educational background in which computers were, at most, a novelty. The person who feels comfortable using computers, who understands the applications possible with the huge library of software, and who feels competent to develop her/his own applications is rare indeed. It is this in-place, working group, the backbone of the nursing profession, who are most in need of instructional programs regarding computers.

First, it is clear that nurses have not been allowed or encouraged to have input when computer systems are to be installed. Despite the fact that nurses use computers more than any other health professionals, they are often overlooked when the developers are soliciting input for system design. One insidious reason may be that the system analysts and developers believe that most women do not understand computers, that there is no reason to consult with women because they could not state their needs. Since nursing is a predominantly female occupation, this sexist attitude is not unexpected. The blame, in this instance, must clearly be placed on the computer specialists.

On the other hand, nursing is also responsible for lack of input because of their admitted inexperience and lack of training in using computers. Since the college and hospital nursing programs have not, in the past, educated their students in using this technology, graduates cannot be held culpable for a failure of the system. This does not, however, lessen the seriousness of the situation. If nurses do not have the information and competence to make their needs and wants known, someone else, most likely someone not connected to nursing, will make that decision for them. If nurses are not prepared to tell the developers what their input will be, how the information must be processed, and what the output should look like, these decisions will be made without them.

The nurses who have been practicing the longest are those who have the experience to contribute substantially to the development of nursing information systems. Sadly, these professionals are those least likely to be consulted because of technical inexperience. This is a loss not only to them individually, but, more importantly, to nursing.

The impact of technology is compounded by other changes in the provision of health care. These include increased operating costs, decreased patient census, and accelerated development of walk-in clinics. All are combining to change the practice of nursing. Instead of large hospitals, there will be more small care centers with reduced staff. Telecommunications will increase the possibility and use of distributed health care.

Those nurses who have developed their management use of computers will be in great demand. The use of technology will provide an opportunity for the entrepreneurial nurse prepared to deal with it.

The Use of Technology in Delivery of Continuing Education (CE)

In addition to providing the opportunities described, whether these are recognized and gained, or ignored and lost, computers will dramatically change the field of continuing education (CE). Again, those nurses who have been prepared to understand and exploit the technology will be the only ones to benefit directly from it. Those incapable of embracing change will benefit from the work of these people indirectly, but the greatest benefits and power will be delegated to those in direct control of the computer.

The use of the computers and attendant software will change the method of development and delivery of CE materials. First, the content developer will team up with the instructional designer and the programmer to develop CE instructional materials. Rather than traveling tens or hundreds of miles for training, nurses will be able to receive training in their own offices on a schedule over which they have control. This technique can incorporate the potential of videodisk through computer-assisted interactive video instruction (CAIVI). Children's Medical Services in Florida has had such programs in place since the early 1980s.

On-site CAI-based CE programs would not only decrease time off nurses must use to travel to CE sites, but would also contain costs. These programs will become increasingly attractive and practical as software becomes easier to use. Authoring systems, like Dr. Richard Pogue's MicroInstructor, will facilitate the development of CE lessons.

Nurses completing their professional education and entering the working world of nursing will expect CAI to be made available to them for both learning and developing their own lessons. For this to occur, however, nurses must leave their primary education environment with certain minimum competencies with regard to computer usage (see Table 6-1).

Summary

One of the most exciting aspects of the computerization of our society has been the increased recognition that there are many leaders and few absolute followers in the use of computers. It is possible, and in fact

Table 6-1
Minimum Exit Competencies

Level I

Conceptual

Be able to:
1. Define basic computer vocabulary.
2. Convert simple (4 place) number from decimal to binary notation.
3. Describe basic system design, including
   a. CPU structure
   b. input devices
   c. output devices
   d. storage devices.
4. Define telecommunications and associated vocabulary, e.g., baud rate, modem, asynchronous and synchronous transmission.
5. Describe telecommunications procedures, including protocols.
6. Define three types of software.
7. Describe function and operation of operating systems.

Applied

Be able to:
1. Apply often-used operating system commands, e.g., for MS DOS, FORMAT, COPY, RENAME, DELETE (ERASE).
2. Format a systems disk and a data disk.
3. Copy programs from disk to disk.
4. Use special function keys on keyboard, e.g., CTRL, Fl, Arrow keys, etc.
5. Copy applications software to a formatted disk (system or data), i.e., backup disk.

Level II

Conceptual

Be able to:
1. Describe the criteria to be used in selecting applications software.
2. Describe the factors to be considered when selecting a software or hardware vendor.
3. Describe use of computers in hospital settings in regard to finance, accounting, administration, patient care, patient recordkeeping, patient teaching, etc.
4. Describe computer use in nonnursing business practices.

Conceptual and Applied

Be able to:
1. Use various applications packages, including one in each of the following categories:

   Word processing
   a. Define the purpose of and processes in word processing.
   b. Load a word processing program.
   c. Create, enter data into, navigate in, modify, save, retrieve, and merge text files.
   d. Print a document on dot matrix, letter-quality, single-feed, and continuous-form feed printers.
   e. Define desktop publishing.

Table 6-1 (*continued*)

Spreadsheets
a. Define the purpose of and processes in spreadsheets.
b. Prepare a manual spreadsheet.
c. Load a spreadsheet program.
d. Create, enter data into, navigate in, modify, develop formulae, save, retrieve, and merge spreadsheets.
e. Print a spreadsheet on dot matrix, letter-quality, single-feed, and continuous-form feed printers.

Data base management
a. Define the purpose of and processes in data base management.
b. Develop a manual form of a data base (file cabinet).
c. Define data base terminology, e.g., file management system, relational data base, tree structure, etc.
d. Load a data base management program.
e. Create, enter data into, save, navigate in, modify, sort, search, and merge records and/or data bases.
f. Print a data base file or report on dot matrix, letter-quality, single-feed, and continuous-form feed printers.

Graphics
a. Define the purpose of and processes in use of graphics software.
b. Load a graphics program.
c. Create, enter data into, save, navigate in, modify, and import data from external source for a graphics package.
d. Print graphic output on dot matrix and ink jet or laser printers.

Telecommunications
a. Define the purpose of and processes in use of telecommunications software.
b. Load a telecommunications package.
c. Enter data into, navigate in, modify parameters of a communications program. Establish communications contact with, upload files from, download files to, capture data during a telecommunications session. Established automatic log on sequences with a remote source. Set modem to answer phone using telecommunications software.
d. Print output captured in a telecommunications session on dot matrix, letter-quality, single-feed, and continuous-form feed printers.
e. Describe purposes of and contact bulletin boards and value-added services like Compuserve.

Networking
a. Define the purpose of, types of, and processes in use of a network and network software.
b. Log on to and use network software, available applications software, and available peripherals.
c. Print output on a remote printer, use a remote modem, use any other remote peripheral on the network.

Level III

Conceptual and Applied
1. Define advantages of and disadvantages of various programming languages.
2. Write code in at least one language.
3. Use a specialized applications package, e.g., statistics, CAD, CAI.

commonplace, for computer users to develop their own software or at least to modify packaged shelf applications software for their specific needs. Perhaps nursing informatics will also escape the curse of self-styled experts. The computer allows the thoughtful person to be his or her own teacher. Individual users have done more than anyone except those with advanced degrees in computer science to promote computer use and devise new applications. This brings home the critical need for basic education and, thus, the need for some authoritative power in nursing education to mandate such training.

We now are recognizing that working with the computer inspires creativity, free thought, and continual exploration of new possibilities and new processes. It challenges old ways of doing things and dogmatic belief systems. There is no more powerful tool in this modern age. It brings new capabilities and new opportunities to the entire profession of nursing.

The fervor and interest in computer delivery of CE will probably fade away as this instrument of CE becomes mundane. There will still be pioneers who develop new techniques. Following close behind will be those pursuing other professional objectives who will learn from the pioneers, and both groups will accept the computer as nothing special. More important, learners will be able to use the computer to promote their own self-education in their profession or any other area by accessing the increasing base of informal computerized education.

Conclusion

There is little doubt that computers will make a major impact on CE in nursing. It should be clear that the computer provides both a source of curriculum delivery and a source of power for nurses. The former point has been made repeatedly; the latter point requires yet one more repetition.

In an increasingly computerized environment, power will belong to those who control information. Within the group controlling information, the greatest power will be assumed by those who control the most information, know how to manipulate it, and use it the most. This last descriptor seems to very clearly define nursing's role in health care informatics. As the great computer-user phalanx marches forward, control will devolve upon the profession with the greatest number of persons who control, use, and manipulate information. Because there are many nurses, and because they use computers more than any other professionals in health care, nurses should exercise the greatest control. In a world of scarce resources and strong pressures for change, nurses will have only themselves to blame if this is not the case.

Questions

1. Will nurses develop a multidisciplinary approach to CAI in CE?

2. Will nursing schools recognize the need for minimum computer competencies for those graduating from undergraduate and graduate programs?

3. Will nursing develop the expertise to exert the necessary control over use of hospital information systems?

4. Will a fully operating nursing AI system be developed by the year 2000?

5. Will nurses recognize the need for self-education in computer use?

Appendices

A—Order Communications/ Nursing System Requirements Questionnaire

Mary Etta Mills

Order Communications/Nursing

Mandatory/Desirable		Available	Not Available

Enter Orders

M   1. Ability to enter all patient care orders via high-level user-oriented data entry methodology and validate

M   2. Ability to restrict the entry of patient care orders to specific personnel based on user identification

M   3. Ability to flash back the order for review before completion of the order entry process and price per test

M   4. Ability to invoke order verification procedures based on the user's authority

M   5. Ability to automatically generate protocol orders and hospital policy orders based on the patient's physician, age, sex, etc.

M   6. Ability to enter multiple department orders and start/stop times for continuing orders following the selection of a single patient on a single screen

		Not
Mandatory/Desirable	Available	Available

Enter Orders (*continued*)

M   7. Ability to enter and modify
     protocol orders

M   8. Ability to enter physician words
     or other special comments

M   9. Ability to modify procedure preps
     based on patient's condition,
     physician orders, etc.

M   10. Ability to cancel verified orders

M   11. Ability to receive hard copy of all
     transactions required to be charted

M   12. Ability to display each selection on
     the subsequent screen

M   13. Ability to validate on line some
     basic orders modifiers (e.g., fre-
     quency, duration, form, route, etc.)

Manage Orders

M   1. Ability to print/display orders for
     professional verification, by patient,
     nursing station, physician, ancillary
     department, etc.

M   2. Ability to hold orders in suspense
     until the appropriate verification
     has been completed

M   3. Ability to require physician verifica-
     tion after the fact for physician
     representative (i.e., nurse) of verified
     orders either on line or by signing a
     printed order

M   4. Ability to automatically direct the
     order for procedures and preps to
     the correct locations

M   5. Ability to generate multiple requisi-
     tions from individual orders, which
     are continuing or have a frequency
     of greater than once per day

Manage Orders (continued)

M   6. Ability to explode orders into
        various procedures and preps to
        the correct locations

M   7. Ability to interface with stand-
        alone computer(s) on a real-time
        basis

M   8. Ability to notify the proper person-
        nel when special handling is required

M   9. Ability to print requisitions
        immediately for
        a. STAT orders
        b. Orders from specific nursing
            units

M   10. Ability to maintain all orders and
        their status on line until purged as
        part of the medical records report-
        ing applications until discharge

M   11. Ability to print/display all orders
        for a patient or ancillary depart-
        ment with its station indicated

M   12. Ability to print all orders scheduled
        to expire within the next 24 hours
        by patient, nursing station, or
        physician

M   13. Ability to print/display all in-
        complete orders for an ancillary
        department on demand or at a
        specified time

M   14. Ability to print/display all in-
        complete orders entered from a
        specified date forward for a
        patient by ancillary department

M   15. Ability to display/print all orders
        sequenced by
        a. Department
        b. Order type

	Mandatory/Desirable	Available	Not Available

Manage Orders (continued)

M   16. Ability to monitor orders. Inquire
     as to status

M   17. Check for duplicate orders

Update Standard Orders Directory

M   1. Ability to establish standard orders
    by physician, nursing care plans,
    service, hospital policy, diagnosis,
    and patient condition

M   2. Ability to update a directory of
    standard order either
    a. On line
    b. Batch

Produce Billing Transactions

M   1. Ability to interface to the patient
    accounting system for automatic
    charging of procedures

M   2. Ability to generate a charge for
    each procedure/test according to
    charging criteria contained in the
    procedure directory (i.e., order
    entry, order verification, procedure/
    test complete, result entry, etc.

M   3. Ability to issue a credit for a test/
    procedure that was not performed
    either
    a. Manually
    b. Automatically when test is
       canceled

D   4. Ability to support point of sale
    billing

Update Procedure Directory

M   1. Ability to update a directory of
    procedures and associated preps
    either
    a. On line
    b. Batch

		Available	Not Available

Mandatory/Desirable

Update Procedure Directory (continued)

M   2. Ability to link specific comment screens to each procedure

M   3. Ability to link procedures that serve as preps to other procedures

M   4. Ability to include the time relationships between the procedure and associated preps

M   5. Ability to indicate the following for each procedure
   a. Frequency of the procedure/prep, if frequency is not selected
   b. Performance times (either available or required)
   c. Whether or not a requisition is to be printed
   d. The standard requisition–print location
   e. Department to perform the procedures/prep
   f. Reports where the procedure is to appear (i.e., nursing care worksheet, care plan, medication plan)
   g. Alternate requisition print location dependent on
      i. Account type

M   6. Provide option, at time of order entry, to review test preparation information or identify other test requirements specific to each other

D   7. Ability to maintain procedure standard price, price required, or no charge with the hospital and professional components

D   8. Ability to maintain STAT and special handling surcharges for each procedure

M   9. Ability to indicate when no charge for each procedure (i.e., order

	Available	Not Available
Mandatory/Desirable		

Update Procedure Directory (continued)

        verification, specimen received, procedure/test complete, result entry, etc.)

M   10. Ability to indicate if professional verification is required and by which categories and authority level before processing the order

M   11. Ability to update standard formats for procedure requisitions either
      a. On line
      b. Batch

Enter Results

M   1. Ability to enter all results via light pen or other high-level user-oriented data entry techniques

M   2. Ability to automatically format the screen to accommodate the results for the ordered procedure

M   3. Ability to interface with stand-alone computer(s) or automated instruments on a real-time basis

M   4. Ability to automatically update the order status on entering results

D   5. Ability to prevent the entry of results without a price for price-required procedures

Manage Results

M   1. Ability to automatically direct test results to the proper location or multiple locations (i.e., nursing station, operating room, emergency room, ancillary department, etc.)

M   2. Ability to print results immediately for STAT orders and patients

Mandatory/Desirable	Available	Not Available

Manage Results (continued)

located in specific units (i.e., ICU, CCU, emergency room, operating room, etc.)

M   3. Ability to print results immediately from specified ancillary departments

D   4. Ability to hold results from specified ancillary departments or specific tests for review and verification before being released for printing or display outside the ancillary department

M   5. Ability to maintain all results on line until purged as part of the medical records reporting application

M   6. Ability to print/display all ancillary results for a specific patient, results from a specified date forward or for a specific order

M   7. Ability to print results suitable for chart

Update Procedure Directory

M   1. Ability to indicate the following additional information on each procedure record
a. Time allowed to obtain result; flag if exceeds maximum time
b. Result format

Update Abstract Code Directories

M   1. Ability to update a directory of abstracting codes for various ancillary department results reporting

| | Mandatory/Desirable | Available | Not Available |

Mandatory/Desirable   Available   Not Available

Print/Display Order/Result Directories

M   1. Ability to print/display the order/
         result directories, in part, in total
         and various sort sequences

Inventory Control

M   1. Ability to maintain inventory
         control system in ancillary area

Patient Scheduling

M   1. Ability to print/display all un-
         scheduled procedures for an ancil-
         lary department with the pertinent
         scheduling information on
         demand or on a scheduled basis

M   2. Ability to schedule a procedure for
         a specific time period for any active
         patient (i.e., preadmitted, in-house,
         preregistered, and registered)

M   3. Ability to automatically pre-
         register a nonactive patient by
         entering the appropriate informa-
         tion when scheduling an ancillary
         department procedure

M   4. Ability to automatically check for
         conflicts in the patient's schedule

M   5. Ability to schedule an appointment
         by
         a. Service
         b. Room/equipment
         c. Personnel
         d. Procedure test

M   6. Ability to indicate where the
         patient is served (i.e., ancillary
         department, patient room, etc.)
         or what procedure is being
         performed

M   7. Ability to reschedule the appoint-
         ment without canceling and
         reentering

		Available	Not Available

Mandatory/Desirable

Patient Scheduling (continued)

M   8. Ability to automatically cancel the appointment when the procedure order is canceled

M   9. Ability to maintain standard hours of availability for services, room/equipment, and personnel

M   10. Ability to modify standard hours on an exception basis

M   11. Ability to maintain an unlimited number of services, room/equipment, and personnel

M   12. Ability to schedule 3 months in advance

D   13. Ability to print/display the schedules for a specific date, procedure, test

D   14. Ability to print/display the room/equipment, physician, and personnel schedules for a specific date, procedure, test

D   15. Ability to print/display future procedures scheduled

D   16. Ability to print/display all procedures requiring scheduling that have not yet been scheduled

D   17. Ability to print time patient tests in and time out

Care Planning

M   1. Ability to enter special activities when standard activities within the care category are inappropriate

M   2. Ability to update a patient's care plan by entering additional phy-

	Mandatory/Desirable	Available	Not Available

Care Planning (continued)

sician and nursing orders or canceling existing orders

D   3. Ability to update all vital signs for each patient

M   4. Ability to indicate compliance with care activities or the justification for noncompliance

D   5. Ability to print/display care activities not complied with and no justification given

D   6. Ability to print/display the entire care plan for a patient

D   7. Ability to print/display the care activities over a specified time period for a patient

D   8. Ability to print care plans limited to activities for a specified time period for a patient

D   9. Ability to group activities by care categories and include pertinent patient data (i.e., allergies, diagnosis, etc.) when printing or displaying care plans

D   10. Ability to print/display a cumulative all-vital-signs summary over a specified time period for a patient

Infection Control

M   1. Ability to print Infection Control notes

Determine Patient Care Requirements

M   1. Ability to interface to a clinical or communication system to obtain acuity classification of all patients in-house

M   2. Ability of Nurse Staffing system to determine the patient's acuity

	Mandatory/Desirable	Available	Not Available

Determine Patient Care Requirements (continued)

                level using nursing input for each acuity criterion

M   3. Ability to computerize the patient care units for a patient based on
        a. Care activity
        b. Its frequency
        c. Patient's acuity level
        d. By nursing stations
        e. For each shift

M   4. Ability to total the patient care units for continuing patients and patients pending discharge from each nursing station by shift on a real-time basis

Compute Nurse Staffing Requirements

D   1. Ability to compute the number of nursing care units required
        a. For each nursing station
        b. By shift
        c. Based on the number of patient care units required on that shift
        d. Scheduled admissions and pending discharges for that shift
        e. Number of patients on the nursing station

D   2. Ability to translate the number of nursing personnel by job category required for each nursing station and assigned preadmitted patients based on a predefined staffing mix specified for that nursing station

D   3. Ability to consider skill mix in computing staffing requirements

D   4. Ability to allow interunit floating

D   5. Ability to report on-call requirements by skill level

| | | Not |
| Mandatory/Desirable | Available | Available |

Print/Display Nurse Staffing Requirements

D   1. Ability to print/display the required nursing personnel according to job category for each nursing station and assigned preadmitted patients for comparison with the scheduled staffing

D   2. Ability to print/display the required nursing care units and available nursing care units for each nursing station as part of the bed assignment procedure

Maintain Patient Care Directories

M   1. Ability to maintain patient care hours for each care activity by acuity level

Maintain Nurse Staffing Conversion Directory

D   1. Ability to maintain nursing care units/factors by nursing station for admissions, discharges, personal time allowances, and nondefined activities

D   2. Ability to maintain factors for each nursing station to convert nursing care units to the appropriate mix of nursing personnel for that nursing station

Performance Reporting

D   1. Ability to interface with the personnel payroll system and pass the required and actual nursing hours by shift for productivity analysis and report patient days

Note: Additional order communications requirements pertaining to the Laboratory System are provided in the original document.

B—Site Visit Checklist*

Karen D. Lafferty

On the Patient Care Unit

___   1. Look at the patient's hardcopy chart. What is manual and what is computer generated?

___   2. Observe an order being transcribed into the system.
___   Is it light-pen entered?
___   What percentage is light-pen?
___   What percentage is keyboard entered?

___   3. Record the time you arrive on the unit.
___   Record the number of phone calls.
___   Record the time you leave the unit.
___   Record the type of unit.

___   4. While on the patient unit, record who is using the system.
___   Pharmacists
___   Ward clerks
___   Physicians
___   Nurses

___   5. Ask the end users (i.e., nurses, pharmacists, ward clerks, etc.) what they like most about the system and what they like least about it. Do not ask your guide.
       Most: _____
       _____
       Least: _____
       _____

*From Lafferty KD: Patient care systems vs. financial systems: the cost justification battle. *Nursing Management* 1987; 18(7):51–55. Reprinted with permission.

——— 6. How many terminals are at the nursing stations?

——— 7. Observe your guide or a user obtaining the following in a live situation:
    ——— a. A medication administration guide
    ——— b. A nursing worksheet
    ——— c. A care plan
    ——— d. A radiology result
    ——— e. A laboratory result
    ——— f. A pharmacy profile complete with medication administration
    ——— g. A diet history
    ——— h. Clinical history
    ——— i. On-line, user-defined reports
    ——— j. Management reports

——— 8. Ask what order entry is performed manually and why.

——— 9. Ask how long orders, results, and demographics are available on line.

——— 10. Ask the hour/patient-day ratio.

——— 11. Ask about explosion of standard order sets.

——— 12. Ask who from the hospital comprised the project team for implementation. _____
_____

——— 13. Ask about the hospital's goals for implementation of an automated system. _____
_____
_____
_____
_____

——— Were they realized?

——— 14. Ask about the knowledge and experience of the vendor's implementation personnel. _____
_____

——— Were health care professionals on the team?

——— 15. Ask about current projects and planned projects for computerization in nursing areas. _____
_____
_____
_____
_____

___   16. Ask about the decision-making process. How did the hospital select the installed vendor? _____

_____

_____

_____

Was nursing involved? _____
Have nursing's needs been met? _____
___   17. What would nursing change about the system? _____

_____

_____

_____

___   18. What would nursing like the system to do that it currently doesn't do? _____

_____

_____

_____

Additional Points:

- Take the time to closely look at screens, content layout, depth and breadth of available information, and ease of use. This is especially important if you make site visits before seeing a demonstration.

- Spend a minimum of 1 hour on the patient care unit. If all your questions are answered in less time, ask to observe.

- Go to at least two patient care areas. The second unit visit may be brief, but be confident that the system is operational on more than one unit.

- If possible, ask to speak to the VP of Nursing to gain an administrative level perspective of the system. This works best if prearranged.

- Pay particular notice to implementation strategies and organizational structures that can assist in your own process.

- An overview of the hospital, its size, programs, objectives, staffing patterns, and administrative support for system installation can be valuable in drawing a parallel to your own environment.

- Do not leave the hospital until you're satisfied that you've seen what you have been sold. "Kick tires" in order to feel confident about the product.

- Many times your site visit and presentations will represent a full package, but a "scaled-down" version has been priced. Be confident of what you are seeing as compared to what has been priced or proposed.

In Ancillary Areas:

___   1. Does the system meet the operational requirements of each ancillary?
       ___   Pharmacy
       ___   Radiology
       ___   Laboratory
       ___   Medical Records
       ___   Central Supply
       ___   Dietary
       ___   All Others

___   2. How many ancillary departments are supported?

___   3. What is the level of support?
       ___   Order Entry
       ___   Results Reporting
       ___   Worklists
       ___   Management Reports

___   4. Are the ancillary departments integrated or interfaced?
       ___   Pharmacy
       ___   Radiology
       ___   Laboratory
       ___   Medical Records
       ___   Central Supply
       ___   Dietary
       ___   All Others

___   5. Can Pharmacy review a nursing data base?

___   6. Can radiology review a medication profile?

___   7. Does pharmacy have a cart refill list for unit/dose dispensing?

___   8. Does pharmacy have reports for drug utilization?

___   9. Does pharmacy have IV and hyperalimentation support?

___   10. Does the automated medication procedure shorten the steps and potential error in a manual medication procedure?

___   11. Does clinical data automatically pass to the medical records system?

___   12. What system support is available for outpatients and clinic patients? _____
_____
_____
_____
_____

(Questions 5–11 are representative of system integration.)

In General:

___   1. What is the response time (time elapsed between probing enter and being able to probe again on the new screen)?

___   2. What is the hardware used to run the system? Size? Relative performance? Downtime?

___   3. What is the total number of terminals operational on the system?

___   4. What is the size of the DP staff? Number of FTEs?

___   5. How long did it take to implement the system?

___   6. How long did it take to obtain benefits from the system?

___   7. What has been the cost per patient-day of the system?

___   8. Does the system offer a user-friendly report writer?

___   9. Are the patient accounting and financial systems interfaced or integrated?

___   10. How much flexibility do you have with your patient accounting and financial systems?

___   11. Do the patient care and financial applications have the same data base?

C—Index to Computer-Assisted Instructional (CAI) Software for Nursing Education

Christine Bolwell

The computer-assisted instructional software listed below is available for viewing by groups or individuals, as part of a hands-on workshop, or for preview before purchase. Christine Bolwell, editor and publisher of the newsletter *Nursing Educators MicroWorld* and author of the *1987 Directory of Educational Software for Nursing* and the *1988 Directory of Educational Software for Nursing* will bring the software to your institution for either purpose. You can request review of the entire collection or just the programs specific for either the Apple or the IBM or IBM-compatible microcomputer. The hands-on workshops are custom designed to fit your needs and to meet your objectives.

The workshops have been enthusiastically received at colleges, universities, hospitals, and as part of larger health care conferences. Institutions have appreciated the convenience of having most of the CAI software for nursing education available at one time for preview before making purchasing decisions.

The listing was current in May 1987. Many additional programs will have been developed and available for review when this book is published. For further information write or call:

Christine Bolwell, RN, MSN
Diskovery: Computer-Assisted Healthcare Education
13740 Harleigh Court
Saratoga, CA 95070
(408) 741-0156

The National League for Nursing's National Forum on Computers in Health Care and Nursing sponsors workshops presented by Christine that include hands-on experience with any or all of these computer-assisted instructional programs. For further information write or call:

Jeanette Lawrence
Division of Continuing Education and Meeting Services
National League for Nursing
Ten Columbus Circle
New York, NY 10019
(800) 847-8480

Index to IBM-Compatible CAI Software by Topic

NAME OF PROGRAM	STYLE	TOPIC	COMPANY
The Ear (see videotape)**	Tutorial	Anatomy	BIO-PSYCH Ed. Tool
Basic Cardiovascular**	Exp/Sim.	Physiol.	J. Randall
Basic Electrophysiology**	Exp/Sim.	Physiol.	J. Randall
Circsyst**	Exp/Sim.	Physiol.	J. Boyle, MD
Gas Exchange**	Exp/Sim.	Physiol.	J. Boyle, MD
Human**	Exp/Sim.	Physiol.	J. Randall
Basic Human—Integrated Systems**	Exp/Sim.	Physiol.	J. Randall
Cardiovascular Systems & Dynamics**	Exp/Sim.	Physiol.	Command App. Tech.
PuFT**	Exp/Sim.	Physiol.	J. Boyle, MD
Pulmonary Mechanics Lab**	Exp/Sim.	Physiol.	Command App. Tech.
Respsyst**	Exp/Sim.	Physiol.	J. Boyle, MD
Starling**	Exp/Sim.	Physiol.	J. Boyle, MD
Building a Med. Vocab.— Fields of Medicine & External Anatomy	D & P	Term.	Saunders
Building a Med. Vocab.— Blood & Circulatory & Lymphatic Systems	D & P	Term.	Saunders
Building a Med. Vocab.— Respiratory & Digestive Systems	D & P	Term.	Saunders
Building a Med. Vocab.— Urinary & Reproductive Systems	D & P	Term.	Saunders

NAME OF PROGRAM	STYLE	TOPIC	COMPANY
Building a Med. Vocab.— Muscular, Skeletal, & Nervous Systems	D & P	Term.	Saunders
Building a Med. Vocab.— Integumentary & Endocrine Systems	D & P	Term.	Saunders
Basic Math & Dosage Calculation	D & P	Calc.	C.V. Mosby
DoseCalc—Fractions	D & P	Calc.	Saunders
DoseCalc—Decimals	D & P	Calc.	Saunders
DoseCalc—Percents	D & P	Calc.	Saunders
DoseCalc—Linear Equations	D & P	Calc.	Saunders
DoseCalc—Ratio & Proportion	D & P	Calc.	Saunders
DoseCalc—Roman Numerals	D & P	Calc.	Saunders
DoseCalc—Systs. of Measurement	D & P	Calc.	Saunders
DoseCalc—Oral Medication Dosages	D & P	Calc.	Saunders
DoseCalc—Parenteral Inj. Dosages	D & P	Calc.	Saunders
DoseCalc—I.V. & Tube Feeding Rates	D & P	Calc.	Saunders
DoseCalc—Pedi Medication Dosages	D & P	Calc.	Saunders
DoseCalc—Test Bank	D & P	Calc.	Saunders
Drug Dosage Calculation Administration	D & P	Calc.	Medi-Sim
Symbols and Abbreviations	D & P	Calc.	Medi-Sim
Systems of Measurement	D & P	Calc.	Medi-Sim
Mathematics of Nursing Pharmacology	Tutor/ D & P	Calc.	MEPC Software
Clinical Simulations in Nursing Pharm.	Simul.	Pharm.	MEPC Software
Antibiotic Therapy, Pt. w/ Fracture	Simul.	Pharm.	MEPC Software
Patient w/ Gastric Pain & Distress	Simul.	Pharm.	MEPC Software

NAME OF PROGRAM	STYLE	TOPIC	COMPANY
Pt. Requiring Anti-arrhythmic Therapy	Simul.	Pharm.	MEPC Software
Patient with Angina Pectoris	Simul.	Pharm.	MEPC Software
Adjuvant Chemotherapy for Breast CA	Simul.	Pharm.	MEPC Software
Client Using Birth Control Pills	Simul.	Pharm.	MEPC Software
Analgesia & Anesthesia —Maternity Pt.	Simul.	Pharm.	MEPC Software
Immunizing Children	Simul.	Pharm.	MEPC Software
Iron Intoxication in a Toddler	Simul.	Pharm.	MEPC Software
Drugs Rx for Pre-schooler w/ Asthma	Simul.	Pharm.	MEPC Software
Psychotropic Drug Rx w/ Schizophrenic	Simul.	Pharm.	MEPC Software
Treating Depressed Pt. w/ Tricyclics	Simul.	Pharm.	MEPC Software
Digitalis: Pharmacology & Clinical Use	Tutorial	Pharm.	Williams & Wilkins
Electronic Drug Reference	Demo	Pharm.	Clinical Ref. Sys.
Pharmacology CAI Series	Tutorial	Pharm.	Medi-Sim
Pharmacology CAI	Tutorial	Pharm.	C.V. Mosby
The Drug Master	Demo	Pharm.	Medical Watch
A-B Game**	Tutorial	ABGs	J. Boyle, MD
ABGee	D & P	ABGs	D. Thompson, RN, MSN
Arterial Blood Gases	Tutorial	ABGs	AJN
Arterial Blood Gases	Tutor/ Sim.	ABGs	Williams & Wilkins
Respiratory Expert	Sim./Anal.	ABGs	Saunders
Arrhythmias I: Pathophys. & Supraventric.	Tutorial	EKG	Williams & Wilkins
Arrhythmias II: Ventric-ular & Heart Block	Tutorial	EKG	Williams & Wilkins
Arrhythmias: Case Studies in Management	Tutorial	EKG	Williams & Wilkins
ECG Primer**	Tutorial	EKG	AJN
EKG Tutor**	Tutorial	EKG	J. Boyle, MD
TACH-MAN**	Simul.	EKG Dx & Rx	MicroTrends
Skills Simulation—Taking a B/P**	D & P	Nurs. Skills	Lippincott

NAME OF PROGRAM	STYLE	TOPIC	COMPANY
Skills Simulation—Calc. & Adjust I. V. Flow Rates**	D & P	Nurs. Skills	Lippincott
Skills Simulation—Calc. & Prep. for Injection**	D & P	Nurs. Skills	Lippincott
Skills Simulation—Urine Testing Sugar & Ketones**	D & P	Nurs. Skills	Lippincott
Skills Simulation—Prep Insulin Injection**	D & P	Nurs. Skills	Lippincott
Physical Assessment**	Tutorial	Nurs. Skills	Lippincott
Head, Face, Mouth & Neck**	Tutorial	Nurs. Skills	Lippincott
Eyes, Ears & Nose**	Tutorial	Nurs. Skills	Lippincott
Breasts & Axillae**	Tutorial	Nurs. Skills	Lippincott
Thorax & Lungs**	Tutorial	Nurs. Skills	Lippincott
Abdomen**	Tutorial	Nurs. Skills	Lippincott
Female Genitalia, Anus & Rectum**	Tutorial	Nurs. Skills	Lippincott
Male Genitalia, Rectum & Hernias**	Tutorial	Nurs. Skills	Lippincott
Cardiovascular: Neck Vessels and Heart**	Tutorial	Nurs. Skills	Lippincott
Cardiovascular: Peripheral Vascular System**	Tutorial	Nurs. Skills	Lippincott
Musculoskeletal System**	Tutorial	Nurs. Skills	Lippincott
Neurological: Cranial Nerves & Sensory System**	Tutorial	Nurs. Skills	Lippincott
Neurological: Motor System & Reflexes**	Tutorial	Nurs. Skills	Lippincott
Diagnostic Test Disk**	Tutorial	Nurs. Skills	Lippincott
Vital Signs and Phys. Assessment	Tutorial	Nurs. Skills	C.V. Mosby
Computer Literacy for Nurses	Tutorial	Computers	Medi-Sim
RNact	Demo	Careplan	RNact
Evaluation of Nursing Interventions**	Tutorial	Nurs. Theory	Medi-Sim
Intro to Nursing Diagnosis**	Tutorial	Nurs. Theory	Lippincott
Intro to Nursing Goals**	Tutorial	Nurs. Theory	Lippincott

NAME OF PROGRAM	STYLE	TOPIC	COMPANY
Intro to Patient Data**	Tutorial	Nurs. Theory	Lippincott
Intro to Patient Problems**	Tutorial	Nurs. Theory	Lippincott
Idea Generator	Analysis	Prob. Solv.	Experience in Soft.
Care of Client with an MI	Simul.	Med. Nurs.	Medi-Sim
Pathophysiology	Simul.	Med. Nurs.	Medi-Sim
Diagnosis	Simul.	Med. Nurs.	Medi-Sim
Immediate care	Simul.	Med. Nurs.	Medi-Sim
Long-term care	Simul.	Med. Nurs.	Medi-Sim
Dietary Intervention in Hypertension	Simul.	Med. Nurs.	Medi-Sim
Gloria Roberts: Retarded Adult w/ Asthma	Simul.	Med. Nurs.	Saunders
Electronic Medical Reference	Demo	Med. Nurs.	Clinical Ref. Sys.
Hypertension Management	Tutorial	Med. Nurs.	Williams & Wilkins
Nursing Care of Patient w/ Alzheimer's	Simul.	Med. Nurs.	Medi-Sim
Mr. Hansie: with Cirrhosis**	Simul.	Med. Nurs.	Lippincott
Mr. Merna: A Patient with Liver Disease	Simul.	Med. Nurs.	Saunders
Mr. Richardson: Man with Diabetes	Simul.	Med. Nurs.	Saunders
Mrs. Shilkraut: Terminal Patient	Simul.	Med. Nurs.	Saunders
UMKC Software Series	Demo	Med. Nurs.	UMKC
Respiratory Failure Tutorial	Tutorial	Med. Nurs.	L. Martin, MD
Mrs. Gates: Elderly Woman	Simul.	Geriatrics	Saunders
Mrs. Pearl: 83-yr-old w/ fx Hip	Simul.	Geriatrics	Saunders
Jerry Burke: Quadriplegic Adolescent**	Simul.	Med/Surg.	Lippincott
Mr. Babain: with Peptic Ulcer**	Simul.	Med/Surg.	Lippincott
Mr. Casey: with Renal Colic**	Simul.	Med/Surg.	Lippincott
Mr. Lewis: with Acute Pancreatitis	Simul.	Med/Surg.	Saunders

NAME OF PROGRAM	STYLE	TOPIC	COMPANY
Mr. Jensen: w/ CAD & Surgery	Simul.	Med/Surg.	Saunders
Mr. Migo: with BPH**	Simul.	Med/Surg.	Lippincott
Mrs. Fiver: Lady with Cystitis**	Simul.	Med/Surg.	Lippincott
Mrs. Mandy: w/ Glomeru- lonephritis**	Simul.	Med/Surg.	Lippincott
Mrs. Pacer: with Cholecystitis**	Simul.	Med/Surg.	Lippincott
Rena Fuller: Renal Crisis**	Simul.	Med/Surg.	Lippincott
Shock: Pathophysiology & Complications	Tutorial	Med/Surg.	Medi-Sim
Shock: Assessment & Pharmacology	Tutorial	Med/Surg.	Medi-Sim
Electronic Surgical Reference	Demo	Surg. Nurs.	Clinical Ref. Sys.
Mr. Petey: w/ Abdomino- perineal Res.**	Simul.	Surg. Nurs.	Lippincott
Mrs. Simms: For Hemor- rhoidectomy	Simul.	Surg. Nurs.	Saunders
Scott Duchess: w/ Appendicitis	Simul.	Surg. Nurs.	Lippincott
Kathy Shaw: Antepartal Care**	Simul.	OB Nurs.	Lippincott
Amy	Simul.	Pedi. Nurs.	UCSF
An Infant	Simul.	Pedi. Nurs.	MEPC Software
A Toddler	Simul.	Pedi. Nurs.	MEPC Software
A Preschooler	Simul.	Pedi. Nurs.	MEPC Software
A School Age Child	Simul.	Pedi. Nurs.	MEPC Software
Beth Popil: Child with V.S.D.**	Simul.	Pedi. Nurs.	Lippincott
Care of Child w/ Cardio- vascular Surgery	Simul.	Pedi. Nurs.	Medi-Sim
Communicable Diseases in Children—Eight Case Studies	Simul.	Pedi. Nurs.	Medi-Sim
Communicable Diseases in Children	Simul.	Pedi. Nurs.	Medi-Sim
Kathy Ortez with Rubeola	Simul.	Pedi. Nurs.	Medi-Sim
Erik Gordon with Mumps	Simul.	Pedi. Nurs.	Medi-Sim

NAME OF PROGRAM	STYLE	TOPIC	COMPANY
Charles Gordon with Scarlet Fever	Simul.	Pedi. Nurs.	Medi-Sim
Nicole Smith with Rubella	Simul.	Pedi. Nurs.	Medi-Sim
Patty Gordon with Chicken Pox	Simul.	Pedi. Nurs.	Medi-Sim
Danny Wong	Simul.	Pedi. Nurs.	UCSF
Developmental Diseases in Children	Simul.	Pedi. Nurs.	Medi-Sim
Keta Smith—Newborn	Simul.	Pedi. Nurs.	Medi-Sim
Matt Lewis—Toddler	Simul.	Pedi. Nurs.	Medi-Sim
Maria Gomez— Preschooler	Simul.	Pedi. Nurs.	Medi-Sim
Melinda George— School Age	Simul.	Pedi. Nurs.	Medi-Sim
Hazel: 6-yr-old with Nephrosis**	Simul.	Pedi. Nurs.	Lippincott
Infant Safety: Anticipatory Guidance**	Simul.	Pedi. Nurs.	Medi-Sim
Infant Nutrition: Newborn to 2 Years**	Simul.	Pedi. Nurs.	Medi-Sim
Jessica Grant: 14-yr-old w/ Sickle Cell	Simul.	Pedi. Nurs.	Saunders
Karen Walcott: 5-yr-old w/ URI	Simul.	Pedi. Nurs.	Saunders
Patient Education— Pediatrics	Data Base	Pedi. Nurs.	Clinical Ref. Sys.
Pediatric Family Assess- ment	Tutorial	Pedi. Nurs.	C.V. Mosby
Ellen Peterson	Simul.	Pedi. Onco- logy	UCSF
Care of Patients w/ Anxiety Disorders	Tutorial	Psych.	Medi-Sim
Mental Health & Community Nursing**	Tutorial	Psych.	Medi-Sim
Mr. Charles: Obsessive- Compulsive**	Simul.	Psych.	Lippincott
Psychiatric Mental Health Nursing	Tutorial	Psych.	C.V. Mosby
Mr. Burke: Open Heart Surgery	Simul.	Crit. Care	UCSF
Critical Care Series: Cardiovascular	Simul.	Crit. Care	Medi-Sim
Myocardial Infarction**	Simul.	Crit. Care	Medi-Sim

NAME OF PROGRAM	STYLE	TOPIC	COMPANY
Angina/Athero-sclerosis**	Simul.	Crit. Care	Medi-Sim
Conduction System Defects**	Simul.	Crit. Care	Medi-Sim
Pulmonary Edema**	Simul.	Crit. Care	Medi-Sim
Cardiogenic Shock**	Simul.	Crit. Care	Medi-Sim
Critical Care Series: Endocrine	Simul.	Crit. Care	Medi-Sim
Thyrotoxic Crisis**	Simul.	Crit. Care	Medi-Sim
Diabetic Ketoacidosis**	Simul.	Crit. Care	Medi-Sim
Syndrome on Inappro-priate ADH**	Simul.	Crit. Care	Medi-Sim
Acute Adrenal Insufficency**	Simul.	Crit. Care	Medi-Sim
Diabetes Insipidus**	Simul.	Crit. Care	Medi-Sim
Critical Care Series: Gastrointestinal	Simul.	Crit. Care	Medi-Sim
Gastroesophageal Varices**	Simul.	Crit. Care	Medi-Sim
Peptic Ulcer Disease**	Simul.	Crit. Care	Medi-Sim
Inflammatory Bowel Disease**	Simul.	Crit. Care	Medi-Sim
Hepatic Failure**	Simul.	Crit. Care	Medi-Sim
Acute Pancreatitis**	Simul.	Crit. Care	Medi-Sim
Critical Care Series: Pulmonary	Simul.	Crit. Care	Medi-Sim
Adult Respiratory Distress Synd.**	Simul.	Crit. Care	Medi-Sim
Pulmonary Embolism**	Simul.	Crit. Care	Medi-Sim
Acute Respiratory Failure**	Simul.	Crit. Care	Medi-Sim
COPD**	Simul.	Crit. Care	Medi-Sim
Chest Trauma**	Simul.	Crit. Care	Medi-Sim
Dx & Management of Pts. w/ Acute MI	Tutorial	Crit. Care	Williams & Wilkins
Fluid & Electrolyte Expert	Sim./Anal.	Crit. Care	Saunders
Hemodynamic Expert	Sim./Anal.	Crit. Care	Saunders
Hemodynamic Monitor-ing—Applied**	Tutorial	Crit. Care	MedSoft
Hypertensive Emergencies	Tutorial	Crit. Care	Williams & Wilkins
Intracranial Pressure Monitoring	Simul.	Crit. Care	Medi-Sim

NAME OF PROGRAM	STYLE	TOPIC	COMPANY
Mr. Jones: Man with Indigestion	Simul.	Emer. Nurs.	Saunders
CPR Training by Computer	Simul.	ACLS	Williams & Wilkins
Call Doc—Cardiovascular	Analysis	SNF Assess.	Clinical Nursing Soft.
Call Doc—Falls	Analysis	SNF Assess.	Clinical Nursing Soft.
Call Doc—U.R.I.	Analysis	SNF Assess.	Clinical Nursing Soft.
Call Doc—U.T.I.	Analysis	SNF Assess.	Clinical Nursing Soft.
Management to the Top	Tutorial	Mgmt.	Career Development
Nursing Leadership: E.S.P. Approach	Tutorial	Mgmt.	Career Development
The Art of Negotiation	Analysis	Mgmt.	Experience in Soft.
The Management Advantage	Analysis	Mgmt.	Thoughtware
M.A.R.T.	Tutorial	Mgmt/Stress	Career Development
Managing Stress	Analysis	Stress	Thoughtware
Stress Assess	Analysis	Stress	National Wellness
Drinking or Not Drinking	Tutorial	Subs. Abuse	Subs. Abuse Education
Keep Off the Grass	Tutorial	Subs. Abuse	Subs. Abuse Education
Compute-A-Life I**	Appraisal	Health	National Wellness
Health Age	Appraisal	Health	Wellsource
Health Analysis Program	Appraisal	Health	MedMicro
Patient Advice—Adult	Data Base	Health	Clinical Ref. Sys.
Heartware	Data Base	Nutrition	Soft Bite
The Balancing Act I	Analysis	Nutrition	Soft Bite
Nursestar	Test	NCLEX	C.V. Mosby
Sandra Smith's Computer Review	Test	NCLEX	Ntl. Nursing Review
Careers in Hospital Nursing	Data Base	Careers	Career Development
Four Stages of Interviewing	Tutorial	Careers	Career Development

NAME OF PROGRAM	STYLE	TOPIC	COMPANY
Micro Guide to Nursing Careers	Data Base	Careers	Career Development
Setting Career Goals the Micro Way	Turtorial	Careers	Career Development
The Right Job Application	Tutorial	Careers	Career Development
Author/Quiz	Demo	Authoring	Brian Jeffreys
Clinical Simulation Authoring System**	Demo	Authoring	DeWitt Data Systems
Microinstructor	Demo	Authoring	C.V. Mosby
Microinstructor (with graphics)**	Demo	Authoring	C.V. Mosby
NEMAS	Demo	Authoring	Lippincott
T.A.P.	Demo	Test Author.	UCSF
Med-Math	Demo	Test Author.	Lippincott
Author/Quiz	System	Quiz Author.	Brian Jeffreys

**Graphics board necessary.

Index to Apple CAI Software by Topic

NAME OF PROGRAM	STYLE	TOPIC	COMPANY
Heart Lab	D & P	Anatomy	Educational Activit.
Human Body Overview	Tutorial	Anatomy	Brain Bank
Neuromuscular Concepts Skeletal muscle contraction	Tutorial	Anatomy	Biosource
	Tutorial	Anatomy	Biosource
Muscle action potentials	Tutorial	Anatomy	Biosource
Disorders of movement	Tutorial	Anatomy	Biosource
Skeletal Muscle A. & P.	Tutorial	Anatomy	Biosource
Microstructure	Tutorial	Anatomy	Biosource
Sliding filament theory	Tutorial	Anatomy	Biosource
Muscle contraction	Tutorial	Anatomy	Biosource
Muscles as levers	Tutorial	Anatomy	Biosource
Skeletal System	Tutorial	Anatomy	Brain Bank
Heart Abnormalities & EKG	Simul.	A. & P.	Focus Media
The Body in Focus	Discovery	A. & P.	CBS Software
The Digestion Simulator	Tutorial	A. & P.	Focus Media
The Digestive System	Tutorial	A. & P.	Marshware
The Endocrine System	Tutorial	A. & P.	Focus Media
The Heart Simulator	Simul.	A. & P.	Focus Media

NAME OF PROGRAM	STYLE	TOPIC	COMPANY
The Muscular System	Tutorial	A. & P.	Focus Media
The Nervous System	Tutorial	A. & P.	Focus Media
The Skeletal System	Tutorial	A. & P.	Focus Media
Basic Cardiovascular	Simul.	Physiol.	J. Randall
Basic Electrophysiology	Simul.	Physiol.	J. Randall
Physiology—Respiratory System	Simul.	Physiol.	Harold Modell
Biology Series	Game	Biology	Academic Hall.
Human cells, organs, & systems	Game	Biology	Academic Hall.
Worms & fish	Game	Biology	Academic Hall.
Birds, mammals, & bacteria	Game	Biology	Academic Hall.
Plant anatomy & physiology	Game	Biology	Academic Hall.
Evolution, genetics, reproduction	Game	Biology	Academic Hall.
Human Genetic Disorders	Tutorial	Genetics	HRM Software
Skills in Electromyography	Tutorial	Myography	Biosource
Prepping skin, reducing artifact	Tutorial	Myography	Biosource
Locating surface electrodes	Tutorial	Myography	Biosource
Preventing shock hazards	Tutorial	Myography	Biosource
Building a Medical Vocabulary	Demo	Term.	Saunders
Medical Terminology Competency Test	D & P	Term.	Educational Software
Exploring Medical Terminology	D & P	Term.	C.V. Mosby
Calculate with Care	D & P	Calc.	Lippincott
Systems of measurement	D & P	Calc.	Lippincott
Fractions	D & P	Calc.	Lippincott
Decimals	D & P	Calc.	Lippincott
Percentages	D & P	Calc.	Lippincott
Roman numerals	D & P	Calc.	Lippincott
Ratio and proportion	D & P	Calc.	Lippincott
Problem solving	D & P	Calc.	Lippincott
Diagnostic & posttest	D & P	Calc.	Lippincott
Calculate—Chemical Conversion Method	Tutorial	Calc.	Computer Ed. Resource

NAME OF PROGRAM	STYLE	TOPIC	COMPANY
Calculation of Drug Dosages	Test	Calc.	T.J. Designs
Dosage Calculation Proficiency Test	Test	Calc.	Educational Software
Dosecalc	Demo	Calc.	Saunders
Drug Calculations—5 modules	Tutorial	Calc.	Computer Ed. Resource
Pretest & review of math	Tutorial	Calc.	Computer Ed. Resource
Systems of measurement	Tutorial	Calc.	Computer Ed. Resource
Oral medications	Tutorial	Calc.	Computer Ed. Resource
Parenteral medications	Tutorial	Calc.	Computer Ed. Resource
Solutions	Tutorial	Calc.	Computer Ed. Resource
Drug Dosage Calculations & Admin.	Tutorial	Calc.	Medi-Sim
Calculating tablets & liquids	Tutorial	Calc.	Medi-Sim
Parenteral dosages	Tutorial	Calc.	Medi-Sim
Nursing Math	D & P	Calc.	Oregon Dept. Ed.
Household—apothecary	D & P	Calc.	Oregon Dept. Ed.
Conversions	D & P	Calc.	Oregon Dept. Ed.
Digitalis: Pharmacology & Clinical Use	Tutor/Sim.	Pharm.	Williams & Wilkins
Drug Interaction Principles	Tutorial	Pharm.	S. Schmidt
Principles of Pharmacology	Tutorial	Pharm.	Biosource
Origins & Pharmacokinetics	Tutorial	Pharm.	Biosource
Pharmacodynamics	Tutorial	Pharm.	Biosource
Drug Safety & Effectiveness	Tutorial	Pharm.	Biosource
ABG Practice	D & P	ABGs	Medsoft
Arterial Blood Gases	Tutorial	ABGs	AJN
Arterial Blood Gases	Tutor/sim.	ABGs	Williams & Wilkins
Interpretation of ABGs	D & P	ABGs	A. Swan

NAME OF PROGRAM	STYLE	TOPIC	COMPANY
Lab Values in Acid-Base Imbalance	Tutorial	ABGs	Oregon Dept. Ed.
Respiratory Expert	Sim./Anal.	ABGs	Saunders
Indirect B/P Measurement	Tutorial	B/P	AJN
Skills Simulation—Taking a B/P	D & P	B/P	Lippincott
ACLS Dysrhythmia Generator	D & P	EKGs	Univ. Osteo. Med.
Arrhythmias Tutorial I: Pathophysiology and Supraventricular Arrhythmias	Tutorial	EKGs	Williams & Wilkins
Arrhythmias Tutorial II: Ventricular Arrhythmias & Heartblock	Tutorial	EKGs	Williams & Wilkins
Arrhythmias: Case Studies in Management	Tutorial	EKGs	Williams & Wilkins
Skills Simulation—Calc. & Adjust I.V. Flow Rates	D & P	Nurs. Skills	Lippincott
Skills Simulation—Calc. & Prep for Injection	D & P	Nurs. Skills	Lippincott
Skills Simulation—Urine Testing Sugar & Ketones	D & P	Nurs. Skills	Lippincott
Skills Simulation—Prep Insulin Injection	D & P	Nurs. Skills	Lippincott
Intro to Nursing Diagnosis	Tutorial	Nurs. Theory	Lippincott
Intro to Behavioral Objectives	Tutorial	Nurs. Theory	Lippincott
Intro to Nursing Orders	Tutorial	Nurs. Theory	Lippincott
Intro to Patient Data	Tutorial	Nurs. Theory	Lippincott
Intro to Nursing Goals	Tutorial	Nurs. Theory	Lippincott
Intro to Patient Problems	Tutorial	Nurs. Theory	Lippincott
Lesson on Developmental Stages (0–65 yr)	Tutorial	Nurs. Theory	Oregon Dept. Ed.
Nursing Diagnosis: Concepts & Cases	Tutorial	Nurs. Theory	McGraw-Hill
Nursing Process	Tutorial	Nurs. Theory	Medi-Sim
Introduction	Tutorial	Nurs. Theory	Medi-Sim
Components of assessment	Tutorial	Nurs. Theory	Medi-Sim
Planning goals & actions	Tutorial	Nurs. Theory	Medi-Sim
Plan implementation	Tutorial	Nurs. Theory	Medi-Sim
Goal evaluation	Tutorial	Nurs. Theory	Medi-Sim

NAME OF PROGRAM	STYLE	TOPIC	COMPANY
Wellness-illness continuum	Tutorial	Nurs. Theory	Heshi Computing
Nursing Research CAI	Tutorial	Research	C.V. Mosby
Research terminology	Tutorial	Research	C.V. Mosby
Sampling	Tutorial	Research	C.V. Mosby
Formulating researchable problem	Tutorial	Research	C.V. Mosby
Systematic approach to critiquing	Tutorial	Research	C.V. Mosby
Tables and graphs	Tutorial	Research	C.V. Mosby
Research Methods	Demo	Research	Heshi Computing
Understanding Concepts of Statistics	Demo	Research	Heshi Computing
The Factory	Discovery	Prob. Solv.	Sunburst
The Incredible Laboratory	Discovery	Prob. Solv.	Sunburst
The Pond	Discovery	Prob. Solv.	Sunburst
Infection Control & Isolation	Tutorial	Inf. Cont.	Heshi Computing
Asepsis: Intro	Tutorial	Inf. Cont.	Medi-Sim
Chain of Infection	Tutorial	Inf. Cont.	Medi-Sim
Medical Asepsis	Tutorial	Inf. Cont.	Medi-Sim
Protective Asepsis: Isolation	Tutorial	Inf. Cont.	Medi-Sim
Surgical Asepsis	Tutorial	Inf. Cont.	Medi-Sim
Pt. Requiring Isolation	Simul.	Inf. Cont.	Educational Software
Clinical Simulations in Nursing I	Simul.	All	M.E.P.C.
Clinical Simulations in Nursing II	Simul.	All	M.E.P.C.
Care of Client with Cirrhosis	Tutorial	Med. Nurs.	Medi-Sim
History & assessment	Tutorial	Med. Nurs.	Medi-Sim
Diagnostic evaluation	Tutorial	Med. Nurs.	Medi-Sim
Crisis of acute cirrhosis	Tutorial	Med. Nurs.	Medi-Sim
Care of Patient with Diabetes	Simul.	Med. Nurs.	Educational Software
Mr. Merna: Pt. w/ Liver Disease	Simul.	Med. Nurs.	Saunders
Mrs. Shilkraut: Terminal Pt.	Simul.	Med. Nurs.	Saunders
UMKC Software Series	Demo	Med. Nurs.	UMKC
Chris Hall: Diabetic	Simul.	Diabetes	Alan Villiers

NAME OF PROGRAM	STYLE	TOPIC	COMPANY
Ketoa	Simul.	Diabetes	Univ. Minnesota
Mr. Richardson: Diabetes	Simul.	Diabetes	Saunders
Sugar	Tutorial	Diabetes	Univ. Minnesota
Mary Dunne	Simul.	Geriatric	Health Sci. Con.
Mrs. Gates: Elderly Woman	Simul.	Geriatric	Saunders
Chest Suction: Pneumothorax	Simul.	Med/Surg.	Univ. Minnesota
Clinical Sims: Med/Surg Nursing I	Simul.	Med/Surg.	MEPC Software
Clinical Sims: Med/Surg Nursing II	Simul.	Med/Surg.	MEPC Software
Inflammation	Tutorial	Med/Surg.	Oregon Dept. Ed.
I.V. One & I.V. Two	Tutorial	Med/Surg.	Univ. Minnesota
Mr. Babain: with Peptic Ulcer	Simul.	Med/Surg.	Lippincott
Mr. Casey: with Renal Colic	Simul.	Med/Surg.	Lippincott
Mr. Hansie: with Cirrhosis	Simul.	Med/Surg.	Lippincott
Mr. Migo: with BPH	Simul.	Med/Surg.	Lippincott
Mrs. Fiver: Lady with Cystitis	Simul.	Med/Surg.	Lippincott
Mrs. Mandy: w/ Glomerulonephritis	Simul.	Med/Surg.	Lippincott
Mrs. Pacer: with Cholecystitis	Simul.	Med/Surg.	Lippincott
Nasogastric Suction	Simul.	Med/Surg.	Univ. Minnesota
Rena Fuller, Renal Crisis	Simul.	Med/Surg.	Lippincott
Shock	Tutorial	Med/Surg.	Oregon Dept. Ed.
Mr. Foley	Simul.	Surg. Nurs.	Concepts Unlimited
Mr. Jay	Simul.	Surg. Nurs.	Concepts Unlimited
Mr. Petey, w/ Abdominoperineal Resec.	Simul.	Surg. Nurs.	Lippincott
Mrs. Simms: Hemorrhoidectomy	Simul.	Surg. Nurs.	Saunders

NAME OF PROGRAM	STYLE	TOPIC	COMPANY
Nursing Care for Surgical Patient	Tutorial	Surg. Nurs.	Medi-Sim
Preoperative Nursing Care	Tutorial	Surg. Nurs.	Medi-Sim
Postoperative Nursing Care	Tutorial	Surg. Nurs.	Medi-Sim
Post-Op Care Simulation	Simul.	Surg. Nurs.	Concepts Unlimited
Wound Healing	Tutorial	Surg. Nurs.	Oregon Dept. Ed.
Kathy Shaw: Antepartal Care	Simul.	OB Nurs.	Lippincott
Nutritional Assess. Pregnant Woman	Tutorial	OB Nurs.	Medi-Sim
Beth Popil, with V.S.D.	Simul.	Pedi. Nurs.	Lippincott
Developmental Concepts #2	Demo	Pedi. Nurs.	Medi-Sim
Hazel: 6-yr-old with Nephrosis	Simul.	Pedi. Nurs.	Lippincott
Home Health Guide for Children	Data Base	Pedi. Nurs.	Clinical Ref. Sys.
I.V. Meds for Kids	Simul.	Pedi. Nurs.	McGraw-Hill
Pediatric Minor Illness	Tutorial	Pedi. Nurs.	Medi-Sim
Pedi. Patient with Head Injury	Simul.	Pedi. Nurs.	Educational Software
Scott Duchess, w/ Appendicitis	Simul.	Pedi. Nurs.	Lippincott
Encephalon: A Neuro Pt. Simulator	Tutorial	Neuro. Nurs.	Andent
Exploring Your Brain	Tutorial	Neuro. Nurs.	Epilepsy Foundation
Neurological Assessment	Tutorial	Neuro. Nurs.	Medi-Sim
Neurosurgical Nursing: Spinal Cord Injury	Tutorial	Neuro. Nurs.	Medi-Sim
Pathophysiology & Diagnosis	Tutorial	Neuro. Nurs.	Medi-Sim
Acute Nursing Care	Tutorial	Neuro. Nurs.	Medi-Sim
Rehabilitation Nursing	Tutorial	Neuro. Nurs.	Medi-Sim
Cognitive Rehabilitation Series	Demo	Rehab/ Neuro.	Hartley
Association	D & P	Rehab/ Neuro.	Hartley

NAME OF PROGRAM	STYLE	TOPIC	COMPANY
Drawing Conclusions and Problem Solving	D & P	Rehab/ Neuro.	Hartley
Categorization	D & P	Rehab/ Neuro.	Hartley
Memory	D & P	Rehab/ Neuro.	Hartley
Sequencing	D & P	Rehab/ Neuro.	Hartley
Jerry Burke, Quadriplegic	Simul.	Rehab/ Neuro.	Lippincott
A Chronic Patient	Simul.	Psych. Nurs.	MEPC Software
A Suicidal Adolescent	Simul.	Psych. Nurs.	MEPC Software
A Patient with Pain & Anxiety	Simul.	Psych. Nurs.	MEPC Software
A Patient with Psychosis & Mania	Simul.	Psych. Nurs.	MEPC Software
Mr. Charles, Obsessive/ Compulsive	Simul.	Psych. Nurs.	Lippincott
Psychology	Game	Psych. Nurs.	Academic Hall.
Communicable Disease	Tutorial	P. Health	Oregon Dept. Ed.
Killer T-Cell	Game	Oncology	Univ. Texas CA Cent
Critical Care Consultant	Analysis	Crit. Care	C.V. Mosby
Dx. & Mgmt. of Acute MI & Complications	Tutorial	Crit. Care	Williams & Wilkins
Fluid & Electrolyte Expert	Sim./Anal.	Crit. Care	Saunders
Hemodynamic Management ICU Pt.	Game	Crit. Care	American Edwards
Hypertensive Emergencies	Tutorial	Crit. Care	Williams & Wilkins
Hypertension Management	Tutorial	Crit. Care	Williams & Wilkins
Hemodynamic Monitoring-Applied	Tutorial	Hemodyn.	Medsoft
Hemodynamic Expert	Sim./Anal.	Hemodyn.	Saunders
Swan-Ganz Catheter Simulation	Simul.	Hemodyn.	American Edwards
Ambulance 10-33	Simul.	Emerg.	Univ. Osteo. Med.
Mr. Jones: Indigestion	Simul.	Emerg. Nurs.	Saunders
Street Medicine	Simul.	Emerg.	Univ. Osteo. Med.
Cardiac Arrest Simulation	Simul.	ACLS	Aspen Publishers

NAME OF PROGRAM	STYLE	TOPIC	COMPANY
CPR Training by Computer	Simul.	ACLS	Williams & Wilkins
Drug Therapy in CPR	Tutorial	ACLS	S. Schmidt
Sudden Death	Simul.	ACLS	Med Ed
The Computer Code	Simul.	ACLS	Univ. Osteo. Med.
Trauma	Simul.	E.R. ACLS	Med Ed
Nursing Examination Review (N.E.R.S.)	Test	NCLEX	Addison-Wesley
Sandra Smith's Computer Review	Test	NCLEX	Ntl. Nursing Review
Careers in Hospital Nursing	Data Base	Careers	Career Development
Micro Guide to Nursing Careers	Data Base	Careers	Career Development
Computer Trivia	Game	Computers	T.J. Design
Welcome to Computer-ville	Simul.	H.I.S.	J. Thiele
Mosbysystems Software			
Teststar	Demo	NCLEX	C.V. Mosby
Administar	Demo	Mgmt.	C.V. Mosby
Mosbysorts	Demo	All-purp.	C.V. Mosby
Nursestar	Demo	TestBank	C.V. Mosby
Questbank			C.V. Mosby
M.A.R.T.	Tutorial	Mgmt./Stress	Career Development
Nursing and Leadership	Tutorial	Mgmt.	Career Development
Alcohol: An Educational Simulation	Simul.	Subs. Abuse	Marshware
Alcoholic Physician	Tutorial	Subs. Abuse	UMKC
American Indian with Alcoholism	Tutorial	Subs. Abuse	UMKC
Blue Color Alcoholic	Tutorial	Subs. Abuse	UMKC
Drugs: Who's In Control	Simul.	Subs. Abuse	Marshware
Drugs: Their Effect on You	Tutorial	Subs. Abuse	Marshware
Geriatric Alcoholic	Tutorial	Subs. Abuse	UMKC
Manic Depressive & Alcoholism	Tutorial	Subs. Abuse	UMKC
Middle-Class, Problem Drinker	Tutorial	Subs. Abuse	UMKC
Patient with Withdrawal Syndrome	Tutorial	Subs. Abuse	UKMC

NAME OF PROGRAM	STYLE	TOPIC	COMPANY
Polydrug Dependent Patient	Tutorial	Subs. Abuse	UMKC
Smoking: It's Up to You	Tutorial	Subs. Abuse	M.E.C.C.
The Smoking Decision	Tutorial	Subs. Abuse	Sunburst
Tobacco: To Smoke or Not to Smoke	Simul.	Subs. Abuse	Marshware
Fit and Trim	Analysis	Fitness	Andent
Fitness: State of Body & Mind	Tutor/ Anal.	Fitness	Marshware
Accident Prevention	Tutorial	Safety	Heshi Computing
Make It Click: Seatbelt Safety	Tutorial	Safety	Sunburst
Caffeine	Tutorial	Nutrition	Oregon Dept. Ed.
Fast Food Micro-Guide	Analysis	Nutrition	Learning Seed
FatJack (daily consumption of fat)	Game	Nutrition	Learning Seed
Food & Nutrition	Tutorial	Nutrition	Heshi Computing
Food Group Puzzles	Tutorial	Nutrition	Marshware
Introductory Nutrition	Tutorial	Nutrition	M.C. Media-Corp.
Nutrition Pursuit	Game	Nutrition	Learning Seed
Salt and You	Analysis	Nutrition	M.E.C.C.
The Eating Machine	Analysis	Nutrition	Muse
The Salt Shaker	Analysis	Nutrition	Learning Seed
WeightWatch	Analysis	Nutrition	Learning Seed
What Did You Eat Yesterday?	Analysis	Nutrition	Learning Seed
You Are What You Eat	Tutorial	Nutrition	Marshware
Health	Game	Health	Academic Hall.
Health Awareness Games	Appraisal	Health	HRM Software
Health Risk Appraisal	Appraisal	Health	Univ. Minnesota
Health Risk Appraisal	Appraisal	Health	HRM Software
Healthstyles	Appraisal	Health	Birdprints
Healthy Living	Appraisal	Health	Heshi Computing
Personal Health Inventory	Appraisal	Health	American Corp. Hlth
Teen Health Advisor	Appraisal	Health	D. Paperny, MD

NAME OF PROGRAM	STYLE	TOPIC	COMPANY
An Apple a Day	Data Base	Health	Avant-Garde
Microinstructor	Demo	Authoring	C.V. Mosby
Simu-Writer	Demo	Authoring	Algorithms Unlmtd
Test Construction Disk I	Tutorial	Test Author.	Heshi Computing
Test Construction Disk II	Tutorial	Test Author.	Heshi Computing
Test Construction Disk III	Tutorial	Test Author.	Heshi Computing
Med-Math	Demo	Test Generat.	Lippincott
Quick Tests	Demo	Test Bank	Seven Hills

Index to CAI Software Vendors

ACADEMIC HALLMARKS
Box 998
Durango, CO 81301
(800) 321-9218

ADDISON-WESLEY
Medical/Nursing Division
2727 Sand Hill Road
Menlo Park, CA 94025
(800) 227-1936

ALGORITHMS UNLIMITED
P.O. Box 3516
Ogden, UT 84409
(801) 546-7546

AMERICAN CORPORATE
HEALTH PROGRAMS, INC.
85 Old Eagle School Road
Strafford, PA 19087
(215) 293-9367

AMERICAN EDWARDS
Customer Service
17221 Redhill Avenue
Santa Ana, CA 92711
(800) 854-6958

AJN (American Journal of
Nursing)

555 West 57th St.
New York, NY 10019
(212) 582-8820

ANDENT
1000 North Avenue
Waukegan, IL 60085
(312) 223-5077

ASPEN PUBLISHERS
1600 Research Blvd.
Rockville, MD 20850
(800) 638-8437

AVANT-GARDE
P.O. Box 30160
Eugene, OR 97403
(503) 345-3043

BIOSOURCE SOFTWARE
2105 S. Franklin, Suite B
Kirksville, MO 63501
(816) 665-5751

BIO-PSYCH EDUCATIONAL
TOOLS
P.O. Box 6436
Reynolds Station
Winston-Salem, NC 27109

BIRDPRINTS
P.O. Box 5053
Vancouver, WA 98668

JOSEPH BOYLE, MD
Department of Physiology
University of Medicine and
   Dentistry of New Jersey
100 Bergen Street
Newark, NJ 07103

THE BRAIN BANK, INC.
220 Fifth Avenue
New York, NY 10001
(212) 686-6565

CAREER DEVELOPMENT
SOFTWARE, INC.
207 Evergreen Drive
Vancouver, WA 98661
(202) 696-3529

CLINICAL NURSING
SOFTWARE, INC.
P.O. Box 172
Middleton, WI 53562
(608) 845-8096

CLINICAL REFERENCE
SYSTEMS
Box 20308
Denver, CO 80220
(303) 220-1661

COMMAND APPLIED
TECHNOLOGY, INC.
400 West Main Street
P.O. Box 511
Pullman, WA 99163
(509) 334-6145

COMPUTER EDUCATION
RESOURCES
2705 N. Bell
Denton, TX 76201
(817) 382-0536

CONCEPTS UNLIMITED
692 S. 450 E
Orem, UT 84058
(801) 378-6088

DeWITT DATA SYSTEMS
617 N. 13th Street
Quincy, IL 62301
(217) 222-5790

EDUCATIONAL ACTIVITIES
P.O. Box 87
Baldwin, NY 11510

EDUCATIONAL IMAGES
P.O. Box 3456
West Side Station
Elmira, NY 14905
(607) 732-1090

EDUCATIONAL SOFTWARE,
INC.
9071 Metcalf
Overland Park, KS 66212

EPILEPSY FOUNDATION OF
AMERICA
4351 Garden City Drive
Landover, MD 20785

EXPERIENCE IN SOFTWARE
2039 Shattuck Ave., Suite 401
Berkeley, CA 94704
(415) 644-0694

FOCUS MEDIA
Microcomputer Software
839 Stewart Avenue, P.O. Box 865
Garden City, NY 11530
(800) 645-8989

HARTLEY COURSEWARE,
INC.
2023 Aspen Glade
Kingswood, TX 77339
(713) 358-0801

HESHI COMPUTING
P.O. Drawer M
Hitchcock, TX 77563

HRM SOFTWARE
175 Tompkins Ave.
Pleasantville, NY 10570

BRIAN JEFFRIES
3841 Northwood Rd.
University Heights, OH 44118
(216) 321-1468

J.B. LIPPINCOTT CO.
East Washington Square
Philadelphia, PA 19105
(800) 523-2945

THE LEARNING SEED
21250 North Andover Rd.
Kildeer, IL 60047

MARSHWARE
P.O. Box 8082
Shawnee Mission, KS 66208
(816) 523-1059

LAWRENCE MARTIN, MD
Pulmonary Division
The Mount Sinai Medical Center
One Mt. Sinai Drive
Cleveland, OH 44106

McGRAW-HILL BOOK
COMPANY
27th Floor
1221 Avenue of the Americas
New York, NY 10020

M.C. MEDIA CORP.
1855 Nelson Street— #405
Vancouver, B.C.
Canada
V6G 1M9
(604) 684-4685

M.E.C.C.
Minesota Educational Computing
   Corporation
3490 Lexington Ave., North
St. Paul, MN 55112
(612) 481-3500

MED ED
Medical Educational Software
   Group
P.O. Box 40592
San Antonio, TX 78229

MEDI-SIM, INC.
P.O. Box 13267
Edwardsville, KS 66113
(913) 441-2881

MEDICAL WATCH SOFTWARE
1620 Ensenada Drive
Modesto, CA 95355

MEDMICRO, INC.
820 W. Wingra Drive
Madison, WI 53715
(608) 798-3002

MEDSOFT CO.
1105 Arondale Drive
Fircrest, WA 98466

MEPC SOFTWARE
52 Vanderbilt Ave.
New York, NY 10017
(212) 370-5520

MICROTRENDS
International, Ltd.
590 California Road
Quakertown, PA 18951
(215) 538-0900

HAROLD I. MODELL
NRCLSE
Mail Stop RC-70
University of Washington
Seattle, WA 98195

THE C.V. MOSBY CO.
Mosbysystems
11830 Westline Industrial Drive
St. Louis, MO 63146
(800) 325-4177

MUSE SOFTWARE
347 North Charles Street
Baltimore, MD 21201
(301) 659-7212

NATIONAL NURSING REVIEW
342 State Street, #6
Los Altos, CA 94022
(800) 221-4093

NATIONAL WELLNESS
INSTITUTE
South Hall—UWSP
Stevens Point, WI 54481
(715) 346-2172

OREGON DEPARTMENT OF
EDUCATION
Wanda Monthey
700 Pringle Parkway, S.E.
Salem, OR 97310

DAVID M. PAPERNY, MD,
FAAP
Project Director
Teen Health Computer Programs
2516A Pacific Heights Road
Honolulu, HI 96813-1027

JAMES RANDALL, PhD
Indiana University
School of Medicine, Myers Hall
Bloomington, IN 47405

RN ACT
1115 N. Ellsworth
Villa Park, IL 60181
(312) 941-0900

W. B. SAUNDERS CO.
West Washington Square
Philadelphia, PA 19105
(212) 750-1330

SHEILA SCHMIDT
5221 N. Kensington
Kansas City, MO 64119

SEVEN HILLS SOFTWARE
2310 Oxford Road
Tallahassee, FL 32304

UNIVERSITY OF CALIFORNIA,
SAN FRANCISCO
School of Nursing, N319Y
University of California
Third & Parnassus Avenues
San Francisco, CA 94143

SOFT BITE, INC.
P.O. Box 5531
Cary, NC 27511

SUBSTANCE ABUSE
EDUCATION (SAE)
670 S. 4th Street
P.O. Box 13738
Edwardsville, KS 66113
(913) 441-1868

SUNBURST COMMUNICA-
TIONS, INC.
39 Washington Ave.
Pleasantville, NY 10570
(800) 431-1934

ANN SWAN, RN, MSN
332 Maplecrest Circle
Jupiter, FL 33458

JOAN THIELE, RN, PhD
Idaho State University
Department of Nursing
P.O. Box 8101
Pocatello, Idaho 83209

DONALD THOMPSON, RN,
MSN
302 Valhalla Drive
Muskogee, OK 74403

T. J. DESIGNS
5905 Ironwood
Rancho Palos Verdes, CA 90274

THOUGHTWARE, INC.
2699 South Bayshore Drive
Suite 1000A
Coconut Grove, FL 33133
(800) 848-9273

UNIVERSITY OF MINNESOTA
Media Distribution
Box 734, Mayo Memorial Building
420 Delaware Street S.E.
Minneapolis, MN 55455

UNIVERSITY OF MISSOURI,
KANSAS CITY
School of Medicine
2411 Holmes, M3-C06
Kansas City, MO 64108

UNIVERSITY OF
OSTEOPATHIC MEDICINE
3200 Grand Avenue
Des Moines, IA 50312
(515) 271-1478

UNIVERSITY OF TEXAS
SYSTEM CANCER CENTER

M.D. Anderson Hospital
MSAH Box 6
6723 Bertner Ave.
Houston, TX 77030

ALAN VILLIERS
1603 Omar Drive
Mesquite, TX 73150

WELLSOURCE
13705 S. E. 142nd
Clackamas, OR 97015
(503) 658-5959

WILLIAMS & WILKINS
428 East Preston Street
Baltimore, MD 21202
(800) 638-0672

Index

Contributors

ELIZABETH E. BALL, B.A.
Senior Systems Analyst, Travenol Healthcare Information Services,
Reston, Virginia, USA

MARION J. BALL, Ed.D.
Associate Vice Chancellor, Information Resources, The University of
Maryland at Baltimore, Baltimore, Maryland, USA

CONSTANCE M. BERG, R.N., M.B.A.
Executive Vice President, MarketGroup, Incorporated, San Francisco,
California, USA

CHRISTINE BOLWELL, R.N., M.S.N.
Education Consultant, Diskovery; Computer Assisted Healthcare
Education, Saratoga, California, USA

PATRICIA FLATLEY BRENNAN, R.N., Ph.D.
Assistant Professor of Nursing and Systems Engineering, Case Western
Reserve University, Cleveland, Ohio, USA

JAMES F. CRAIG, Ed.D.
Associate Professor, Chairman, Department of Educational and
Instructional Resources, Director, Dental Informatics, Dental School,
University of Maryland at Baltimore, Baltimore, Maryland, USA

NOEL DALY, M.A., H.D.E.
Chief Executive, Irish Nursing Board, Dublin, Ireland

SHIRLEY P. DAMROSCH, Ph.D.
Associate Professor, School of Nursing, The University of Maryland at
Baltimore, Baltimore, Maryland, USA

CAROLYNE K. DAVIS, Ph.D.
National and International Health Care Advisor, Ernst and Whinney,
Cleveland, Ohio, USA

ELIZABETH C. DEVINE, Ph.D.
Assistant Professor, School of Nursing, The University of Wisconsin-Milwaukee, Milwaukee, Wisconsin, USA

JUDITH V. DOUGLAS, M.H.S.
Associate Director for Planning and Management, Information Resources, The University of Maryland at Baltimore, Baltimore, Maryland, USA

JAMES M. GABLER, M.S.
Vice President, Management Systems, The Moses H. Cone Memorial Hospital, Greensboro, North Carolina, USA

ULLA GERDIN JELGER, R.N.
Stockholm County Council, Health Care Information Systems, Stockholm, Sweden

SUSAN J. GROBE, R.N., Ph.D., F.A.A.N.
Associate Professor of Nursing, The University of Texas at Austin, School of Nursing, Austin, Texas, USA

MARK S. GROSS
Principal, Ernst and Whinney, National Office, Cleveland, Cleveland, Ohio, USA

GARY D. HALES, Ph.D.
Editor in Chief, Computers in Nursing, Houston, Texas, USA

GARY L. HAMMON
President, Hammon Associates, San Antonio, Texas, USA

KATHRYN J. HANNAH, R.N., Ph.D.
Professor, Faculty of Nursing, The University of Calgary, Calgary, Alberta, Canada

BARBARA R. HELLER, R.N., Ed.D.
Professor and Chairman, Department of Nursing Education, Administration and Health Policy, School of Nursing, The University of Maryland at Baltimore, Baltimore, Maryland, USA

BETSY S. HERSHER
President, Hersher Associates, Ltd., Northbrook, Illinois, USA

SHIRLEY HUGHES
Director of Marketing, Clinicom, Incorporated, Boulder, Colorado, USA

ADA K. JACOX, R.N., Ph.D.
Professor and Director of the Center for Research, School of Nursing, The University of Maryland at Baltimore, Baltimore, Maryland, USA

BETH JAEKLE, R.N., M.S.N.
Application Support Analyst, The Moses H. Cone Memorial Hospital, Greensboro, North Carolina, USA

SUZANNE JENKINS, R.N.
Operations Manager of CareScan, HCS, Washington, D.C., USA

THOMAS JENKINS, Ph.D.
Principal, Morse Learning Systems, Elkton, Maryland, USA

KRISTEN H. KJERULFF, Ph.D.
Research Assistant Professor, School of Nursing, The University of Maryland at Baltimore, Baltimore, Maryland, USA

KAREN D. LAFFERTY, R.N., B.S.N.
Coordinator, Patient Care Information Systems, Roanoke Memorial Hospitals, Roanoke, Virginia, USA

DARLENE LARSON, R.N., M.Ed.
Independent Consultant, Minneapolis, Minnesota, USA

MARY R. MCCARTHY, S.C., R.N., Ed.D.
Assistant Professor, School of Nursing, The University of Maryland at Baltimore, Baltimore, Maryland, USA

KATHLEEN A. MCCORMICK, Ph.D., R.N.
Commander, U.S.P.H.S.; Research Nurse, Gerontology Research Center, Baltimore, Maryland, USA

KERRY E. MEYER-PETRUCCI, C.N.P.
Doctoral Candidate, School of Nursing, The University of Maryland at Baltimore, Baltimore, Maryland, USA

MARY ETTA MILLS, R.N., Sc.D.
Vice President for Nursing, University of Maryland Hospital, Baltimore, Maryland, USA

ROBERT I. O'DESKY, Ph.D.
President, RIO Consultants, Columbia, Missouri, USA

MARCIA ORSOLITS, Ph.D., R.N.
Senior Manager, Ernst and Whinney, National Office, Cleveland, Cleveland, Ohio, USA

MAUREEN OSIS, R.N., M.N.
Osis Consulting, Calgary, Alberta, Canada

JUDY G. OZBOLT, Ph.D., R.N.
Associate Professor, School of Nursing, The University of Michigan,
Ann Arbor, Michigan, USA

HANS PETERSON, M.D.
Director, Health Care Information Systems, Stockholm County Council,
Stockholm, Sweden, USA

MARY PETERSON, B.N.
Coordinator, Nursing Management Information Systems, Calgary General
Hospital, Calgary, Alberta, Canada

CHERYL PLUMMER, R.N., B.Sc.N.
Nursing Systems Coordinator, Shaughnessy Hospital, Vancouver, British
Columbia, Canada

DENIS PROTTI, M.Sc.
Professor and Director, Health Information Science, University of Victoria,
Victoria, Canada

CAROL A. ROMANO, R.N., M.S.
Director, Information Systems and Quality Assurance, Clinical Center,
National Institutes of Health, Bethesda, Maryland, USA

S. DENNI SHEFFIELD, R.N., B.S.N., M.S.P.H.
Director, Operations Analysis, Strong Memorial Hospital, Rochester,
New York, USA

BARBARA S. THOMAS, Ph.D.
Professor, College of Nursing, The University of Iowa, Iowa City,
Iowa, USA

RUSSELL E. TRANBARGER, R.N., C.N.A.A., M.S.N.
Administrator for Nursing, The Moses H. Cone Memorial Hospital,
Greensboro, North Carolina, USA

ANN WARNOCK-MATHERON, R.N., B.N.
Coordinator, Nursing Systems, Calgary General Hospital, Calgary,
Alberta, Canada

HARRIET H. WERLEY, Ph.D.
Distinguished Professor, School of Nursing, University of Wisconsin-
Milwaukee, Milwaukee, Wisconsin, USA

CECELIA R. ZORN, M.S.N.
Project Assistant, School of Nursing, University of Milwaukee-Wisconsin,
Milwaukee, Wisconsin, USA

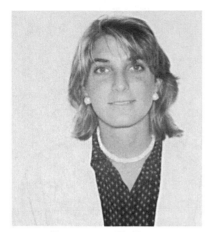

Elizabeth E. Ball

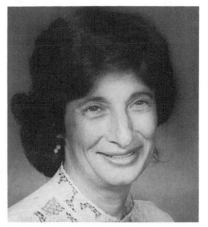

Marion J. Ball

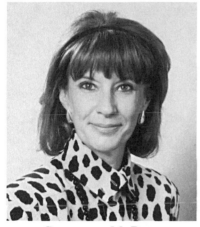

Constance M. Berg

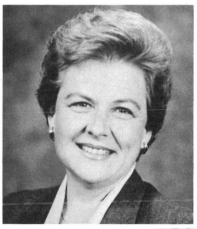

Christine Bolwell

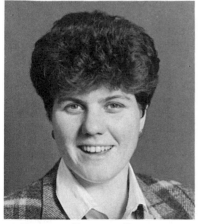

Patricia Flatley Brennan

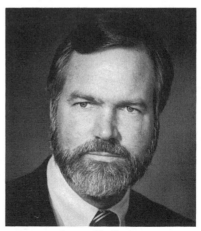

James F. Craig

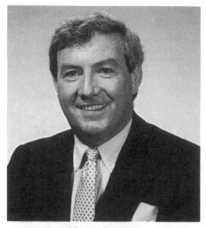

NOEL DALEY

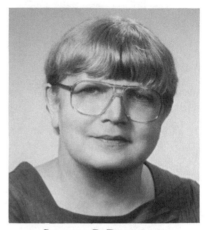

SHIRLEY P. DAMROSCH

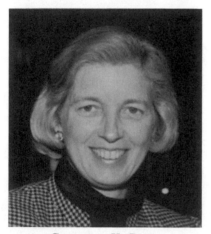

CAROLYNE K. DAVIS

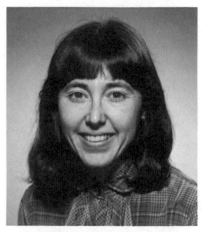

ELIZABETH C. DEVINE

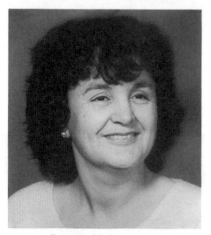

JUDITH V. DOUGLAS

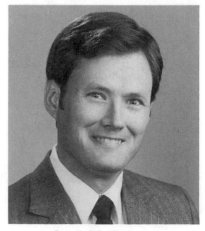

JAMES M. GABLER

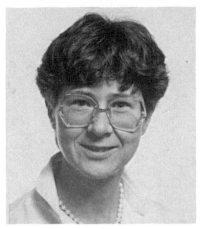

ULLA GERDIN JELGER

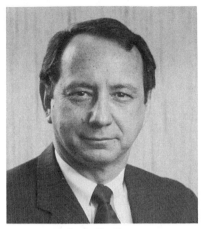

MARK S. GROSS

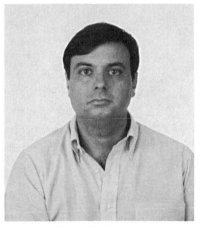

GARY D. HALES

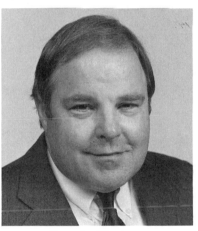

GARY L. HAMMON

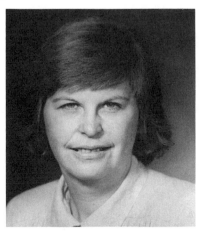

KATHRYN J. HANNAH

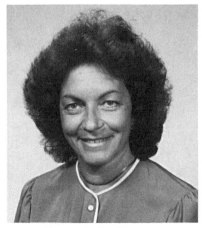

BARBARA R. HELLER

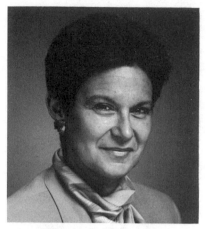

BETSY S. HERSHER

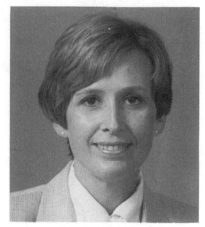

SHIRLEY HUGHES

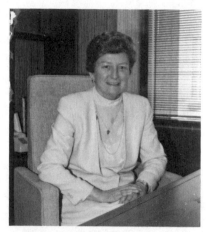

ADA K. JACOX

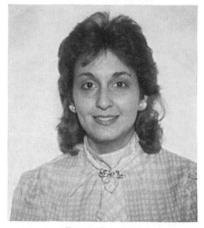

BETH JAEKLE

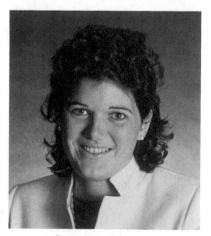

SUZANNE JENKINS

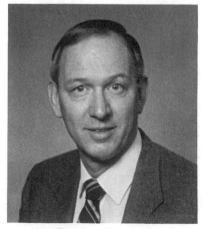

THOMAS JENKINS

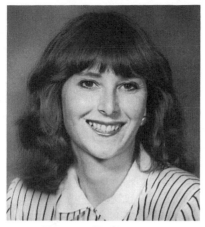

Kristen H. Kjerulff

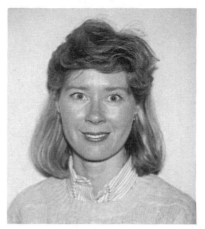

Karen D. Lafferty

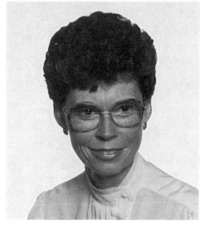

Darlene Larson

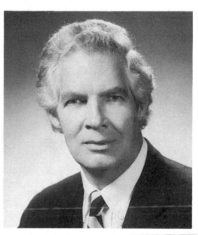

Donald A.B. Lindberg

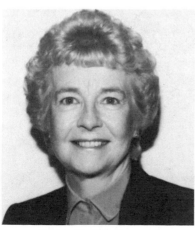

Mary R. McCarthy

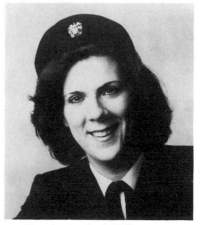

Kathleen A. McCormick

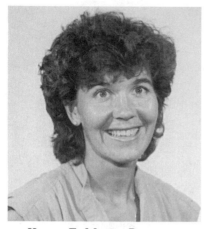

KERRY E. MEYER-PETRUCCI

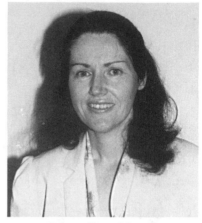

MARY ETTA MILLS

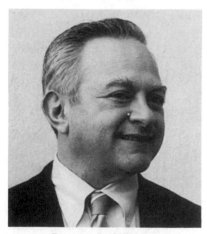

ROBERT I. O'DESKY

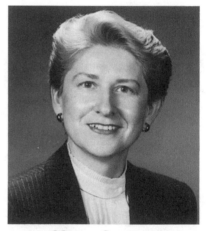

MARCIA ORSOLITS

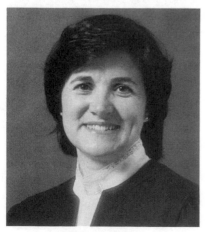

MAUREEN OSIS

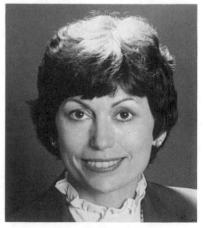

JUDY G. OZBOLT

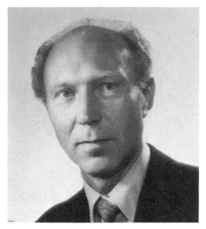

Hans Peterson

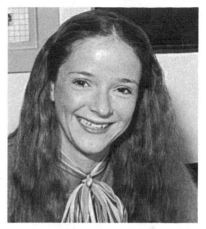

Mary Peterson

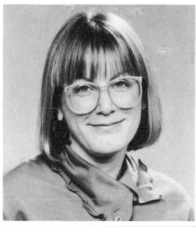

Cheryl Plummer

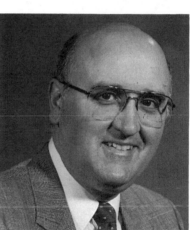

Denis Protti

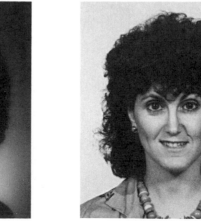

Carol A. Romano

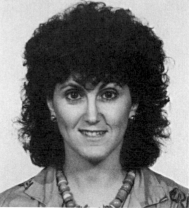

S. Denni Sheffield

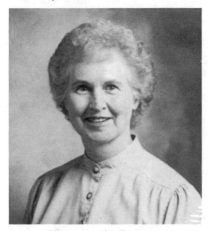

Barbara S. Thomas

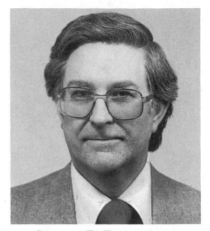

Russell E. Tranbarger

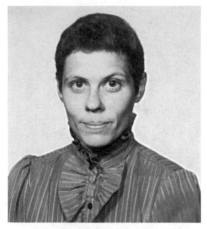

Ann Warnock-Matheron

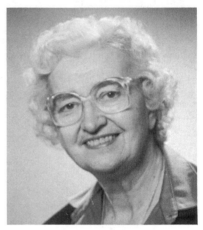

Harriet H. Werley

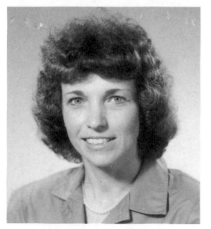

CeCelia R. Zorn